EDUCATION, SOCIAL FACTORS, AND HEALTH BELIEFS IN HEALTH AND HEALTH CARE SERVICES

RESEARCH IN THE SOCIOLOGY OF HEALTH CARE

Series Editor: Jennie Jacobs Kronenfeld

Recent Volumes:

RESEARCH IN THE SOCIOLOGY OF HEALTH CARE
VOLUME 33

EDUCATION, SOCIAL FACTORS, AND HEALTH BELIEFS IN HEALTH AND HEALTH CARE SERVICES

EDITED BY

JENNIE JACOBS KRONENFELD
Department of Sociology, Arizona State University, Tempe, AZ, USA

Emerald

United Kingdom – North America – Japan
India – Malaysia – China

Emerald Group Publishing Limited
Howard House, Wagon Lane, Bingley BD16 1WA, UK

First edition 2015

Reprints and permissions service
Contact: permissions@emeraldinsight.com

British Library Cataloguing in Publication Data
A catalogue record for this book is available from the British Library

ISBN: 978-1-78560-367-9
ISSN: 0275-4959 (Series)

Printed and bound by CPI Group (UK) Ltd, Croydon, CR0 4YY

CONTENTS

LIST OF CONTRIBUTORS

Brad Barber	School of Social Work, University of Alabama, Tuscaloosa, AL, USA
Chloe E. Bird	RAND Corporation, Santa Monica, CA, USA
Celeste Campos-Castillo	Department of Sociology, University of Wisconsin-Milwaukee, Milwaukee, WI, USA
Claudia Chaufan	Institute for Health & Aging, University of California, San Francisco, CA, USA
I-Chien Chen	Department of Sociology, Michigan State University, East Lansing, MI, USA
Catherine Chesla	Department of Family Health Care Nursing, University of California, San Francisco, CA, USA
Cara A. Chiaraluce	Department of Sociology, University of California, Davis, CA, USA
Neale R. Chumbler	Department of Public Health, Western Kentucky University, Bowling Green, KY, USA
Arthur Culbert	Health Literacy Missouri, St. Louis, MO, USA
Samir P. Desai	Department of Health Policy and Management, University of Georgia, Athens, GA, USA
Kevin K. Dobbin	Department of Epidemiology and Biostatistics, University of Georgia, Athens, GA, USA

Aileen A. Duldulao	Community Epidemiology Services, Multnomah County Health Department, Portland, OR, USA
Marc N. Elliott	RAND Corporation, Santa Monica, CA, USA
José J. Escarce	RAND Corporation, Santa Monica, CA, USA
Alicia Fernandez	School of Medicine, University of California, San Francisco, CA, USA
Hegla Fielding	Institute for Health & Aging, University of California, San Francisco, CA, USA
Allen Fremont	RAND Corporation, Santa Monica, CA, USA
Charles Gasper	Missouri Foundation for Health, St. Louis, MO, USA
Bonnie Ghosh-Dastidar	RAND Corporation, Arlington, VA, USA
Justin B. Ingels	Department of Health Policy and Management, University of Georgia, Athens, GA, USA
Jennie Jacobs Kronenfeld	Sanford School of Social and Family Dynamics, Arizona State University, Tempe, AZ, USA
Bronwen Lichtenstein	Department of Criminal Justice, University of Alabama, Tuscaloosa, AL, USA
Nicole Lurie	RAND Corporation, Arlington, VA, USA
Laurie T. Martin	RAND Corporation, Arlington, VA, USA
Ethel G. Nicdao	Department of Sociology, University of the Pacific, Stockton, CA, USA
Aggie J. Noah	Department of Sociology, Pennsylvania State University, State College, PA, USA
Michael Polgar	Department of Sociology, Pennsylvania State University, Hazleton PA, USA

Thomas Christian Quinn	Department of Sociology, University of Utah, Salt Lake City, UT, USA
Rashawn Ray	Department of Sociology, University of Maryland, College Park, MD, USA
Teague Ruder	RAND Corporation, Arlington, VA, USA
Jason Schnittker	Department of Sociology, University of Pennsylvania, Philadelphia, PA, USA
Abigail A. Sewell	Department of Sociology, Emory University, Atlanta, GA, USA
Daniel Sherman	American Institutes for Research, Washington, DC, USA
Heeju Sohn	Department of Sociology, University of Pennsylvania, Philadelphia, PA, USA
David T. Takeuchi	School of Social Work, Boston College, Chestnut Hill, MA, USA
Rebecca L. Utz	Department of Sociology, University of Utah, Salt Lake City, UT, USA
Tse-Chuan Yang	Department of Sociology, University at Albany, State University of New York, Albany, NY, USA

PART I
INTRODUCTION TO VOLUME

EDUCATION, OTHER SOCIAL FACTORS, AND HEALTH BELIEFS AND HEALTH CARE SERVICES

Jennie Jacobs Kronenfeld

ABSTRACT

Purpose – *This chapter provides both an introduction to the volume and a brief review of literature on education and other social factors and health beliefs in health care services.*

Methodology/approach – *Literature review.*

Findings – *The chapter argues for the importance of greater examination of education, other social factors, and health beliefs in the use of health care services.*

Originality/value – *Reviews the issues of education, social factors, and beliefs and previews this volume.*

Keywords: Health care disparities; education; social factors; health beliefs

Education, Social Factors, and Health Beliefs in Health and Health Care Services
Research in the Sociology of Health Care, Volume 33, 3–13

ISSN: 0275-4959/doi:10.1108/S0275-495920150000033001

This chapter provides an introduction to Volume 33 in the Research in the Sociology of Health Care series, *Education, Social Factors, and Health Beliefs in Health and Health Care Services*. The beginning of this chapter will review some of the more important material about education, other social factors, and health beliefs as related to health care. The second part of this chapter will review the overall contents of the volume and the structure of the volume.

EDUCATION, OTHER SOCIAL FACTORS, AND HEALTH BELIEFS

Many social factors are important in health and health care utilization. This includes some straight-forward social factors such as education or income as well as more complex factors such as health beliefs. Among the most important factors are aspects of socio-economic status (SES) such as education, income, and occupation, because these factors often create and shape patterns of disease and patterns of health care utilization. People who have greater advantages in SES live longer than those without such advantages (Kunst, Feikhe, Mackenbach, & the EU Working Group on Socioeconomic Inequalities in Health, 1998). This is true at the beginning of life in terms of differences in infant mortality as well as across the life-span (Gortmaker & Wise, 1997). It has also been true across time and is true in many different countries, not just the United States.

Education has often been viewed as the key to position in the SES system, because education is so strongly linked with the likelihood of being employed, the types of jobs people obtain, and income. Thus, in the health area, education has a fundamental influence on adult health because it generates social inequalities in employment, job, and occupational status (Mirowsky, Ross, & Reynolds, 2000). In addition to the impact through work and economic conditions, education also impacts social psychological resources and health lifestyle. Thus, the literature supports that the well-educated are less likely to smoke (Winkleby, Jatulis, Frank, & Fortmann, 1992), drink more moderately, and avoid obesity (Hayes & Ross, 1986). They are also more likely to use preventive medical care such as immunizations, screenings, and physician services (Ross & Wu, 1995).

More recent research in medical sociology has especially focused on some broader approaches to SES and other social factors, an approach now known as the fundamental cause approach (Link & Phelan, 1995,

1996). This is a sociologically based explanation for persistent associations between SES and disease. The argument is that the reason SES is so consistently associated with disease is that resources such as knowledge, money, power, and prestige, all factors embodied in the SES concept, can be used in many different ways and in many different situations to avoid risks for diseases and even death. More socioeconomically advantaged people can better avoid risks and also take up protective strategies to improve health and well-being and can modify these over time to take advantage of new knowledge and approaches in the medical arena. This means that this relationship is a dynamic one, and the associations change as knowledge and conditions change. If new risk factors emerge, for example, such as lack of exercise or changes in nutritional information, those with the most resources are better able to avoid those risks and take advantage of protective factors. The same is true for knowledge about new treatments; the most advantaged people not only often have the best health insurance that allows people to use the treatments but also are more likely to learn about the treatments, seek out health providers who make those treatments available, and be able to cover the costs with their own resources if the new treatments are not yet covered by standard health insurance.

This approach is different from the risk factor epidemiology approach, because that approach views more distal social conditions as less relevant and focuses on proximal risk factors and argues that once proximal risk factors are addressed via interventions that social patterns and even social disparities in health and health services use will disappear. In contrast, the fundamental cause approach points out why this is unlikely to occur, because of the dynamic relationship between social factors such as SES and risk factors. In addition, this approach also shows why stress can also become one of many health risks that more advantaged people are better able to avoid.

In addition, there has been research that shows that communities or societies with low-income inequality have higher levels of social capital, such as positive feelings of community trust, and more social cohesion (Kawachi & Kennedy, 1997; Wilkinson, 1996). One of the interesting questions is whether the impact of community or societal income inequality on individual mortality operates primarily through individual SES or through aggregate levels of social capital (Gravelle, 1998).

Moving away from these broader SES measures, fundamental cause approaches, and issues of social capital, there is also literature on more specific examples of education and related factors such as health literacy. These ideas link to some of the articles in this research annual and also grow out of some of the earlier wok on social factors as fundamental determinants of health disparities. The chapter in this volume by Laurie T. Martin, Teague Ruder, José J. Escarce, Bonnie Ghosh-Dastidar, Daniel Sherman, Marc N. Elliott, Chloe E. Bird, Allen Fremont, Charles Gasper, Arthur Culbert, and Nicole Lurie discusses the concept of health literacy and argues that it has emerged as a potentially critical pathway through which education, income, and other fundamental determinants affect health care quality and disparities. The most common definition of health literacy is "the degree to which individuals have the capacity to obtain, process, and understand basic health information and services needed to make appropriate health decisions" (Ratzen & Parker, 2000). In an emerging health care system in which consumers are expected to make decisions about their health insurance choices as well as the choices about what care to actually receive, health literacy becomes an even more important aspect of social factors, especially since recent data indicate that about one-third of the adult US population have health literacy skills that can be classified as basic or below basic (National Center for Education Statistics, 2003). These skill levels raise important questions about whether such consumers are able to make informed choices about health care insurance and health system use. Many recent reforms in health care delivery make assumptions about health literacy of most citizens. The creation of the health care marketplace as a way to help people choose a health care insurance plan assumes both health literacy, overall literacy and some ability to use computers to locate different choices of health insurance options. The need to use computers and understand the complexities of different choices of health care plans as part of the ACA affordable health care insurance options makes these issues of lack of health literacy more important within the American context, in contrast to an earlier era when a person's employment often provided a person's health insurance and gave people few if any options in making those choices.

In addition to basic SES factors and education-related factors, beliefs especially such factors as perception of the health care system and the trust of individuals in the health care system are another type of factor that impacts health and health care services use. Polling data in the United States as well as research in the last decade or so has shown that individuals' trust in the health care system has decreased in the United States. According to the Harris Poll, about 73 percent of respondents reported "a great deal of confidence" in the US health care system in 1966 but this has declined to 34 percent of respondents by 2012 (Harris Interactive Polls, 2012). Lack of trust in the health care system can lead to negative impacts on a person's health behavior such as the use of health care services (Armstrong et al., 2006; Yang, Matthews, & Hillemeier, 2011). Several chapters in this volume examine issues related to lack of trust in the health care system and health beliefs, adding to the literature in this area.

REVIEW OF CONTENTS OF THE VOLUME

The volume contains six parts, and most (other than this introductory chapter which makes up Part I of this volume) contain 2–4 chapters per part. This first part contains only one chapter, this introductory chapter to the volume. Part II of this volume is entitled "Beliefs and Health Beliefs" and contains two chapters. The first chapter in this part is entitled "The Politics of Health Beliefs: Cross-National Evidence" and is written by Jason Schnittker. He points out that there has been little research from a comparative perspective on health beliefs. This study evaluates cross-national differences in public beliefs about the causes of health and the role of these beliefs in shaping attitudes regarding health policy.

The chapter uses data from the 2011 International Social Survey Program, which includes questions on health and health care, asked in 29 countries. Respondents were asked about four specific causes of poor health (i.e., genes, behavior, the environment, and poverty) and also about their attitudes regarding three aspects of health policy: their support for government-provided care, the perceived fairness of income disparities in medical treatment, and their support for providing health care to non-citizens. The study reveals the global reach of a multicausal view. The four beliefs about the causes of poor health are positively correlated in all countries but there is considerable cross-national variation in the average support for specific causes. Although in some countries proximate causes, such as genes, are endorsed more frequently than distal causes, such as poverty, this is by no means a uniform pattern. Support for genetic causes is high, but genetic reductionism is rare. In addition, the study points out that health beliefs are fundamentally political beliefs. The single most important determinant of beliefs about the causes of health is the country in which the respondent resides. The study demonstrates the importance of national context in shaping health beliefs, as well as the role of beliefs regarding the causes of health in setting the stage for public receptivity to government-provided care.

The second chapter in this part is authored by Tse-Chuan Yang, I-Chien Chen, and Aggie J. Noah and is titled "Examining the Complexity and

Variation of Health Care System Distrust across Neighborhoods: Implications for Preventive Health Care." In contrast to the first chapter that deals with comparative data and beliefs broadly, this chapter focuses on one aspect of belief, distrust, and examines the impact of neighborhood environment factors and the linkages with preventive care. The data are from one city, Philadelphia, and there is information from 9,497 respondents in 914 census tracts which are used as the neighborhood context in this study. The chapter identifies four different distrust patterns: believers, doubters, competence skeptics and value skeptics. More than half of the people evaluated competence and values distrust coherently, with believers reporting low levels and doubters reporting high levels of distrust. Competence and values skeptics assessed distrust inconsistently. Overall, the chapter shows that distrust patterns are functions of neighborhood conditions and are associated with preventive care.

Part III of the volume is titled "Education" and includes two chapters. The first is by Laurie T. Martin, Teague Ruder, José J. Escarce, Bonnie Ghosh-Dastidar, Daniel Sherman, Marc N. Elliott, Chloe E. Bird, Allen Fremont, Charles Gasper, Arthur Culbert, and Nicole Lurie and is titled "Identifying and Mapping 'Hot Spots' of Low Health Literacy: A Potential Tool to Guide Intervention." This chapter focuses specifically on literacy and views low health literacy as an important barrier that needs to be overcome to eliminate health care disparities and improve health care quality and health outcomes. The chapter focuses on communities, not individuals, and identifies geographic areas with large numbers of individuals with low health literacy. The chapter applies regression coefficients from a predictive model of health literacy to US census data and then creates health literacy scores for census geographic areas in the state of Missouri. The authors also compare areas identified by the predictive model with those identified on the basis of educational attainment. There were substantial differences between the two approaches with the multivariate approach being more accurate. The chapter also raises some issues about ways to use this approach from a policy perspective.

The second chapter in this part is by Heeju Sohn and focuses on Education and Self-Awareness of Health: Toward a Better Understanding of Self-Rated Health. The focus of this chapter is to evaluate the extent to which a person's educational attainment moderates the relationship between objective markers of health and self-rated health. The chapter uses 10 years of data from the Health and Nutrition Examination Survey to explore, with regression analyses, how diagnosed medical conditions, health behaviors, and biomarkers are differentially associated with self-rated health by educational attainment. While medical conditions are negatively associated with self-rated health equally across educational levels, behaviors, and biomarkers have stronger associations with self-rated health for people with greater education attainment. This shows that education may play a role in how people interpret and evaluate their health.

The next two chapters in Part IV focus on one particular type of health concern, mental health concerns. Part V focuses on other social factors as explanatory factors beyond health beliefs and education. The final part focuses on special types of care settings. Mental health concerns are very important aspects of today's health care system and each of the three chapters in this part focuses on different aspects of mental health issues. The first chapter in this part is by Ethel G. Nicdao, Aileen A. Duldulao, and David T. Takeuchi. The chapter covers Psychological Distress, Nativity and Help-Seeking among Filipino Americans. The chapter uses data from the Filipino American Community Epidemiological Study of 2,285 Filipino adults living in the United States. The chapter uses OLS regression to examine the association between psychological distress and help-seeking among US born Filipinos and immigrants. Lay people were the major source of help for psychological distress. Important predictors for help-seeking were years spent in the United States, ethnic identity, and discrimination. Those born in the United States were more likely to seek help. People with low ethnic identity and who had experienced medium to high discrimination were less likely to seek help. The chapter suggests the importance of examining factors such as social support and acculturation in future research.

The second chapter in this part is by Michael Polgar and discusses Connections and Transitions in Mental Health Care Organizations and Systems. The chapter summarizes sociological research on mental health care organizations and systems and illustrates the macro-social perspective by applying it to the problem of transitions in care for young adults. The chapter points out that the scope and management of care involves a focus on modes of treatment supported by research evidence and delivered effectively by people with cultural competences. Care and continuity of care are delivered through systems of inter-organizational networks.

The third mental health-oriented chapter is by Thomas Christian Quinn and Rebecca L. Utz. This chapter examines Personal Religiosity and Mental Health Care Utilization among Adolescents. The study examines whether personal religiosity in any way associated with adolescents' propensity to seek out formal mental health care. The chapter uses data from the National Longitudinal Study of Adolescent Health (Add Health) and applies logistic regression models to test for an association between personal religiosity and mental health services use net of depressive symptomology and demographic controls. The authors find a negative, statistically significant relationship between personal religiosity and mental health services use. Highly religious adolescents had lower odds of having seen a mental health professional compared to their less religious counterparts even after controlling for depressive symptomology. The authors point out that religiosity represents a potentially important consideration in addressing the mental health needs of adolescents. This is one of the first studies in which a nationally representative sample of adolescents is used to examine the relationship between personal religiosity and mental health services use.

Part V examines other social factors besides education and health beliefs and how they impact health and health care. The two major other factors the four different chapters in this part include are racial and ethnic issues. Each chapter deals with some aspect of race and ethnicity, often combined with SES and other social factors. The first chapter by Celeste Campos-Castillo looks at racial and ethnic differences in trust in sources of health information, with a particular focus on trust in physicians. Past research has found that racial and ethnic minorities have lower levels of trust than whites. The chapter uses data from the Health Information National Trends Survey and uses multivariable logistic regression to assess whether racial and ethnic differences in distrust are equivalent among health care users and non-users and how this links to variation in the health of respondents and their SES status. The chapter finds that racial and ethnic minorities have less trust in physicians as health information sources and that these differences are the same among both health care users and non-users, regardless of health and SES. Celeste Campos-Castillo also finds that the racial and ethnic patterns are not there when predicting trust in other health information sources such as the internet, family, friends, and government health agencies.

Claudia Chaufan, Hegla Fielding, Catherine Chesla, and Alicia Fernandez have included a chapter with the title "'It's Not the Doctor – It's Me': How Self-Blame Obscures Language and Other Structural Barriers to Diabetes Care among Low-Income Latinos with Limited English Proficiency." The chapter examines how professional interpreter use improves care in patients with limited English proficiency, although some disparities still remain. The authors conducted 20 in-depth interviews with 20 low-income Latino patients with diabetes and limited English proficiency. The patients themselves report that they do not think the language discordance impacts their outcomes because these are more linked to whether they comply with the recommendations of physicians. They point out how self-blame ends up being encouraged by physicians in some ways due to their emphasis on praise of favorable outcomes. Despite the limitations of the small, convenience sample these are important findings that also bring up the need for more studies on this topic.

The third chapter in this part is by Neale R. Chumbler, Samir P. Desai, Justin B. Ingels, and Kevin K. Dobbin and looks at the issues of race and SES as related to public perceptions toward quality and access to care in the Affordable Care Act (ACA). The focus is on determining whether race is independently associated with perceptions of quality of care and access to care after the implementation of the ACA. The data are from a telephone survey of a representative sample of Georgia adults. The chapter uses quality of care and access to care as dependent variables and fits three different models, one with only race, one with race and SES, and one with a number of additional characteristic such as self-rated health status, sense of coherence, travel time to doctor's office, importance of short waits in the doctor's office and whether rural or non-rural. They find that race was significantly associated with both quality of care and access to care. People with higher education or income were also more likely to perceive improvements in quality and access due to the implementation of the ACA. These associations were partially explained by a person's self-reported political affiliation. Because the more general parts of the ACA have only been in place in the United States for a year or so, there are not yet that many studies on this topic, and this chapter raises important issues linked to quality and access of care and policy issues for the future.

The last chapter in this part is by Abigail A. Sewell and Rashawn Ray and looks at issues related to the Celeste Campos-Castillo's chapter. This chapter looked at differences in trust of sources of health information with a particular focus on physician trust. This chapter looks at issues of trust in personal physicians and links it to black Protestant affiliation. Making a similar point as did the Celeste Campos-Castillo's chapter about blacks being less trusting of physicians than whites, this chapter focuses more heavily on within group differences. Using data from the 2002 and 2006 General Social Surveys, the chapter examines heterogeneity in trust levels among black associated with religious groups and compares black Protestants with those from other religious groups. Black-white differences in physician trust are found only when religious affiliation is considered but not when it is omitted. Blacks affiliated with black Protestant churches are more trusting than other religious groups including those of Evangelical Protestants, Mainline Protestants and blacks affiliated with other faiths.

There ends up being more heterogeneity in trust levels among blacks than between blacks and whites. The chapter also points out that religion can have an important impact on issues linked to health care use.

The last part of this volume, Part VI, looks at special types of care settings. One of the chapters looks at offenders who are under probation or parole in an American state and the other focuses on caregivers of children with an autism diagnosis. Brad Barber and Bronwen Lichtenstein examine whether laws for mandatory HIV disclosure to sexual partners are a barrier to HIV testing among offenders under community supervision. Using data from 197 probationers and parolees surveyed on two reporting days in Alabama, they specifically gathered information on what offenders know about HIV, what they know about the laws for mandatory disclosure, and if they support mandatory HIC disclosure and testing. Testing and criminalization of non-disclosure were supported as part of HIV prevention. This was linked to the idea of HIV as a killer disease and of people with HIV as serious risks to other people. These approaches lead to a conclusion that disclosure laws legitimate HIV stigma and may undermine test and treatment strategies in communities at risk for HIV.

The last chapter in this volume is by Cara A. Chiaraluce and is titled "Becoming an Expert Autism Caregiver: Health Literacy and Community Catalysts." The purpose of the study was to investigate the informal micro-level mechanisms through which caregivers maximize their health literacy and caregiving skill set. This includes an exploration of the role of factors such as lay self-education and local community networks in caring for a child with autism. Qualitative research methods were used. These involved 50 individual intensive interviews with primary caregivers of at least one child under the age of eighteen years with an official autism diagnosis. In addition to the interviews, the author was involved in two years of participant-observation at two primary sites for autism parent and caregiver local resource meetings in northern California. The study demonstrated the major institutional limits and gaps involved in health related caregiving for children with autism. It finds that caregivers develop and rely upon a sophisticated set of health literacy skills and key local community based ties.

All these chapters make important contributions to the literature in medical sociology and research in the sociology of health care. Most relate to important social factors such as education, SES, race and ethnicity, and health beliefs. Some look at unusual populations such as those on parole from prisons or those with autism and a variety of mental health related concerns.

REFERENCES

Armstrong, K., Rose, A., Peters, N., Long, J. A., McMurphy, S., & Shea, J. A. (2006). Distrust of the health care system and self-reported health in the United States. *Journal of General Internal Medicine*, *21*(4), 292–297. doi:10.1111/j.1525-1497.2006.00396.x

Gortmaker, S. L., & Wise, P. H. (1997). The first injustice: Socioeconomic disparities, health services technology and infant mortality. *Annual Review of Sociology*, *23*, 147–170.

Gravelle, H. (1998). How much of the relation between population mortality and unequal distribution of income is a statistical artifact? *British Medical Journal*, *316*, 382–385.

Harris Interactive Polls. (2012). *Confidence in Congress stays at lowest point in almost fifty years*. Retrieved from http://www.harrisinteractive.com/vault/Harris%20Poll%2044%20-%20Confidence%20Index_5%2021%2012.pdf. Accessed on January 20, 2013.

Hayes, D., & Ross, C. E. (1986). Body and mind: The effect of exercise, oversight and physical health on psychological well-being. *Journal of Health and Social Behavior*, *27*(4), 3874–3900.

Kawachi, I., & Kennedy, B. P. (1997). Health and social cohesion: Why care about income inequality? *British Medical Journal*, *314*, 1037–1040.

Kunst, A. E., Feikhe, G., Mackenbach, J. P., & the EU Working Group on Socioeconomic Inequalities in Health. (1998). Occupational class and cause specific mortality in 11 European countries: Comparison of population based studies. *British Medical Journal*, *316*, 1636–1642.

Link, B. G., & Phelan, J. C. (1995). Social conditions as fundamental causes of disease. *Journal of Health and Social Behavior*, Extra issue, *36*, 80–94.

Link, B. G., & Phelan, J. C. (1996). Understanding socioeconomic differences in health – The role of fundamental social causes. *American Journal of Public Health*, *86*, 471–473.

Mirowsky, J., Ross, C. E., & Reynolds, J. (2000). Links between social status and health status. In E. Chloe, P. C. Bird, & A. M. Fremont (Eds.), *Handbook of medical sociology* (5th ed., pp. 47–67). Upper Saddle River, NJ: Prentice-Hall.

National Center for Education Statistics. (2003). National Assessment of Adult Literacy (NAAL). Retrieved from nces.ed.gov/naal.

Ratzen, S. C., & Parker, R. (2000). Introduction. In C. Selden, M. Zorn, S. Ratzan, & R. Parker (Eds.), *National library of medicine current bibliographies in medicine: Health literacy*. Bethesda, MD: National Institutes of Health, U.S. Department of Health and Human Services.

Ross, C. E., & Wu, C.-L. (1995). The links between educational attainment and health. *American Sociological Review*, *60*, 719–745.

Wilkinson, R. G. (1996). *Unhealthy societies: The afflictions of inequality*. New York, NY: Routledge.

Winkleby, M. A., Jatulis, D. E., Frank, E., & Fortmann, S. P. (1992). Socioeconomic status and health: How education, income and occupation contribute to risk factors for Cardiovascular disease. *American Journal of Public Health*, *82*, 816–820.

Yang, T. C., Matthews, S. A., & Hillemeier, M. M. (2011). Effect of health care system distrust on breast and cervical cancer screening in Philadelphia, Pennsylvania. *American Journal of Public Health*, *101*(7), 1297–1305.

PART II
BELIEFS AND HEALTH BELIEFS

THE POLITICS OF HEALTH BELIEFS: CROSS-NATIONAL EVIDENCE

Jason Schnittker

ABSTRACT

Purpose – *This study evaluates cross-national differences in public beliefs about the causes of health and the role of these beliefs in shaping attitudes regarding health policy.*

Methodology/approach – *The study uses data from the 2011 International Social Survey Program, which includes questions on health and health care, asked in 29 countries. Respondents were asked about four specific causes of poor health (i.e., genes, behavior, the environment, and poverty). Respondents were also asked about their attitudes regarding three aspects of health policy: their support for government-provided care, the perceived fairness of income disparities in medical treatment, and their support for providing health care to noncitizens.*

Findings – *The study has three findings. First, the study reveals the global reach of a multicausal view. The four beliefs about the causes of poor health are positively correlated in all countries. However, there is considerable cross-national variation in the average support for specific causes.*

Education, Social Factors, and Health Beliefs in Health and Health Care Services
Research in the Sociology of Health Care, Volume 33, 17–42

ISSN: 0275-4959/doi:10.1108/S0275-495920150000033002

Although in some countries proximate causes, such as genes, are endorsed more frequently than distal causes, such as poverty, this is by no means a uniform pattern. Support for genetic causes is high, but genetic reductionism is rare. Second, the study reveals that health beliefs are fundamentally political beliefs. The single most important determinant of beliefs about the causes of health is the country in which the respondent resides, exceeding in influence religion, education, and even personal experiences with health and health care. Third, the study reveals that the political connotations of health beliefs vary between countries, especially beliefs regarding genes. In general, those who endorse behavioral arguments favor less government involvement in health care and are more accepting of income disparities in the quality of care. Those who endorse the environment and poverty, meanwhile, tend to support a stronger role of government. Yet, the magnitude of these associations varies and, in the case of genetic arguments, even the direction of the association varies. Genetic arguments are frequently associated with support for a stronger role of government, but genetic arguments also are occasionally associated with support for the exclusion of noncitizens from the health care system.

Research limitations/implications – *International survey research is valuable for exploring the scope of patterns revealed in a limited set of countries, but it is difficult to pinpoint the source of cross-national differences.*

Originality/value – *The study demonstrates the importance of national context in shaping health beliefs, as well as the role of beliefs regarding the causes of health in setting the stage for public receptivity to government-provided care. The study also illustrates the value of thinking about beliefs about genes as reflecting larger projects of biocitizenship, at least in some countries.*

Keywords: Health beliefs; cross-national research; genetics; health policy

A good deal is known about health beliefs generally, but very little research adopts an explicitly comparative perspective. This is unfortunate for a number of reasons. For one, there has been considerable interest in the connections between national culture and health beliefs. One implication of this line of research is that health beliefs are influenced by a large number of factors, well beyond a simple consideration of the actual determinants of health or a reflection upon personal experiences with disease. Another implication is that health beliefs have a wide range of connotations. Indeed, religious and political factors often emerge as the most powerful determinants of beliefs about health, suggesting a close association between health beliefs and more general philosophical orientations (Furnham, 1994). In all, health beliefs might reflect a schema for interpreting how societies should respond to misfortune, elevating their relevance for a wide variety of political attitudes (Helman, 2007).

In particular, health beliefs could play a pivotal role in explaining cross-national differences in public receptivity to national health policy. In particular, health beliefs could explain support for government-provided care, especially given the intersection between the perceived causes of poor health and attitudes regarding who is responsible for its treatment. At least in the United States there is a tight connection between perceived personal responsibility for poor health and reduced support for government-provided health care (Mechanic, 2006; National Research Council and Institute of Medicine, 2013). In countries where the public is more receptive to publicly funded care, the foundation of this support could be a public that sees poor health in terms of natural misfortune rather than personal guilt and, in turn, sees health care as a right more than an entitlement. However, the political connotations of health beliefs do not stop with support for publicly funded care. Some recent frameworks, for instance, link support for genetic arguments regarding health to larger projects of nation-building and health promotion (Rose, 2007). Perspectives along these lines bring health beliefs to entirely new fields of relevance, including questions of equality, citizenship, and peoplehood. Given the global scope of these frameworks, only a truly comparative approach can provide an adequate empirical assessment.

In this study, I used data from the 2011 International Social Survey Program (ISSP) health module to explore cross-national differences in health beliefs, as well as the consequences of these beliefs for policy-related attitudes. The ISSP provides a valuable addition to the literature, allowing for, among other things, cross-national comparisons based on a consistently worded survey instrument. The ISSP also provides high-quality data collection within each of the participating countries, based on a set of best-practice agreements. Although there has certainly been *international* research on health beliefs, much of this work has been conducted on a country-by-country basis, allowing for only implicit comparisons between countries or regions. In contrast, 29 countries participated in 2011 ISSP, spanning regions (e.g., the United Kingdom, the Philippines, Russia, and Israel) and levels of economic development (e.g., Norway, Croatia, and Chile). The health module contains questions on the perceived causes of poor health, as well attitudes regarding publicly funded health care, treatment disparities, and access to health care for noncitizens. The United States is included in the ISSP, permitting a crucial comparison given how much of the research on health beliefs was generated in the United States. But the true value of the ISSP is in providing data from countries that have received considerably less attention and differ in history and culture. A brief review of the literature suggests that the United States might be unusual.

BACKGROUND

Understanding the actual causes of health is a crucial scientific enterprise, but the public holds its own beliefs about the causes of health. Although these beliefs need not be a faithful representation of reality, they are nonetheless consequential in various ways. Most research finds that health beliefs reflect how individuals understand misfortune more generally and, furthermore, that health beliefs have a complex set of connotations (Helman, 2007). The source of health beliefs reflects some mix of knowledge, personal experience, and inference. In this vein, much of the literature regards health beliefs as an explanation for *personal* illness, thereby casting health beliefs as a tool for illness management. For instance, research regularly situates patient explanatory models in sharp contrast to physician explanatory models (Kleinman, 1980). By this logic, health beliefs are highly individualistic and holistic and, therefore, tend to depart from the more impersonal and entity-based understandings of modern medicine, setting the stage, in turn, for doctor-patient conflict.

Yet lurking in the background of the literature is a growing appreciation of cross-national differences in health beliefs, as well as an appreciation of the complex political implications of such beliefs. Health beliefs reflect more than we realize. Perhaps as much as individual experience or knowledge, health beliefs could reflect a nation's history and culture and, therefore, health beliefs could have considerable coherence at the level of the country. The most immediate expression of this idea can be found in the assorted explanations for health that emerge in specific contexts, including explanations related to supernatural forces (Helman, 2007). These explanations have a significant geographic component in that they tend to be popular in certain regions and entirely absent in others. Yet research also recognizes the possibility of significant cross-national variation in support for even the most basic social, behavioral, or biological explanations for health. For instance, there may be considerable cross-national variation in support for biological arguments, even among countries of similar economic development (see, e.g., Saguy, Gruys, and Gong (2010) for evidence regarding obesity in France and the United States).

Furthermore, some health beliefs – including whether one regards health as the product of genes or behavior – might have connotations that are impossible to separate from the cultural context in which they emerge. For instance, whereas genetic arguments might imply fatalism in the United States, they might imply social and personal responsibility in other countries. By the same token, behavioral explanations for poor health might be equated with personal responsibility, but this association need not exist or be especially strong in countries where medical care is regarded as a right. In short, health beliefs may be fundamentally political beliefs situated in a specific setting, but at this point the literature has more speculation in this regard than deliberate comparative analysis. Furthermore, there remains a tendency to regard public beliefs in the United States as emblematic of beliefs in other countries. It is entirely possible, however, the political overtones of health beliefs are much sharper in the United States because health tends to be seen through a more moral frame (Leichter, 2003). Below I review the literature and end with some general propositions, which can be evaluated empirically.

Public Beliefs about the Causes of Health

Public beliefs about the causes of health usually begin with the individual (Gordon, 1988). When asked to describe the causes of poor health, individuals routinely cite diet, exercise, and other personal health behaviors, moving toward more distal causes only when they see a clear path from these causes through the individual (Robert & Booske, 2011). Although culture plays an important role in determining this emphasis – and, for this reason, some argue the focus on behavior is more pronounced in Western cultures (Gordon, 1988) and especially the United States (Goldberg, 2012; Leichter, 2003) – the importance of behavior also rests with personal experience. Those with the most control over their lives, for instance, are more likely to endorse behavioral causes, whereas those with less control grant the environment more influence (Pill & Stott, 1982). In short, when the public can plainly appreciate the consequences of the environment, they recognize its significance.

Even so, the public is not blind to the environment. This is especially true when it is clear how the environment gets under the skin, again showing how the public regards proximate causes as more compelling than distal ones. This is certainly the case in the United States, as several studies have demonstrated. In a public opinion survey, Robert and Booske (2011) find that most adults appreciate the role of living in a neighborhood where there are options for healthy food and exercise, even if most adults do not cite where a person lives per se as having a strong effect on health. Similarly, stress is a very popular explanation for poor health, even if some of the most common sources of stress, such as whether one has a job or the type of job one has, are not seen as especially significant (Robert & Booske, 2011). In both of these cases, public appreciation of a particular cause requires that cause to operate plainly through the individual.

Given this apparent tendency toward reduction and proximate causes, it is perhaps no surprise that genetic explanations are increasingly popular. Scientific knowledge of the genetic causes of health has, of course, grown enormously over time and the public absorbs new information about these causes from a variety of sources (Bates, 2005). Public opinion has followed apace: based on the limited data that is available, it appears public support for genetic causes has increased over time (Pescosolido et al., 2010; Schnittker, 2008; Singer, Corning, & Lamias, 1998). Furthermore, it appears public enthusiasm for genetic causes is quite broad. Most Americans endorse genetic arguments for a wide variety of outcomes and behavior, although, once again, outcomes closer to the body, like health, are seen as more strongly genetic than outcomes further away, like success in life (Shostak, Freese, Link, & Phelan, 2009). In accounting for the appeal of genetics, some research argues that genes provide a uniquely resonant explanation: genetic arguments carry scientific authority, they provide an apparently simple explanation for otherwise complex phenomena, and they clearly inhere to the individual (Nelkin & Lindee, 1996). With their scientific allure and credibility, genetic arguments might eventually supersede behavioral arguments, although genetic arguments also carry significant political weight. Indeed, it is with the political connotations of health beliefs that perhaps the greatest controversies still lie.

The Political Connotations of Health Beliefs

Although health beliefs can be categorized as internal or external to the individual, the political connotations of health beliefs belie a neat dichotomy.

To be sure, a number of themes have informed previous research, but there have been few absolute claims, and the literature becomes even more complex once it moves to an international focus. For instance, much of the research suggests that endorsing behavioral causes implies personal responsibility, whereas endorsing genetic causes implies fate. Accordingly, individuals who endorse genetic causes might favor a stronger role of government involvement in health care, reasoning that medical care is a necessary corrective to the inequities of birth. Similarly, explanations focusing on the social environment are often cast in contradistinction to explanations focused on personal choice, with only choice regarded as blameworthy (see Helman, 2007, chapter 5 for a review). Several studies of public beliefs are largely consistent with this claim. For example, in the United States, endorsing behavioral causes for poor health significantly reduces support for government-provided health care (Gollust & Lynch, 2011). Conversely, casting poor health in terms of unfairness – that is, seeing poor health as the result of misfortune – increases support (Lynch & Gollust, 2010). By the same token, most political liberals identify income as a cause of health – indeed, they regard it as parallel in influence to genes – but among conservatives income is a less popular explanation (Robert & Booske, 2011).

Although the political dimensions of these beliefs seem clear, it is increasingly apparent that conventional understandings of health behavior – pitting personal responsibility against natural misfortune – mask some complexity. For instance, some scholars conclude that genetic beliefs are essentially conservative in nature and help to advance conservative political projects (Nelkin & Lindee, 1996). In this framework, genetic explanations map just as well onto categories of deserving and undeserving as do behavioral explanations, especially once one appreciates the historical role of genetic arguments in naturalizing group differences in life chances. Contrary to this, however, Shostak et al. (2009) find no relationship between political orientation and the willingness to endorse genetic arguments. More generally, some scholars have questioned whether genetic arguments necessarily imply fatalism. Indeed, much to the contrary, some argue that genetic frameworks generate even more tools for the personal management of health and, thus, engender personal responsibility just as much as, say, strong admonitions for better health behavior. In this way, knowledge of genetic risk might obligate individuals to act in precisely the same way as an awareness of the importance of diet or exercise (Novas & Rose, 2000; Rose, 2007). This logic has other implications. For instance, support for genetic explanations might be positively correlated with support for behavioral explanations, even though most research contrasts the two. At a minimum, the fact that individuals almost always embrace a multicausal framework – that is, they endorse multiple causes simultaneously – is inconsistent with the idea that the public respects a sharp distinction between nature and nurture and favors one over the other. Although early research feared genetic reductionism as one possible outcome of the growth of genetic knowledge, there is little evidence, at least in the United States, the public endorses *only* genetic causes (Shostak et al., 2009).

More recent frameworks argue that genetic arguments intersect with a different political dimension, one that cuts across political lines. If genetic arguments reflect a type of biosociality, for instance, in which people organize concepts of citizenship around a shared genetic heritage, then support for genetic arguments might be associated with support for policies that exclude noncitizens from the health care system, even if the same arguments are associated with strong support for government-provided care (Rabinow, 2008). These two orientations are not ordinarily associated, but they are consistent once one draws a link between beliefs about genes and larger projects surrounding improving the health of a nation and its people. In the same vein, Rose (2007) discusses the intersection between the modern practice of health promotion and managing population health, linking enthusiasm for personal health projects with a parallel interest in the collectivity. In some countries, citizenship may be increasingly organized along genetic lines, becoming a key dimension upon which state-based obligations to its people are organized (Heath, Rapp, & Taussig, 2008). If these arguments are correct, support for genetic arguments regarding health might be inseparable from a broader mindset regarding citizenship and who does or does not deserve public goods.

The Importance of Cross-National Comparisons

As the above suggests, the literature on health beliefs contains a variety of conflicting claims, especially with respect to those beliefs' intersection with politics, but it also points to the possibility of between-country variation and the limits of focusing on the United States. In the United States, there remains an unusually strong moral dimension to health and health care, reflected in the strong distinction between "sinners" and "victims" and the obligation to help one but not the other (Mechanic & Tanner, 2007; Morone, 2003). With this in mind, it is possible the political connotations of health beliefs are simply much stronger in the United States than elsewhere. Consistent with this idea, Saguy et al. (2010) find the French endorse behavioral explanations for obesity just as much as Americans do, but they also find that this endorsement does not translate into the same lack of support for national health care as it does in the United States (see also Saguy & Gruys, 2010). More generally, European policy analysts emphasize a culture of solidarity, wherein the public supports efforts to improve everyone's health, regardless of the perceived causes of health (Morone, 2003). By this reasoning, environmental explanations for health might be more popular in Europe than in the United States, but all beliefs about the causes of health – whether behavioral, biological, or environmental – might be positively related to support for public health care in Europe.

In what follows I use data from the ISSP to explore health beliefs and their correlates. The ISSP contains questions assessing the extent of respondents' support for the government provision of health care. Specific questions ask about providing care for different sorts of conditions and to different types of people, including noncitizens. The same granularity applies to health beliefs. The ISSP asks about four separate causes, including genes, behavior, the environment, and poverty. With this information, I will examine the cross-national validity of a series of propositions drawn from the existing literature:

1. Proximate causes should be endorsed more frequently than distal causes.
2. Genetic explanations should be especially popular in developed countries, superseding behavioral explanations.
3. Behavioral explanations should have mixed associations with support for government-provided health care.
4. Social explanations for health should be associated with less acceptance of inequality in health care.
5. Genetic explanations will have variable political connotations, conservative in some countries but progressive in others.
6. Genetic reductionism will be rare, even when the endorsement of genetic explanations is not.

DATA

The International Social Survey Program (ISSP) is a long-running cross-national collaborative program that administers annual topical surveys in a set of member countries (International Social Survey Programme Research Group, 2011). The value of the ISSP is in allowing for cross-national comparison, based on identical questions and similar administration. The ISSP has developed best-practices guidelines for member countries, although each country fields its survey independently. In most countries, the survey is administered either face-to-face or through self-completion with interviewer involvement. Variation in the administration of the 2011 survey is described by Gendall (2013), although participating countries recognize the importance of consistency. The topics for the annual survey are decided by committee and pre-tested in several countries prior to their general administration. In developing the instrument, the focus is on questions that will be meaningful in all member countries and can be expressed in an equivalent manner regardless of language or culture. Of course, this ideal might not be achieved in each and every country. The same questions can connote very different associations, as previous research has shown (Heath, Martin, & Spreckelsen, 2009). For my analysis, however, I make this bug a feature: I will explicitly evaluate between-country variation in the associations between health beliefs and political attitudes.

The 2011 topical module was on health and health care. Data were collected largely in 2011, but spilled over into 2012 and 2013 for a few countries. For simplicity, I refer only to the year 2011. The countries included in the 2011 ISSP are Australia, Belgium, Bulgaria, Chile, Croatia, Czech Republic, Denmark, Finland, France, Germany, Great Britain, Israel, Japan, South Korea, Lithuania, the Netherlands, Norway, Philippines, Poland, Portugal, Russian Federation, Slovakia, Slovenia, South Africa, Sweden, Switzerland, Taiwan, Turkey, and the United States. The universe of respondents consists of adults, although the definition of adult differs slightly between countries: it was those age 18 and over in most countries, except for Finland, which included those 15 and older; Japan and South Africa, which included those 16 and older; and Norway which included those 19 and older. Participating countries used sampling designs appropriate for their context, with the number of stages ranging from one to four. The response rate ranged from 30% in West Germany to 86% in South Africa, although most countries reported a response rate of over 50%. Sample weights were developed to render each sample more representative within each country, and these weights are used in calculating country-specific descriptive statistics.

HEALTH BELIEFS

Four questions were asked in response to the stem, "Severe health problems may have many causes. How much do you agree or disagree with the following statements? People suffer from severe health problems ...." Four statements followed the stem: "because they behave in ways that damage their health," "because of the environment they are exposed to at work or where they live," "because of their genes," and "because they are poor." Respondents were provided with five response categories, ranging from strongly agree to strongly disagree, but I code responses simply whether they agree or not, reflecting the skewed distribution. In order to preserve a consistent sample size and minimize the consequences of listwise deletion, respondents who selected "can't choose" or did not provide an answer were coded as not endorsing the cause. At most this represented 5.4% of respondents (for the genetic question). For the other causes, it represented a little over 3%.

ATTITUDES TOWARD HEALTH POLICY

Respondents were asked a series of questions designed to assess the depth of their support for the public provision of health care. Questions were selected to assess overall support for government-provided care, as well as two basic dimensions of access and equality. Respondents were asked how much they agree with the following: "the government should provide only limited health care services" and "people should have access to publicly funded health care even if they do not hold citizenship of [country]." Response categories ranged from "strongly agree" to "strongly disagree" on a five-point scale. In another question respondents were asked, "Is it fair or unfair that people with higher incomes can afford better health care than people with lower incomes," with response categories ranging from "very fair" to "very unfair" on a five-point scale. In all three cases, I retained all the response categories rather than dichotomizing, given the much wider spectrum of responses for these questions than was found for the questions regarding the causes of poor health. I coded the variables such that higher values reflect more support for government-provided care, more perceived unfairness of income disparities, and more support for providing care to noncitizens. In short, higher values reflect a greater commitment to a strong, fair, and open public sector. A small number of respondents (less than 5% in each case) reported that they "can't choose" or didn't provide an answer, and they were assigned the midpoint value of three, the value most consistent in meaning with the proffered response categories (e.g., "neither agree nor disagree" or "neither fair nor unfair").

INDEPENDENT VARIABLES

A number of covariates are included as independent variables, selected for their thematic relevance for my research questions and because they form the core covariates of prior studies. The models include sex, age, religion (none, Catholic, Protestant, Orthodox, Other Christian, Jewish, Islamic, and other), education (combined into three categories: no formal education, only primary, or only secondary; post-secondary or lower tertiary; and upper tertiary), and whether the respondent voted for a leftist candidate in the last general election. In addition, three variables were designed to capture personal experiences with health and health care: whether the respondent had insurance or not (in countries where "no insurance" is an appropriate response); whether the respondent reported receiving no medical treatment because they could not pay for it, there was no treatment available in the area, or there was a long waitlist; and whether the respondent reported fair or poor health. This latter set of variables is particularly important, as beliefs about the causes of poor health and its appropriate treatment often develop in light of personal experiences and frustrations. With this set of variables, the goal is to determine the best predictor of health beliefs and, furthermore, to discern the impact of health beliefs on political attitudes once these variables are inserted as controls. The results and tables progress sequentially toward this goal.

RESULTS

The tables explore the following in sequence: descriptive differences between countries in health beliefs; the determinants of health beliefs; descriptive differences between countries in health policy attitudes; the determinants of these attitudes; and the relationship between health beliefs and policy attitudes, including between-country variation in this relationship. Table 1 starts with mean support for the four health beliefs across all the countries. The columns are arrayed from proximate (genes) to distal (poverty), allowing for an easy assessment of the idea that the public prefers the former over the latter. The table also presents the percent within each country that *only* endorse the specific cause. Expressed as a sample-wide average, the environment is the most popular cause, but the overall pattern is one of multicausality. In the United States, for example, the four causes are each endorsed by most people, although genes remains the most

Table 1. Percent Endorsing Each of Four Explanations for Poor Health by Country, 2011 ISSP.

Country	Explanation for What Causes Poor Health			
	Genes (genes only)	Behavior (behavior only)	Environment (environment only)	Poverty (poverty only)
Australia	62 (7)	55 (7)	50 (2)	42 (2)
Belgium	60 (4)	52 (4)	66 (4)	52 (3)
Bulgaria	68 (1)	62 (1)	70 (2)	78 (6)
Chile	55 (3)	62 (7)	63 (7)	47 (2)
Taiwan	65 (4)	61 (3)	80 (6)	29 (1)
Croatia	65 (7)	51 (3)	63 (3)	49 (1)
Czech Republic	81 (5)	63 (3)	77 (2)	33 (1)
Denmark	66 (6)	71 (10)	57 (2)	31 (1)
Finland	70 (5)	72 (8)	51 (1)	47 (2)
France	63 (4)	50 (3)	77 (6)	52 (2)
Germany	69 (2)	72 (4)	77 (3)	48 (2)
Israel	74 (7)	58 (3)	63 (2)	49 (1)
Japan	39 (3)	47 (6)	62 (9)	28 (2)
Korea	70 (3)	54 (2)	74 (3)	66 (3)
Lithuania	80 (2)	81 (1)	82 (2)	54 (1)
The Netherlands	75 (13)	54 (4)	52 (1)	33 (1)
Norway	57 (7)	57 (8)	53 (4)	30 (1)
Philippines	64 (2)	73 (3)	73 (3)	66 (3)
Poland	84 (2)	63 (1)	80 (1)	74 (2)
Portugal	75 (7)	60 (3)	67 (2)	53 (3)
Russia	62 (1)	61 (2)	83 (5)	62 (2)
Slovak Republic	78 (5)	59 (2)	74 (2)	57 (2)
Slovenia	64 (3)	61 (3)	78 (5)	61 (2)
South Africa	53 (2)	65 (6)	70 (3)	52 (2)
Sweden	49 (2)	67 (11)	57 (3)	38 (2)
Switzerland	64 (7)	60 (6)	54 (3)	45 (2)
Turkey	70 (1)	80 (2)	76 (1)	77 (3)
The United Kingdom	59 (5)	61 (6)	59 (3)	43 (1)
The United States	72 (6)	58 (4)	62 (3)	54 (2)
Overall average	65 (4)	60 (4)	67 (3)	49 (2)

Notes: Total $N = 45{,}563$, country-specific sample sizes range from 936 (the United Kingdom) to 3,319 (France). All percents calculated using country-specific sample weights.

commonly endorsed cause. In all countries, it is rare to endorse only one cause and, at that, genetic reductionism (endorsed by 4% of people on average) is no more popular than behavioral reductionism (also 4%). Furthermore, the most popular cause varies considerably by country.

Indeed, all four causes appear as the most popular cause in at least one country. Poverty, for example, is the most popular cause in Bulgaria (78%), behavior in Turkey (80%), the environment in Russia (83%), and genes in Poland (84%). Genes are the most popular explanation in 11 countries, as is the environment (counting ties). In the four East Asian countries (Taiwan, Japan, Korea, and the Philippines), the environment is the most popular explanation, suggesting one aspect of regional consistency.

Although the endorsement level varies considerably across countries, all four explanations are positively correlated with each other. Table 2 presents tetrachoric correlations among the four beliefs, presenting the overall correlation as well as the highest and lowest correlation for each health-belief pairing (denoting also which country that correlation appeared in). In no country is there a single negative correlation. In this way, environmental explanations in no way compete with genetic explanations, as would be indicated by a negative correlation. The correlations are also quite strong. Notably the weakest correlation between behavior and genes – two explanations that are usually pitted against each other – is found in the United States (.132), suggesting some independence. But this correlation is unusual. Overall the weakest correlation is between poverty and behavior. Remarkably, the largest overall correlation is found between genes and the environment. There is also no unusually strong affinity between the two

Table 2. Tetrachoric Correlations among Four Beliefs about the Causes of Poor Health in 29 Countries, 2011 ISSP.

	Behavior	Environment	Genes
Environment			
Overall	.426		
Highest	.708, Turkey		
Lowest	.164, Switzerland		
Genes			
Overall	.330	.494	
Highest	.653, Turkey	.662, Bulgaria	
Lowest	.132, the United States	.394, France	
Poverty			
Overall	.258	.457	.382
Highest	.531, Croatia	.705, Croatia	.566, Croatia
Lowest	.057, South Korea	.320, Taiwan	.204, France

Note: Total $N = 45{,}563$, country-specific sample sizes range from 936 (the United Kingdom) to 3,319 (France).

proximate ($r = .330$) or the two distal causes ($r = .457$) relative to the other correlations in the matrix. Rather than regarding explanations as competing in some fashion, the results point to the global reach of a multicausal view and the lack of a conceptually clean set of underlying factors. The public readily accepts heterogeneous interpretive frameworks.

Table 3 turns to the determinants of health beliefs. The table presents a series of BIC statistics, as derived from logit models predicting each of four health beliefs (Raftery, 1995). The BIC statistic assesses overall model fit and allows for easy comparison between models, including between non-nested models. In this table, variables are inserted in sets, corresponding to types of influences, as described in the first column. The BIC statistic formally prefers a more parsimonious model by imposing a penalty for additional parameters, meaning the BIC would ceteris paribus prefer a model with leftist voting (which has only one coefficient) over a model with country dummy variables (which has 28 coefficients). Among models with the same dependent variable, the lowest value indicates the best fit. Table 3 presents the BIC statistic for five models for the four health beliefs and indicates the best fitting model with an asterisk. The results are plain. For each belief, the best fitting model is a model that simply includes the country dummy variables. By the criteria outlined by (Raftery, 1995), the preference for this model is "very strong" (a difference of more than 10 points relative to its nearest competitor). In each case, religion is the next most important influence, but in no case is it a truly close competitor. Similarly, education is important for endorsing genetic arguments, as one would anticipate if one regarded genetic beliefs as one feature of a scientifically sophisticated

Table 3. BIC Statistics from Logit Models Predicting Four Health Beliefs Using Thematic Covariate Sets, 2011 ISSP.

Variable Sets	Explanation for What Causes Poor Health			
	Behavior	Environment	Genes	Poverty
Country	59,957[a]	55,524[a]	57,491[a]	60,255[a]
Religion	60,820	57,002	58,807	62,088
Leftist voting	61,030	57,338	58,988	63,077
Education	61,041	57,232	58,919	63,002
Health and health care	61,031	57,172	59,008	62,471

Note: Total $N = 45{,}563$, country-specific sample sizes range from 936 (the United Kingdom) to 3,319 (France).
[a]Preferred model.

public, but education is still not as important as the country in which the respondent resides.

Table 4 presents the mean values for the three political attitudes by country. The subsequent tables link health beliefs to these attitudes, but Table 4 sets the stage. Recall that each of the variables ranges from one to five. In general, there is strong support for government-provided care (if we regard a score of three as denoting the point of indifference), although the level of support varies by country. This variation reflects some well-known patterns. For instance, support is tightly related to the extent to which the government of that country, in fact, provides insurance: support is high in Scandinavian countries, France, and the United Kingdom (which have robust government systems); low in the Philippines (which relies mostly on a private system); and moderate in the United States (which has a mix of public and private). Support is also low in Switzerland, which has compulsory insurance system offered through private insurers.

When the three variables are interpreted as a set, however, they reveal more political nuance. In countries where there is strong support for government-provided care, there also tends to be more perceived unfairness of income disparities in care. Yet this concern over disparities does not always translate into a willingness to extend care to noncitizens. For instance, while France shows high support for government-provided care and a concern over income disparities, there is considerably less support for providing health care to noncitizens. A similar pattern is observed in the United Kingdom and Australia. To a more limited degree, the United States fits the same pattern, although without the same level of support for government-provided care. Among the items, the lowest correlation is between support for government-provided care and support for providing care to noncitizens ($r = .015$, correlation not shown). In nine countries, this correlation is actually negative. These patterns could be interpreted through the lens of biocitizenship, an interpretation that becomes even more compelling in subsequent tables.

Table 5 turns to the determinants of these attitudes. The table again presents BIC statistics corresponding to models that include variables related to the thematic categories listed on the left (in this case, all the models control for country). Of all the influences shaping attitudes regarding health policy, beliefs about the causes of health matter the most. For two of the three attitudes, a model that includes only health beliefs is the best fitting model. In the case of support for access to noncitizens, a model including only leftist voting fits somewhat better than a model including

Table 4. Country-Specific Means for Three Health Policy Attitudes, 2011 ISSP.

Country	Health Policy Attitudes		
	Support for government-provided health care	Perceived unfairness of income disparities in health care	Support for health care access to noncitizens
Australia	3.81	3.40	2.55
Belgium	3.82	4.06	3.05
Bulgaria	3.58	4.08	3.66
Chile	3.80	3.60	3.98
Taiwan	3.15	2.99	2.56
Croatia	3.72	4.13	3.31
Czech Republic	3.74	4.00	2.86
Denmark	4.05	3.74	3.55
Finland	3.68	3.05	3.06
France	3.96	4.22	2.80
Germany	3.78	4.03	3.63
Israel	3.69	3.93	3.44
Japan	3.50	3.75	3.24
Korea	3.21	3.31	3.70
Lithuania	3.58	3.16	3.27
The Netherlands	3.66	4.23	3.36
Norway	3.91	4.01	3.05
Philippines	2.18	2.11	3.38
Poland	3.47	3.85	3.51
Portugal	3.70	3.78	4.07
Russia	3.58	3.86	4.07
Slovak Republic	4.00	3.90	3.37
Slovenia	3.77	4.45	4.00
South Africa	3.39	2.91	3.43
Sweden	3.65	4.15	3.72
Switzerland	2.97	3.78	3.63
Turkey	3.45	3.60	3.78
The United Kingdom	3.88	3.29	2.31
The United States	3.31	3.48	2.45

Notes: Total $N = 45{,}563$, country-specific sample sizes range from 936 (the United Kingdom) to 3,319 (France). All means calculated using country-specific sample weights. Each variable ranges from 1 to 5 with higher values indicating more support or more perceived unfairness.

health beliefs, although subsequent models show that this is partly due to the highly contingent effects of genetic beliefs by country. In a model that estimates all the beliefs except genetics, the BIC drops to 143,675, rendering it the preferred model.

Table 5. BIC Statistics from Logit Models Predicting Three Health Policy Attitudes Using Thematic Covariate Sets, 2011 ISSP.

Variables	Health Policy Attitudes		
	Support for government-provided health care	Perceived unfairness of income disparities in health care	Support for health care access to noncitizens
Health beliefs	138,578[a]	145,417[a]	143,685
Religion	138,679	146,044	143,916
Leftist voting	138,847	145,823	143,677[a]
Education	138,857	145,928	143,990
Health and health care	138,968	145,762	144,062

Notes: Total $N = 45{,}563$, country-specific sample sizes range from 936 (the United Kingdom) to 3,319 (France). All models include controls for country. Each dependent variable ranges from 1 to 5 with higher values indicating more support or more perceived unfairness.
[a]Preferred model.

Table 6 unpacks this finding further. The table presents the relationship between health beliefs and health policy attitudes. The coefficients are from multilevel mixed-effects linear regression models (see Searle, Casella, & McCulloch, 1992). The coefficients themselves can be interpreted as simple linear regression coefficients. The addition of a mixture component allows for the direct estimation of between-country variation in the coefficient for each of the four health beliefs (referred to, per convention, as "random" effects, whereas the other coefficients remain "fixed"). The random effects are summarized in the bottom panel of the table, presented as standard deviations in the coefficients. The table reveals generally robust relationships between health beliefs and support for specific health policies. Environmental and poverty-related explanations have the most consistent associations, increasing support for government-provided care, increasing the perceived unfairness of income disparities in care, and increasing support for access to noncitizens. Endorsing behavioral explanations reduces support for government-provided care and reduces the perceived unfairness of income disparities in care. Genetic beliefs, however, have more complex associations, as revealed by the small and mixed average effects (the coefficient itself is not statistically significant) and large variance components. Genetic beliefs are positively associated with support for government-provided care, negatively associated with the perceived unfairness of income disparities in care, and unassociated with support for access to noncitizens.

Table 6. Mixture Models Predicting Health Policy Attitudes and Estimating Between-Country Variation in Health-Belief Coefficients, 2011 (ISSP).

	Health Policy Attitude		
	Support for government-provided care	Perceived unfairness of income disparities in care	Support for access to noncitizens
Health belief			
Behavior	−.176***	−.133***	−.003
Environment	.100***	.133***	.089***
Genes	.038*	−.046*	−.001
Poverty	.086***	.200***	.169***
Between country standard deviation of coefficients			
Behavior	.105	.072	.075
Environment	.087	.080	.028
Genes	.078	.100	.100
Poverty	.099	.140	.095

Notes: Total $N = 45{,}563$, country-specific sample sizes range from 936 (the United Kingdom) to 3,319 (France). Coefficients from linear regression mixture models. All models include controls for sex, religion, leftist voting, educational attainment, age, poor health, health insurance, difficulty with health care, and country.
*$p < .05$; **$p < .01$; ***$p < .001$ (two-tailed test).

Table 7 presents this variation in its specific forms. The table presents the coefficient for genetic beliefs for each of the 29 countries across the three dependent variables. The coefficients are from linear regression models that also control for the other factors considered in the preceding discussion. The table reveals the remarkable complexity surrounding beliefs about genes. Although the overall relationship is positive between the endorsement of genetic beliefs and support for government-provided care, the size and even the direction of the relationship varies between countries. In Bulgaria and the Philippines, the relationship is negative. In Israel and the Czech Republic, however, the relationship is positive. In no country is the relationship across the three outcomes uniformly progressive or conservative – that is, in no country are the three coefficients significant and also signed in the same direction. Indeed, in both Israel and Czech Republic, endorsing genetic causes is *positively* associated with support for government-provided care, but *negatively* associated with support for providing that care to noncitizens. The relationship with genes is especially

Table 7. Country-Specific Relationship between Endorsement of Genetic Causes of Poor Health and Three Health Policy Attitudes, 2011 ISSP.

Country	Health Policy Attitudes		
	Support for government-provided health care	Perceived unfairness of income disparities in health care	Support for health care access to noncitizens
Australia	.016	.149**	−.038
Belgium	.071	.054	−.147***
Bulgaria	−.240***	−.093	−.002
Chile	.163**	−.091	.153**
Taiwan	.014	−.250***	−.142**
Croatia	.038	.079	.304***
Czech Republic	.240***	.075	−.198**
Denmark	.032	−.001	.040
Finland	.092	−.071	−.015
France	.038	.044	−.099*
Germany	.166**	−.062	.115
Israel	.213**	.042	−.155*
Japan	.070	−.061	−.049
Korea	−.058	−.123	.025
Lithuania	−.041	−.292***	−.074
The Netherlands	.031	.199**	.019
Norway	.063	.073	.123*
Philippines	−.239***	−.385***	.154*
Poland	.206*	.108	.005
Portugal	.082	−.023	−.028
Russia	−.104	−.104	.137*
Slovak Republic	.014	−.053	.098
Slovenia	.024	−.005	.010
South Africa	.089*	−.355***	−.076
Sweden	.009	−.060	.050
Switzerland	−.092	−.085	−.202**
Turkey	.055	.034	.125
The United Kingdom	.038	−.068	−.055
The United States	−.012	.057	−.105

Notes: Total $N = 45{,}563$, country-specific sample sizes range from 936 (United Kingdom) to 3,319 (France). All coefficients from linear regression models predicting dependent variable controlling for sex, religion, leftist voting, educational attainment, age, poor health, health insurance, difficulty with health care, and country.

$^{*}p < .05$; $^{**}p < .01$; $^{***}p < .001$ (two-tailed test).

contingent with respect to providing care to noncitizens. When significant, the relationship is positive nearly as often as it is negative (5 vs. 6). Previous research has shown no strong connection between political orientation and genetic beliefs within the United States (Shostak et al., 2009), a result that is replicated here in finding a coefficient in the United States that is statistically indistinguishable from zero. However, this finding is not duplicated in other countries, suggesting the complex political connotations of genetic arguments is a global pattern.

The results regarding behavior, presented in Table 8, reveal more consistent patterns. These patterns vary more in magnitude than direction, but it is still notable that behavioral arguments are not more politicized in the United States than elsewhere, despite speculation to the contrary. In general, behavioral arguments are negatively associated with support for government-provided care and with the perceived unfairness of income disparities in care. The magnitude of the association varies a great deal, but the association is negative in all but two cases. The strongest negative relationship is in Poland ($b = -.393$), while the United States is intermediary between this and zero ($b = -.252$). The association between behavioral beliefs and perceived unfairness of income disparities in health care is generally negative as well, although it also varies in magnitude. As with genetics the most variable associations pertain to support for health care access to noncitizens. The association is statistically zero in the United States, but positive in two countries and negative in five. The strongest negative association is found in the United Kingdom.

DISCUSSION

In interpreting these patterns, it is useful to return to the propositions that motivated the analysis. The results confirm some patterns heretofore observed only in the United States, but also suggest some complexities when moving to a more global perspective. First, genetic explanations are, indeed, very popular. Support for genetic explanations falls below 50% for only two countries (Sweden at 49% and Japan at 39%) and reaches as high as 84% (in Poland). Yet environmental explanations are also popular and, in fact, slightly exceed the popularity of both genetic and behavioral explanations when expressed as an overall average. Proximate explanations may, in general, be popular, but worldwide the social environment is still viewed as a strong cause of poor health. In no country is there an overwhelming

Table 8. Country-Specific Relationship between Endorsement of Behavioral Causes of Poor Health and Three Health Policy Attitudes, 2011 ISSP.

Country	Health Policy Attitudes		
	Support for government-provided health care	Perceived unfairness of income disparities in health care	Support for health care access to noncitizens
Australia	−.202***	−.123*	−.026
Belgium	−.168***	−.077	−.090*
Bulgaria	−.284***	−.010	−.171*
Chile	−.048	−.018	.098
Taiwan	−.145**	−.156**	−.041
Croatia	−.322***	−.078	.358***
Czech Republic	.134*	−.223***	.011
Denmark	−.243***	−.158*	.016
Finland	−.218***	−.148*	−.157*
France	−.276***	−.132***	−.092*
Germany	−.150*	−.114	.041
Israel	−.368***	−.062	−.016
Japan	−.216***	−.225***	−.001
Korea	−.331***	−.032	.082
Lithuania	−.177*	−.338***	−.036
The Netherlands	−.163**	−.045	−.037
Norway	−.052	−.144**	.008
Philippines	−.209**	−.071	−.012
Poland	−.393***	−.135	.059
Portugal	−.207**	−.075	−.009
Russia	−.318***	−.366***	.096
Slovak Republic	−.189**	−.089	.035
Slovenia	−.113	−.041	.026
South Africa	.003	−.277***	.041
Sweden	−.015	−.151*	−.032
Switzerland	−.197**	−.240***	−.133
Turkey	−.164*	−.044	.249***
The United Kingdom	−.062	−.044	−.199**
The United States	−.252***	−.218***	−.019

Notes: Total $N = 45{,}563$, country-specific sample sizes range from 936 (United Kingdom) to 3,319 (France). All coefficients from linear regression models predicting dependent variable controlling for sex, religion, leftist voting, educational attainment, age, poor health, health insurance, difficulty with health care, and country.

$^{*}p < .05$; $^{**}p < .01$; $^{***}p < .001$ (two-tailed test).

tendency toward genetic reductionism or, indeed, reductionism of any sort. The percent of people who endorse *only* genetic explanations for poor health is less than 8% in all but one country (the Netherlands, at 13%). Furthermore, behavioral reductionism is, on average, just as popular as genetic reductionism. All four explanations are positively correlated in all 29 countries. Even the least popular (and probably most politically charged) cause, poverty, is endorsed by most people in 14 of the 29 countries.

These patterns also suggest there is no obvious competition in the mind of the public between genes and the environment. One might argue that countries will eventually accept genetic arguments to the exclusion of the environment, but even in countries that have the highest overall endorsement of genetic arguments (e.g., Czech Republic and Poland) the correlation between these two beliefs is, if anything, higher than the sample-wide average (.632 and .642, respectively). If there is an "evolution" in public beliefs, it is toward a multicausal view rather than toward a genetic view that obviates the relevance of the environment.

This study confirms previous research in demonstrating the importance of religion and personal experiences in shaping health beliefs. Yet the best fitting model is one that simply includes dummy variables for country of residence. Similarly, national context strongly shapes the political connotations of health beliefs, although across the countries health beliefs remain a foundation to policy-related attitudes. Beliefs about the causes of health exert more influence than any other factor explored here. In general, the environment and poverty have the most consistent relationships with policy-related attitudes, encouraging stronger support for government-provided care and a greater emphasis on equality. In this sense, distal causes have more uniform political connotations than proximate causes. Behavioral and genetic explanations, meanwhile, have highly contingent relationships with policy attitudes. To be sure, behavioral explanations encourage individual responsibility for health, but the strength of this association varies. This interpretive framework is stronger, for example, in the United States ($b = -.252$) than in Norway ($b = -.052$) or Sweden ($b = -.015$) (coefficient differences significant at $p < .01$), suggesting a robust "cause neutral" health care safety net in the latter two countries. Yet the United States is not alone in aligning behavioral explanations with less support for government-provided care. The relationship is negative and significant in 22 of 29 countries. Similarly, genetic explanations have highly contingent political associations and, if anything, these connotations are weaker in the United States. Genetic arguments are not associated with any of the three political attitudes in the United States. In some other countries, however, they assume strong political resonance. In the Czech Republic and Israel, where support for genetic explanations is particularly high, endorsing genetic arguments is associated with more support for government-provided care but also more support from excluding noncitizens from that care. In all, genetic arguments are associated with exclusionary attitudes in six countries. It is also notable that in only two countries is support for genetic arguments negatively associated with support for government-provided care. Although some speculate that genetic arguments are associated with fundamentally conservative projects, this is not uniformly the case across countries.

The ISSP provides an invaluable resource for comparative research, but a number of features of the module likely shaped my conclusions. As in any survey of this sort, framing effects are particularly important. It is possible the close relationship between health beliefs and political attitudes reflects the ordering of the questions in the instrument. Because the health-belief questions were asked shortly after questions about the health care system, respondents may have responded to questions about the causes of health in light of how they regard the health care system, producing a natural affinity. Nevertheless, I find the relationship between these health beliefs and policy attitudes varies even in its direction across countries, suggesting that any uniform pattern due to priming does not result in an overwhelming single-direction bias. Other framing effects might also affect my interpretations. Respondents were asked about the causes of "severe health problems" rather than, say, a specific problem or a mild problem. What respondents believe cause severe problems probably reflects what severe problems come to mind first. This might vary between countries. In places where smoking is still common, for example, the perceived relevance of behavior might be higher. Responses might be anchored in other ways as well. For example, support for government-provided care might be interpreted in terms of whether respondents support *more* government-provided care relative to what is provided for them already. The purpose of my study was to see whether health beliefs tap similar policy-related schema in different countries. To some degree, they do, and this study provides some certainty regarding claims about specific health beliefs. But for those beliefs where the association varies in direction, the reasons for this heterogeneity are likely complex. It is also possible, of course, that cross-national differences reflect differences in the administration of the survey, even though an effort was made to minimize these differences.

CONCLUSION

Although it is popular to regard health beliefs as a reflection of personal experiences with health or health care or as a reasoned reflection on the actual determinants of health, the current study shows that health beliefs are fundamentally political beliefs. They vary enormously between countries and, indeed, in absence of other information, knowing where someone lives is the best predictor of what they believe causes poor health. Furthermore, beliefs about the causes of health do more to predict political attitudes regarding health care than many other influences, including leftist voting, education, or even personal experiences with health and health care. A modern mindset regarding the causes of health might encourage better health behaviors or a more active approach to promoting personal health. Yet the results of this study suggest that health beliefs perhaps do more to shape what you think a government should do for its citizens than what you might do personally for your well-being.

REFERENCES

Bates, B. R. (2005). Public culture and public understanding of genetics: A focus group study. *Public Understanding of Science*, *14*, 47–65.

Furnham, A. (1994). Explaining health and illness: Lay perceptions on current and future health, the causes of illness, and the nature of recovery. *Social Science & Medicine*, *39*, 715–725.

Gendall, P. (2013). *International social survey programme, study monitoring 2011, health.* Dunedin: University of Otago.

Goldberg, D. S. (2012). The difficulties of enhancing public understanding of the social determinants of health in the United States: A commentary on Pesce, Kpaduwa, Danis (2011). *Social Science & Medicine*, *74*, 1139–1142.

Gollust, S. E., & Lynch, J. (2011). Who deserves health care? The effects of causal attributions and group cues on public attitudes about responsibility for health care costs. *Journal of Health Politics, Policy and Law*, *36*, 1061–1095.

Gordon, D. R. (1988). Tenacious assumptions in western medicine. In M. Lock & D. R. Gordon (Eds.), *Biomedicine examined* (pp. 19–56). Dordrecht: Kluwer.

Heath, A., Martin, J., & Spreckelsen, T. (2009). Cross-national comparability of survey attitude measures. *International Journal of Public Opinion Research*, *21*, 293–315.

Heath, D., Rapp, R., & Taussig, K.-S. (2008). Genetic citizenship. In D. Nugent & J. Vincent (Eds.), *A companion to the anthropology of politics* (pp. 152–167). Oxford: Blackwell Publishing Ltd.

Helman, C. G. (2007). *Culture, health, and illness*. New York, NY: Hodder Arnold.

International Social Survey Programme Research Group. (2011). Health and health care, 2011. Cologne Germany, ZA 5800, Data Version 2.0 (2014-1-8) Distributor: GESIS.

Kleinman, A. (1980). *Patients and healers in the context of culture*. Berkeley, CA: University of California Press.

Leichter, H. M. (2003). "Evil Habits" and "Personal Choices": Assigning responsibility for health in the 20th century. *Milbank Quarterly*, *81*, 603–626.

Lynch, J., & Gollust, S. E. (2010). Playing fair: Fairness beliefs and health policy preferences in the United States. *Journal of Health Politics, Policy and Law*, *35*, 849–887.

Mechanic, D. (2006). *The truth about health care: Why reform is not working in America*. New Brunswick, NJ: Rutgers University.

Mechanic, D., & Tanner, J. (2007). Vulnerable people, groups, and populations: Societal view. *Health Affairs*, *26*, 1220–1230.

Morone, J. (2003). *Hellfire nation: The politics of sin in American history*. New Haven, CT: Yale University.

National Research Council and Institute of Medicine. (2013). In S. H. Woolf & L. Aron (Eds.), U.S. health in international perspective: *Shorter lives*, poorer health. Washington, DC: The National Academies Press.

Nelkin, D., & Lindee, M. S. (1996). "Genes Made Me Do It": The appeal of biological explanations. *Politics and the Life Sciences*, *15*, 95–97.

Novas, C., & Rose, N. (2000). Genetic risk and the birth of the somatic individual. *Economy and Society*, *29*, 485–513.

Pescosolido, B. A., Martin, J. K., Long, J. S., Medina, T. R., Phelan, J. C., & Link, B. G. (2010). 'A Disease Like Any Other'? A decade of change in public reactions to schizophrenia, depression, and alcohol dependence. *American Journal of Psychiatry*, *167*, 1321–1330.

Pill, R., & Stott, N. C. H. (1982). Concepts of illness causation and responsibility: Some preliminary data from a sample of working class mothers. *Social Science & Medicine*, *16*, 43–52.

Rabinow, P. (2008). Artificiality and enlightenment: From sociobiology to biosociality. In J. X. Inda (Ed.), *Anthropologies of modernity: Foucault, governmentality, and life politics* (pp. 179–193). Oxford: Blackwell Publishing Ltd.

Raftery, A. E. (1995). Bayesian model selection in social research. *Sociological Methodology*, *25*, 111–163.

Robert, S. A., & Booske, B. C. (2011). US opinions on health determinants and social policy as health policy. *American Journal of Public Health*, *101*, 1655–1663.

Rose, N. (Ed.). (2007). *The politics of life itself: Biomedicine, power, and subjectivity in the twenty-first century*. Princeton, NJ: Princeton University.

Saguy, A. C., & Gruys, K. (2010). Morality and health: News media constructions of overweight and eating disorders. *Social Problems*, *57*, 231–250.

Saguy, A. C., Gruys, K., & Gong, S. (2010). Social problem construction and national context: News reporting on "Overweight" and "Obesity" in the United States and France. *Social Problems*, *57*, 586–610.

Schnittker, J. (2008). An uncertain revolution: Why the rise of a genetic model of mental illness has not increased tolerance. *Social Science and Medicine*, *67*, 1370–1381.

Searle, S. R., Casella, G., & McCulloch, C. E. (1992). *Variance components*. New York, NY: Wiley.

Shostak, S., Freese, J., Link, B. G., & Phelan, J. C. (2009). The politics of the gene: Social status and beliefs about genetics for individual outcomes. *Social Psychology Quarterly*, *72*, 77–93.

Singer, E., Corning, A., & Lamias, M. (1998). Trends: Genetic testing, engineering, and therapy: Awareness and attitudes. *Public Opinion Quarterly*, *62*, 633–664.

EXAMINING THE COMPLEXITY AND VARIATION OF HEALTH CARE SYSTEM DISTRUST ACROSS NEIGHBORHOODS: IMPLICATIONS FOR PREVENTIVE HEALTH CARE

Tse-Chuan Yang, I-Chien Chen and Aggie J. Noah

ABSTRACT

Purpose – *Recently, the institutional performance model has been used to explain the increased distrust of health care system by arguing that distrust is a function of individuals' perceptions on the quality of life in neighborhood and social institutions. We examined (1) whether individuals assess two dimensions of distrust consistently, (2) if the multilevel institutional performance model explains the variation of distrust across neighborhoods, and (3) how distrust patterns affect preventive health care behaviors.*

Methodology – *Using data from 9,497 respondents in 914 census tracts (neighborhoods) in Philadelphia, we examined the patterns of how individuals evaluate the competence and values distrust using the Multilevel Latent Class Analysis (MLCA), and then investigated how neighborhood environment factors are associated with distrust patterns. Finally,*

Education, Social Factors, and Health Beliefs in Health and Health Care Services
Research in the Sociology of Health Care, Volume 33, 43–66

ISSN: 0275-4959/doi:10.1108/S0275-495920150000033003

we used regression to examine the relationships between distrust patterns and preventive health care.

Findings – *The MLCA identified four distrust patterns: Believers, Doubters, Competence Skeptics, and Values Skeptics. We found that 55 percent of the individuals evaluated competence and values distrust coherently, with Believers reporting low levels and Doubters having high levels of distrust. Competence and Values Skeptics assessed distrust inconsistently. Believers were the least likely to reside in socioeconomically disadvantaged and racially segregated neighborhoods among these patterns. In contrast to Doubters, Believers were more likely to use preventive health care, even after controlling for other socioeconomic factors including insurance coverage.*

Practical implications – *Our findings suggest that distrust patterns are a function of neighborhood conditions and distrust patterns are associated with preventive health care. This study provides important policy implications for health care and future interventions.*

Keywords: Health care system distrust; preventive health care; multilevel latent class analysis; neighborhood

INTRODUCTION

Individuals' trust of the health care system has important implications for individuals as it can influence individuals' perception and utilization of the health care system (Musa, Schulz, Harris, Silverman, & Thomas, 2009). In the last five decades, individuals' trust of the health care system dropped significantly in the United States. According to the Harris Poll, about 73 percent of respondents reported "a great deal of confidence" in the U.S. health care system in 1966; however, only 34 percent of respondents maintained the same level of confidence in 2012 (Harris Interactive Polls, 2012). In the past decade, this low confidence rate remained roughly constant (Harris Interactive Polls, 2012). Such decrease and persistently low rates of individuals' trust of the health care system warrant the need for more public policy efforts to improve individuals' trust in the U.S. health care system. Thus, it is important to systematically investigate the multiple factors influencing individuals' trust of the health care system.

To understand individuals' perception of the health care system, the distrust of the health care system (hereafter, "distrust") – rather than trust – provides more information because the conceptualization of distrust includes the belief that the trustee will act against the individual's interest (Armstrong et al., 2008; Hall, Dugan, Zheng, & Mishra, 2001; Shoff & Yang, 2012). Distrust is a belief status with a greater possibility of negative consequences than "no trust" (Shoff & Yang, 2012). Negative belief creates adverse impacts on an individual's health behaviors and outcomes, like the use of preventive health services (Musa et al., 2009; Yang, Matthews, & Hillemeier, 2011) and self-rated health (Armstrong et al., 2006; Yang, Matthews, & Shoff, 2011). Furthermore, it can be a barrier to quality health care processes (LaVeist, Isaac, & Williams, 2009).

Distrust is a concept that comprises multiple dimensions (Hall et al., 2001). Rose and colleagues attempted to construct a single dimension measure of distrust but found that the reliability of their scale was low (Rose, Peters, Shea, & Armstrong, 2004). In 2008, Shea, Micco, Dean, McMurphy, Schwartz, & Armstrong, (2008) identified two dimensions of distrust – competence and values – and developed a reliable and valid distrust scale. *Competence* refers to the technical skills necessary for successful health care, whereas *values* indicate the ethics a health care system should possess such as respect and integrity. In another study, scholars discussed the individual-level determinants of competence and value distrust separately (Armstrong et al., 2008). For example, values distrust varied significantly across various individual demographic and socioeconomic features such as race-ethnicity, educational attainment, income, and insurance status. However, the variations in competence distrust across these characteristics were not statistically significant (Armstrong et al., 2008). Though both dimensions were designed to capture the concept of distrust, little is known about how individuals assess these dimensions together. Understanding such assessment process is critical as there are potential implications of the inconsistent assessment for the use of preventive health care service along these two dimensions.

Among the plausible explanations for the formation of distrust of the health care system in the United States (Norris, 2007), this study focuses on the institutional performance model. Blendon (2007) explained the institutional performance model with a detailed discussion of the increasing distrust of a range of social institutions in the United States including the federal government, churches, banking, and airlines. He argued that the soaring distrust of these social institutions parallels the general increase in the distrust of the health care system. Specifically, the institutional performance model implies that the poor performances of social institutions contribute to the process of shaping distrust, as individuals' distrust may not be directly relevant to personal experience with the health care system.

That is, distrust is not solely a consequence of actual health care system performance and individuals' experience but also a product of the perceptions of other social institutions or environment (Blendon, 2007; Norris, 2007). Recently, researchers have started to use the institutional performance model to explain racial differences in distrust (Shoff & Yang, 2012) and to investigate the interaction effect between distrust and neighborhood social environment on self-rated health (Yang et al., 2011). These studies found that the institutional performance model is an adequate framework to explain individuals' distrust by demonstrating that distrust is a function of individuals' perceptions on the quality of life in neighborhood and social institutions. Despite the important findings guided by this model, we argue that previous studies have adopted this model without critically examining its validity. Furthermore, we argue that it is important to examine the validity of the model and if institutional performance model explains the variations in the distrust of the health care system.

The goal of this study is to fill the gaps mentioned above by answering three related questions. First, how do individuals assess two dimensions of distrust together? Specifically, does an individual's competence distrust correspond to values distrust? Previous research has not extensively discussed whether both distrust dimensions of distrust are related to each other. Should an individual assess competence and values distrust coherently, one would observe that high (or low) competence distrust is always accompanied with high (or low) values distrust. Second, does the institutional performance model explain the variations in distrust patterns? Moving beyond the institutional performance model that predominantly focused on individual-level factors, we extend the scope to include neighborhood-level factors because individuals' high levels of competence and values distrust may be the consequences of the perceptions of their neighborhood environment in which individuals and social institutions are embedded. Should this perspective stand, those living in a neighborhood with poor living conditions would have higher competence and values distrust than their counterparts in a better-off community. Finally, what are the potential implications of different assessment patterns of distrust – from the second part of the chapter – for the use of preventive health care service? The previous literature suggested that overall high levels of distrust discourage the use of preventive health care (Musa et al., 2009; Yang et al., 2011); however, it remains underexplored whether different assessment patterns alter the relationship between distrust and the use of preventive health care service. We have three hypotheses: (H1) Most individuals evaluate competence and values distrust in a coherent fashion, while others may report in an incoherent fashion (e.g., high level in one dimension but low level in the other), (H2) when considering neighborhood-level factors such as racial composition, living condition, and socioeconomic status (SES), individuals with high levels of competence and values distrust are more likely to reside in socioeconomically disadvantaged (i.e., poor housing condition and low SES) and racially segregated neighborhoods (i.e., high concentration of minority) than other patterns, and (H3) individuals who consistently report high competence and values distrust are the least likely to use preventive health care service, whereas those who persistently report low competence and values distrust are the most likely to engage in preventive health care activities.

METHODS

Data Sources and Measures

To test our hypotheses, we draw from two data sources to construct both individual- and neighborhood-level factors. The individual-level data comes from the Public Health Management Corporation's (PHMC) 2008 Household Health Survey. The PHMC survey covered five counties in southeastern Pennsylvania (Bucks, Chester, Delaware, Montgomery, and Philadelphia counties) and used both stratified sampling and the random-digit dialing methodology to conduct interviews (PHMC, 2008). The validity of this data set was discussed in previous research (Matthews & Yang, 2010; Shoff & Yang, 2012). There were 9,497 adult respondents in this study. They were asked to answer how much they agree or disagree with the following six statements: (1) the health care system makes patients' health better, (2) patients receive high quality care from the health care system, (3) the health care system gives excellent medical care, (4) patients get the same medical treatment regardless of race, (5) the health care system puts making money above patients' needs, and (6) the health care system lies to make money. These questions were rated on a five-level Likert scale ("strongly disagree," "disagree," "neither agree nor disagree," "agree," and "strongly agree"), and all questions were coded to reflect that high values indicate high distrust. The first four questions were associated to competence distrust and the last two questions were associated with values distrust. The reliability of this scale was 0.795 (Cronbach's Alpha) and the multilevel latent class analysis approach (MLCA, discussed below) used respondents' answers to these questions to understand whether individuals consistently assess the competence and values distrust.

In addition to the distrust scale, the PHMC also collected information on respondents' utilization of preventive health care services. Three screening tests were considered: blood cholesterol, Papanicolaou smear test (Pap test), and prostate cancer screening. More specifically, respondents were asked how long it has been since blood cholesterol has been checked and the answers range from one (less than one year) to six (never) where larger values indicating longer time since last blood cholesterol check. Female participants were first asked how long it has been since the last Pap test and the PHMC compared the answers with the cervical cancer screening guidelines – which differ by age groups – to create a dichotomous variable where those who follow the guidelines were coded 1, otherwise 0. Similarly, male respondents reported how long it has been since last prostate cancer screening and the PHMC created a binary variable where those followed the cancer screening guidelines were coded 1, otherwise 0. These three variables served as the dependent variables in this study. The ordinary least square (OLS) regression was applied to blood cholesterol test and the logistic regression was used for the Pap and prostate cancer tests. The blood cholesterol test measure assessed how both female and male respondents utilize the general preventative health care service, and Pap test and prostate cancer screening assessed how individuals utilize the gender-specific preventative health care services.

Six additional individual characteristics were included in the analysis. *Gender* was coded 1 for females and 0 for males, and this variable was only applied to the blood cholesterol test. An individual's *age* was treated as a continuous variable. *Educational attainment* was categorized into five groups: less than high school (reference), high school graduate, some college education, college graduate, and post-college degree. Three *race/ethnicity* groups were identified: non-Hispanic white, non-Hispanic black, and others. As the Philadelphia metropolitan area had relatively small Hispanic population, we combined Hispanics with other racial/ethnicity groups. With respect to one's socioeconomic status, a respondent was determined to be impoverished based on the Federal poverty line. The *poverty* variable was coded as 1, otherwise 0. Individuals who had any health insurance coverages were coded 1 and those without any insurance were coded 0.

Beyond the individual-level covariates, we included neighborhood-level factors to examine the institutional performance model. Neighborhood-level factors were operationalized at the Census tract level, which is a common approach in health research (Wight et al., 2013). We draw our neighborhood-level data from the American Community Survey (ACS) 2006–2010 five-year estimates (US Census Burean, 2011). The 9,497 respondents resided in 914 neighborhoods (tracts) in the survey area, and we used three measures of the neighborhood environment. First, *racial composition* comprises of four variables: percent of non-Hispanic white percent of non-Hispanic black, percent of non-Hispanic other races, and percent of Hispanics. The race/ethnicity was self-reported and the group of non-Hispanic other races included those who reported more than two races. Second, *living conditions* were measured with four variables: percent of households with more than one person per room, percent of households without telephone service, percent of households without vehicles, and percent of household without plumbing systems. Third, *SES* included six variables: percent of single-parent households with children, percent of population with at least a high school diploma, unemployment rate, median family income, percent of owner-occupied housing units, and percent of family in poverty. These neighborhood variables were used to profile the neighborhoods where individuals in different distrust evaluation patterns live.

Analytic Strategies and Methods

Our analytic strategy had three stages. The first stage was to identify the patterns of assessing competence and values distrust questions with MLCA, and to label the patterns based on the results. The second stage was to compare the neighborhood variables across different distrust patterns and test if individuals in different evaluation patterns reside in different neighborhoods. It is important to note that the MLCA specification in the previous stage only included the neighborhood-level random effect and the neighborhood covariates were not included. This specification aligns recent studies (Henry & Muthén, 2010; Vermunt, 2003) and justifies the second stage of analysis. The third stage was to understand the relationships between the patterns identified by MLCA and the three preventive health care tests with the OLS and logistic regressions. We elaborate on each stage in greater details:

Stage 1: As discussed previously, the respondents in the PHMC survey were linked to their neighborhoods to constitute a hierarchical data set using Census tract as a common geographic identifier. We used the MLCA to identify the number and structure of latent profiles that emerged from this hierarchical data set. The traditional latent class analysis (LCA) approach fails to address the potential dependence among respondents from the same neighborhood (Clogg, 1988; Lazarsfeld & Henry, 1968) and does not fit the hierarchical data structure. Addressing these limitations, the MLCA approach (Henry & Muthén, 2010; Vermunt, 2003) has improved this shortcoming by taking the neighborhood-level random effects into account in recent years. More specifically, the MLCA allows the latent classes to account for both neighborhood- and individual-level variations.

The MLCA approach improves the traditional LCA approach. The LCA approach provides an important foundation for understanding the MLCA approach. LCA converts continuous variables into dichotomous variables by using a probability-based approach (Lazarsfeld & Henry, 1968). LCA used Expectation-Maximization algorithm to complete the process. The MLCA approach further includes the random errors at the neighborhood level into the LCA probability-based procedure in order to account for the potential clustering within neighborhoods (Vermunt, 2008). Our MLCA assumed that respondents' latent distrust of health care system was a random variable, which overcame the shortcoming of assuming the probability of the outcome was constant within each neighborhood (Asparouhov & Muthén, 2008; Snijders & Bosker, 2001). For example, our MLCA model included six indicators which can be written as follows. The conditional probability of P given a latent class for each respondent in each neighborhood is

$$P=\left(U_{ij1}=s_1, U_{ij2}=s_2 \ldots U_{ijk}=s_k\right)=\sum_{w=1}^{W} P\left(C_{ij}=w\right) \prod_{k=1}^{K} P\left(U_{ijk}=S_K | C_{ij}=w\right)$$

where U_{ijk} represent the distrust of individual i in the neighborhood j on the indicator k and s_1 represents the specific response for the first indicator. C_{ij}refers to the latent class membership and the total number of latent classes are referring as w. The probability of a specific respondent pattern, such as P $\{k_1 = 1, k_2 = 1, k_3 = 1, k_4 = 1, k_5 = 0, k_6 = 0\}$, is the weighted average of the probabilities conditional on class membership (Henry & Muthén, 2010).

To fully utilize the data structure of the unique hierarchical data constructed from the PHMC and ACS, this study employed the MLCA approach to identify potential patterns of how individuals rated competence and values distrust, and the variations of distrust patterns across neighborhoods. For example, some individuals may experience similar competence and values distrust patterns, but the probability and the mean level of distrust patterns that these individuals belong to a certain latent class may be more concentrated in neighborhoods with certain characteristics. The features of MLCA with random coefficient allow more flexibility to assess the institutional performance model and the impacts of neighborhood on distrust patterns.

Stage 2: Using the MLCA results, we employed neighborhood-level analysis by comparing the mean values of the neighborhoods across different latent classes. The main analytic approach included the analysis of variance and post-hoc pairwise comparisons, consistent with previous studies (Montgomery, 2008). These analyses aim to examine whether there are any significant differences in neighborhood environments across latent classes and if yes, to investigate whether the difference support the institutional performance model as discussed previously.

Stage 3: The OLS and logistic regressions were used to understand if the latent classes have different implications for the use of preventive health care service even after accounting for other individual sociodemographic characteristics. We opt not to discuss the details of these methods due to their popularity in research but they are available upon request.

Fig. 1 summarizes the analytic stages. To reiterate, we first used MLCA to identify the underlying distrust patterns and then examined whether the neighborhood conditions varied significantly across different patterns. The last stage is to include the distrust patterns and other covariates to understand if the distrust patterns have implications for preventive health care utilization, namely blood cholesterol test, Pap test, and prostate cancer screening.

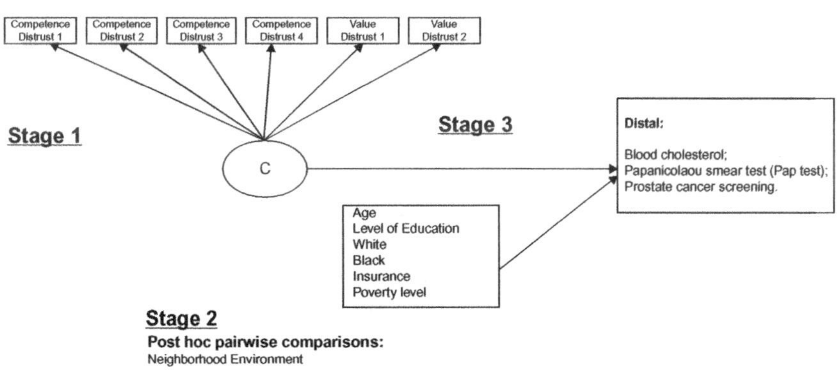

Fig. 1. Summary of the Analytic Strategy and Key Variables.

RESULTS

Our MLCA suggests that there are four distrust patterns (latent classes) of responses to the six distrust questions; the results are summarized in Table 1. We added each subsequent model to include an additional profile until the Vuong-Lo-Mendell-Rubin likelihood ratio test was non-significant indicating that additional profile did not improve model fit. We then evaluated model fit by examining Akaike's information criterion (AIC), Baysian information criterion (BIC), the adjusted Baysian information criterion (ABIC), and entropy. Our model fit statistics – especially the Bayesian Information Criterion (BIC) and entropy – strongly suggested the four-class typology fit the data best. Explicitly, the entropy value was the highest (0.896) in the four-class analysis, compared to the two-, three-, and five-class analyses (see Table 1).

The MLCA identified four distrust patterns: Believers, Doubters, Competence Skeptics, and Values Skeptics. The first group showed low distrust scores in all six items and thus was labeled as "Believers." Roughly 25 percent of the respondents were classified into this category. The second group of participants reported high scores for all questions and accordingly was named "Doubters," which accounted for about 30 percent of our data. Believers and Doubters rated competence and values distrust coherently meaning if one rated high competence distrust then he or she also rated high values distrust, vice versa. In other words, their evaluation of distrust did not vary across two dimensions of distrust. However, they only explain 55 percent of individuals' assessments of distrust, and nearly 45 percent of

Table 1. Results of the Multilevel Latent Class Analysis (Mean Values in Cells).[a]

	Believers	Doubters	Competence Skeptics	Values Skeptics
Distrust Q(1): Competence	2.06	3.60	2.94	2.57
Distrust Q(2): Competence	1.90	4.04	3.94	2.20
Distrust Q(3): Competence	2.05	3.66	3.21	2.51
Distrust Q(4): Competence	2.49	3.85	3.35	3.15
Distrust Q(5): Values	2.10	4.40	2.13	4.06
Distrust Q(6): Values	2.21	3.74	2.62	3.17
Total number of respondents	*2374 (25%)*	*2873 (30%)*	*543 (6%)*	*3707 (39%)*

Bayesian Information Criterion (BIC) = 162.022; Entropy = 0.896.

[a]The entropy values for 2, 3, and 5 groups are 0.826, 0.826, and 0.874, respectively. Similarly, the BICs are 167.895, 164.716, and 167.595.

individuals assessed distrust in incoherent manner. The third subtype only included 543 respondents (six percent) who had high competence distrust but low values distrust. This type was called "Competence Skeptics." Despite the relative small group size, it represents a qualitatively distinct type of assessing distrust. The last, and the largest, category embraced almost 40 percent of the participants and was labeled as "Values Skeptics." They had high values distrust but low competence distrust. For the last two subtypes, rating competence distrust seemed to be independent of assessing values distrust as they evaluated them incoherently.

Overall, in contrast to competence distrust, the values of the health care system received higher distrust among all participants. That is, almost 70 percent (30 percent Doubters and 39 percent Values Skeptics) of the respondents had high values distrust. For example, they suspected that making money is the first priority of the system (see questions (5) and (6) above). On the other hand, respondents in the PHMC survey largely trusted the technical abilities of the health care system to make patients' health better (about 65 percent). The four subtypes not only confirmed that distrust has both competence and values dimensions, but also have suggested that a significant number of people in fact assess them independently.

After identifying four patterns, we compared and tested whether neighborhood characteristics varied significantly across the patterns. The analytic results of multiple comparison tests are summarized in Table 2. We found statistically significant differences in all neighborhood variables except one (i.e., percent of non-Hispanic other races). The key findings are summarized as follows: First, Doubters and Competence Skeptics seemed to share similar neighborhoods in terms of racial composition in which they reside in neighborhoods with high concentrations of non-Hispanic blacks. On the other hand, Believers lived in neighborhoods dominated by non-Hispanic white with less concentration of any minority populations. Second, in terms of living conditions, Doubters and Competence Skeptics tended to live in neighborhoods with more households lacking in room space, telephone service, vehicles, and/or plumbing systems compared to Believers. Furthermore, comparing the neighborhoods of Doubters with those of Values Skeptics, the latter seemed to be better off in all four indicators of living conditions. Third, with respect to SES, the neighborhoods where Believers lived had the highest SES compared to any other subtypes. Explicitly, Believers were exposed not only to the lowest percent of single-parent households with children and unemployment rate, but also to the highest levels of educational attainment and family income. However, no significant differences

Table 2. Descriptive Statistics and Group Significance Comparisons (Mean Values in Cells).

Neighborhood Variables	Overall Sample	Believers	Doubters	Competence Skeptics	Values Skeptics	Comparisons
Racial composition						
Percent of non-Hispanic white	63.18	69.29	56.34	59.35	65.06	a, b, c, d, e
Percent of non-Hispanic black	24.70	19.04	30.87	28.48	23.07	a, b, c, d, e
Percent of non-Hispanic other races	5.95	5.88	6.04	5.72	5.95	
Percent of Hispanics	5.90	5.58	6.43	6.45	5.63	a, d
Living conditions						
Percent of households with more than 1 person per room	1.48	1.25	1.77	1.59	1.39	a, b, d
Percent of households without telephone service	3.48	3.05	3.98	3.77	3.33	a, b, c, d
Percent of households without vehicles	17.12	14.68	20.32	19.65	15.86	a, b, d, e
Percent of household without plumbing system	1.76	1.46	2.15	2.25	1.59	a, b, d, e
SES						
Percent of single-parent households with children	12.40	10.81	14.19	13.85	11.83	a, b, c, d, e
Percent of population with at least a high school diploma	86.13	87.60	84.37	84.97	86.70	a, b, c, d, e
Unemployment rate	5.19	4.68	5.81	5.54	5.01	a, b, c, d, e
Median family income	76010.32	83511.25	68344.34	72116.30	77623.24	a, b, c, d, e
Percent of owner-occupied housing units	68.91	70.96	66.19	67.48	69.87	a, b, d
Percent of family below poverty line	20.65	17.92	23.93	23.46	19.49	a, b, c, d, e

a: Believers and Doubters are significantly different; b: Believers and Competence Skeptics are significantly different; c: Believers and Values Skeptics are significantly different; d: Doubters and Values Skeptics are significantly different; e: Competence skeptics and Values Skeptics are significantly different ($p < 0.05$).

were found in poverty and the percent of owner-occupied housing units between the neighborhoods of Believers and those of Value Skeptics. In comparison with Doubters, Values Skeptics' neighborhoods were significantly better in all six SES variables. In other words, Believers were less likely to reside in socioeconomically disadvantaged and racially segregated neighborhoods than other patterns. Fourth, a notable trend in Table 2 was that the neighborhoods of Doubters were not significantly different from those of Competence Skeptics. Fourth, Competence Skeptics and Values Skeptics were found to live in very different neighborhoods. Specifically, the former's exposure to minorities, households in poor living conditions (e.g., no vehicles and/or plumbing systems), and disadvantaged SES (e.g., high poverty and low income) were significantly greater than the latter. However, the similarity between these two subtypes lied in the percentages of households that were crowded and without telephone service, as well as the percentages of non-Hispanic other races and Hispanics. In summary, neighborhood characteristics of four different patterns of distrust vary significantly.

In the last stage of the analysis, the relationships between the distrust patterns (latent classes) and the use of preventive health care service were examined with a series of regression models. We used Doubters as our reference group throughout the analyses in this stage. Table 3 presents the OLS results of the blood cholesterol test and one major finding was observed. The associations between latent classes and the time since last blood cholesterol test were not apparent (see Models 1 and 3) until we took the interactions between insurance coverage and latent classes into account (Models 2 and 4). In Model 2, all other variables being equal, among those respondents who had insurance, Values Skeptics had a slightly shorter time period ($-1.14-0.214+0.213=-1.141$) since their last blood cholesterol than Doubters (-1.14). This gap increased to 0.214 between uninsured Doubters and uninsured Values Skeptics. Similar patterns could be observed between Competence Skeptics and Doubters, though the differences were marginally significant. Surprisingly, we did not observe any significant time differences for blood cholesterol test between Doubters and Believers.

With respect to whether a female respondent followed the guidelines to have a Pap smear test, the logistic regression results (see Table 4) suggested a clear disadvantage for Doubters. Specifically, in Model 1 of Table 4, *ceteris paribus*, Believers were approximately 20 percent more likely to have a Pap test within a recommended time period than Doubters. Despite a slight decrease, Values Skeptics were about 15 percent more likely to follow

Table 3. OLS Regression Results of Blood Cholesterol Test (All Respondents).

Variables	Model 1		Model 2		Model 3		Model 4	
	Estimates	S.E.	Estimates	S.E.	Estimates	S.E.	Estimates	S.E.
Distrust latent class (ref = Doubters)								
Believers	0.006	(0.032)	0.024	(0.139)	−0.013	(0.036)	0.000	(0.142)
Competence Skeptics	−0.044	(0.053)	−0.366^{+}	(0.200)	−0.045	(0.063)	−0.373^{+}	(0.203)
Values Skeptics	−0.016	(0.028)	−0.214*	(0.106)	−0.047	(0.033)	−0.262*	(0.109)
Demographics								
Gender (female = 1)	−0.046^{+}	(0.025)	−0.045^{+}	(0.025)	−0.047^{+}	(0.025)	−0.047^{+}	(0.025)
Age	−0.219***	(0.009)	−0.220***	(0.009)	−0.220***	(0.009)	−0.220***	(0.009)
Educational attainment								
High school graduate	−0.027	(0.049)	−0.028	(0.049)	−0.027	(0.049)	−0.027	(0.049)
Some college education	−0.068	(0.053)	−0.069	(0.053)	−0.066	(0.053)	−0.067	(0.053)
College graduate	−0.100^{+}	(0.053)	−0.101^{+}	(0.053)	−0.098^{+}	(0.053)	−0.099^{+}	(0.053)
Post-college degree	−0.141*	(0.056)	−0.143*	(0.056)	−0.140*	(0.056)	−0.142*	(0.056)
Race/ethnicity (ref = others)								
Non-Hispanic white	0.045	(0.041)	0.045	(0.041)	0.046	(0.041)	0.046	(0.041)
Non-Hispanic black	−0.233***	(0.045)	−0.234***	(0.045)	−0.287***	(0.057)	−0.291***	(0.057)
Socioeconomic status								
Insurance coverage (yes = 1)	−1.045***	(0.050)	−1.140***	(0.075)	−1.044***	(0.050)	−1.145***	(0.075)
Poverty status (poor = 1)	0.007	(0.014)	0.007	(0.014)	0.007	(0.014)	0.007	(0.014)
Interaction terms								
Insurance × Believers			−0.014	(0.143)			−0.008	(0.143)
Insurance × Competence Skeptics			0.348^{+}	(0.207)			0.352^{+}	(0.208)
Insurance × Values Skeptics			0.213^{+}	(0.110)			0.229*	(0.111)
NH black × Believers					0.065	(0.076)	0.062	(0.077)
NH black × Competence Skeptics					−0.003	(0.118)	0.002	(0.118)
NH black × Values Skeptics					0.116^{+}	(0.064)	0.126^{+}	(0.065)
Constant	3.240***	(0.077)	3.329***	(0.094)	3.257***	(0.078)	3.353***	(0.095)
R-squared	0.113		0.114		0.114		0.114	

***$p < 0.001$; *$p < 0.05$; $^{+}p < 0.10$.

Table 4. Logistic Regression Results of Pap Smear Test (Female Respondents, 1 = Following Guidelines to Have a Pap Smear Test).

Variables	Model 1		Model 2		Model 3		Model 4	
	Odds ratio	C.I.	Odds ratio	C.I.	Odds ratio	C.I.	Odds ratio	C.I.
Distrust latent class (ref = Doubters)								
Believers	1.219*	(1.026–1.450)	1.688	(0.849–3.356)	1.311**	(1.083–1.589)	1.913^{+}	(0.944–3.878)
Competence Skeptics	1.052	(0.787–1.407)	1.401	(0.530–3.701)	1.382^{+}	(0.979–1.951)	2.095	(0.773–5.682)
Values Skeptics	1.163*	(1.001–1.352)	1.101	(0.671–1.806)	1.286**	(1.087–1.522)	1.305	(0.779–2.184)
Demographics								
Age	0.624***	(0.591–0.658)	0.624***	(0.591–0.658)	0.622***	(0.590–0.657)	0.623***	(0.590–0.657)
Educational attainment								
High school graduate	1.151	(0.905–1.464)	1.154	(0.907–1.467)	1.143	(0.899–1.454)	1.145	(0.900–1.457)
Some college education	1.325*	(1.019–1.725)	1.331*	(1.023–1.732)	1.298^{+}	(0.996–1.690)	1.303*	(1.000–1.696)
College graduate	1.889***	(1.431–2.493)	1.900***	(1.439–2.507)	1.866***	(1.413–2.464)	1.877***	(1.421–2.479)
Post-college degree	2.134***	(1.577–2.888)	2.142***	(1.582–2.899)	2.093***	(1.545–2.834)	2.101***	(1.551–2.845)
Race/ethnicity (ref = others)								
Non-Hispanic white	0.881	(0.700–1.110)	0.885	(0.703–1.115)	0.880	(0.699–1.108)	0.884	(0.702–1.114)
Non-Hispanic black	1.653***	(1.285–2.127)	1.660***	(1.290–2.136)	2.248***	(1.612–3.136)	2.278***	(1.630–3.183)
Socioeconomic status								
Insurance coverage (yes = 1)	3.489***	(2.740–4.442)	3.658***	(2.568–5.211)	3.512***	(2.757–4.475)	3.852***	(2.688–5.520)
Poverty status (poor = 1)	0.901**	(0.841–0.965)	0.900**	(0.840–0.965)	0.901**	(0.841–0.966)	0.901**	(0.841–0.966)
Interaction terms								
Insurance × Believers			0.708	(0.348–1.440)			0.672	(0.328–1.374)
Insurance × Competence Skeptics			0.730	(0.263–2.020)			0.636	(0.231–1.753)
Insurance × Values Skeptics			1.060	(0.630–1.782)			0.982	(0.580–1.661)
NH black × Believers					0.721	(0.464–1.119)	0.701	(0.451–1.091)
NH black × Competence Skeptics					0.345**	(0.182–0.654)	0.338***	(0.178–0.639)
NH black × Values Skeptics					0.629*	(0.434–0.911)	0.628*	(0.432–0.912)
Constant	3.219***	(2.186–4.740)	3.062***	(1.934–4.849)	3.039***	(2.059–4.486)	2.770***	(1.735–4.420)
AIC	6071.233		6075.651		6064.402		6068.478	

C.I.: confidence interval.
***$p < 0.001$; **$p < 0.01$; *$p < 0.05$; $^{+}p < 0.10$.

the guidelines to have a cervical cancer test than Doubters. Moreover, unlike the findings of blood cholesterol tests, the distrust latent patterns seemed to be independent of insurance coverage but were related to race/ethnicity. Doubters who identified themselves as other race/ethnicity groups had the lowest odds of having a Pap test on time (Model 3). Across the latent patterns, non-Hispanic black respondents consistently had higher odds of receiving a cervical cancer screening test than other race/ethnicity groups.

Though the associations between distrust latent classes and Pap test were not moderated by insurance coverage, whether women had health insurance is a crucial factor for utilizing the regular Pap tests. This relationship remained valid after considering other sociodemographic characteristics such as educational attainment and poverty. More importantly, our findings indicated that as long as the competence distrust was low, respondents were willing to use this specific screening test. That being said, whether an individual believe that health care system is capable of making patients healthy is a key facilitator for cervical cancer screening.

As for male respondents, the associations between distrust latent classes and prostate cancer screening were summarized in Table 5. In contrast to Doubters, Believers were almost 40 percent more likely to have a prostate cancer test during a recommended time period (Model 1 of Table 5). Though the estimated relationships between Values and Competence Skeptics and prostate cancer screening followed the expectations, they were marginally significant across the four models in Table 5. Several findings were different from those in the blood cholesterol and cervical cancer screening analyses. First, the associations between distrust patterns and prostate cancer screening did not vary across insurance coverage or race/ethnicity. Including these interactions neither improved our model fits nor unveiled any nuanced relationships. Second, race/ethnicity was not a determinant of receiving a prostate cancer screening test, though race/ethnicity contributes to our understanding of why individuals have blood cholesterol and Pap tests.

In addition to the findings about how distrust latent classes were associated with the use of preventive health care services, we observed several patterns shared across Tables 3–5. First, an individual's age was associated with the preventive health behaviors but the associations varied by the dependent variables. As age increases, the time between two blood cholesterol tests would be shorter, and older men were more likely to have a prostate cancer screening test than their younger counterparts. However, the odds of having a Pap test actually decreased with the increase in age among women.

Table 5. Logistic Regression Results of Prostate Cancer Test (Male Respondents, 1 = Following Guidelines to Have a Prostate Cancer Test).

Variables	Model 1		Model 2		Model 3		Model 4	
	Odds ratio	C.I.	Odds ratio	C.I.	Odds ratio	C.I.	Odds ratio	C.I.
Distrust latent class (ref = Doubters)								
Believers	1.385*	(1.070–1.794)	1.964	(0.542–7.120)	1.310⁺	(0.979–1.752)	1.828	(0.493–6.772)
Competence Skeptics	1.514⁺	(0.939–2.439)	1.441	(0.215–9.635)	1.381	(0.812–2.350)	1.357	(0.202–9.107)
Values Skeptics	1.165	(0.919–1.476)	1.591	(0.518–4.882)	1.089	(0.827–1.435)	1.455	(0.466–4.539)
Demographics								
Age	1.816***	(1.638–2.012)	1.816***	(1.639–2.013)	1.812***	(1.634–2.009)	1.812***	(1.635–2.009)
Educational attainment								
High school graduate	1.534*	(1.066–2.206)	1.531*	(1.065–2.202)	1.537*	(1.069–2.211)	1.535*	(1.067–2.208)
Some college education	1.884**	(1.273–2.786)	1.880**	(1.270–2.782)	1.892**	(1.278–2.799)	1.887**	(1.275–2.795)
College graduate	2.448***	(1.660–3.609)	2.446***	(1.658–3.607)	2.460***	(1.668–3.628)	2.457***	(1.666–3.625)
Post-college degree	2.137***	(1.428–3.196)	2.134***	(1.426–3.193)	2.145***	(1.434–3.210)	2.142***	(1.432–3.206)
Race/ethnicity (ref = others)								
Non-Hispanic white	0.898	(0.632–1.276)	0.906	(0.638–1.288)	0.902	(0.635–1.280)	0.909	(0.639–1.292)
Non-Hispanic black	1.144	(0.771–1.698)	1.151	(0.775–1.709)	0.981	(0.592–1.624)	0.992	(0.598–1.646)
Socioeconomic status								
Insurance coverage (yes = 1)	3.343***	(2.073–5.393)	4.081**	(1.732–9.616)	3.339***	(2.068–5.390)	4.030**	(1.710–9.497)
Poverty status (poor = 1)	0.832**	(0.740–0.935)	0.831**	(0.739–0.934)	0.830**	(0.738–0.934)	0.829**	(0.737–0.933)
Interaction terms								
Insurance × Believers			0.694	(0.186–2.584)			0.707	(0.189–2.650)
Insurance × Competence Skeptics			1.058	(0.149–7.521)			1.027	(0.143–7.379)
Insurance × Values Skeptics			0.721	(0.229–2.270)			0.739	(0.234–2.331)
NH black × Believers					1.222	(0.623–2.398)	1.206	(0.613–2.371)
NH black × Competence Skeptics					1.481	(0.430–5.103)	1.451	(0.418–5.044)
NH black × Values Skeptics					1.284	(0.743–2.217)	1.275	(0.737–2.205)
Constant	0.031***	(0.015–0.064)	0.025***	(0.009–0.069)	0.032***	(0.015–0.068)	0.027***	(0.010–0.074)
AIC	2704.43		2709.922		2709.418		2714.992	

C.I.: confidence interval.

***$p < 0.001$; **$p < 0.01$; *$p < 0.05$; $^{+}p < 0.10$.

Second, insurance coverage was a consistent facilitator for the use of preventive health care service and this finding was not altered by including other covariates. This finding became even more critical when we investigated whether and how distrust latent classes affect the use of screening tests. Specifically, even when individuals have the access to health care providers (i.e., being insured), their competence or values distrust would undermine their willingness to use screening tests. Finally, the protective effect of high educational attainment was persistent across models, particularly among those who have at least a bachelor degree. Our finding suggests that it is important to target individuals with certain education background to facilitate greater understanding of the importance of regular screening or preventive health care service.

DISCUSSION

Our chapter had three goals. First, we examined the dimensions of distrust by identifying different subgroups (patterns) related to two distrust dimensions – competence and values distrust. Second, we examined how neighborhood characteristics of individuals in different distrust subgroups vary. Third, we assessed the relationships between distrust subgroups and individuals' preventive health care behaviors. The results provide empirical evidence for our hypotheses. We first hypothesized that the most individuals evaluate competence and values distrust in a coherent fashion. The MLCA results appear to partially confirm this hypothesis as only about 55 percent of the respondents consistently reported their competence and values distrust (i.e., Doubters and Believers). Values Skeptics – comprising almost 40 percent of the participants – was the largest group, and it suggests that individuals have strong confidence in the ability of the health care system to make their health better, yet they have less confidence in the integrity or honesty of the health care system. This divergent pattern suggests that the etiologies of developing competence and values distrust are different, and future research should investigate on exploring the factors that lead to the divergent patterns of distrust.

We then hypothesized that individuals with high distrust were more likely to reside in economically disadvantaged (measured by poor living conditions and lower SES) and racially segregated (measured by high concentrations of minorities) neighborhoods. The multiple comparison results provided strong evidence for this hypothesis. As several previous studies have found (Armstrong et al., 2008; Shoff & Yang, 2012), the non-Hispanic black population reported significant higher distrust compared to other race/ethnic groups. Our own findings that Doubters' neighborhoods had the highest percent of non-Hispanic black echoes the literature. Similarly, Doubters, as well as Competence and Values Skeptics, tend to live in socioeconomically disadvantaged neighborhoods indicated by higher rates of crowded housing units and poverty. Distinct from other three patterns, Believers reside in economically better neighborhoods characterized by better living conditions and higher SES and but highly segregated neighborhoods (i.e., lower concentration of minorities). In addition to the structural characteristics of neighborhoods we have tested in our study, future studies should investigate different dimensions of neighborhoods. Namely, more scholarly investigations are needed to investigate the social and physical characteristics of neighborhoods. For example, future studies should investigate whether individuals in a neighborhood with high collective efficacy (e.g., the combination of trust and cohesion among residents in a neighborhood that allows for social control) (Sampson, Raudenbush, & Earls, 1997) are more likely to have lower distrust.

Lastly, we hypothesized that Doubters are the least likely to use preventive health care services, whereas Believers are the most likely to use preventive health care services. Although we have obtained evidence to bolster this hypothesis from the analyses of Pap test and prostate cancer screening, this hypothesis did not hold for the blood cholesterol test. We found that the relationships between distrust latent classes and the use of preventive health care services may differ by the screening test of interest because there are different thresholds for obtaining these services. For example, it is more time consuming and invasive to receive a Pap test compared to blood cholesterol test; thus, individuals' physical and emotional costs related to these two types of test may differ. In addition, as long as individuals reported low competence distrust, individuals may still be more likely to adopt preventive health care services in contrast to those who do not believe that health care systems are able to make patients healthy. Our results are consistent with the previous studies in that individuals who distrust health care system are less likely to engage in preventive health care behaviors (Shoff & Yang, 2012). However, the associations between distrust patterns and preventive health care behaviors differ in a meaningful way that distrust was associated with lower engagement in Pap test and prostate cancer screening only. We suspect that different associations between distrust and types of preventive services may be attributable to varying costs and benefits associated with different types of preventive services.

Our findings above convey several important messages to health researchers. Particularly, the institutional performance model implies that an individual's distrust is not only associated with personal experience with the health care system, but also related to the individual's social and residential environments. That is, the changes in the neighborhood social environment would "trickle down" to an individual's assessment of distrust. Since distrust plays a key role in health interventions and research (Corbie-Smith & Ford, 2006; Corbie-Smith, Thomas, & St George, 2002), individual health behaviors (Musa et al., 2009; Yang et al., 2011), and self-reported health outcomes (Armstrong et al., 2006; Cunningham, Sohler, Korin, Gao, & Anastos, 2007; Yang et al., 2011), it is important to reduce the high distrust among Americans to improve population health and promote health research. More importantly, the neighborhood-level characteristics and individual's attitudes are generally more amendable than other individual-level characteristics (e.g., educational attainment, race/ethnicity, and age) (Consedine, Christie, & Neugut, 2009). Our findings provide a plausible approach to improving the neighborhood conditions for lowering individuals' health care distrust. Policies targeted to improve the neighborhood conditions can potentially influence more people (e.g., all neighborhood residents) than those targeting individuals.

Moreover, relatively few people had the competence dimension of health care system distrust, but the high values distrust warrants further attention. Others have argued that modernization and cultural shifts would naturally encourage the development of critical views on authorities (Norris, 2007); however, if this knowledge stream holds, why does the literature, especially in the United States, suggest that values distrust is higher than competence distrust (Armstrong et al., 2008; Rose et al., 2004; Shoff & Yang, 2012)? One should expect that the difference between competence and values distrust is minimal as these critical views should be applied to both dimensions. A plausible explanation may come from Putnam's social capital argument (Putnam, 2001), which indicates that mutual trust, reciprocity, and civil participation among individuals in a community have collapsed in the past few decades in the United States. The overall decrease in these social norms, civil involvement, and social trust led to high distrust of various social institutions, especially their values of providing services. Due to data limitations, this study could not test this statement, but future research should further clarify the role of social capital in the formation of distrust. Future research should also investigate whether individual-level and neighborhood-level factors influence competence dimension of distrust and value dimension of distrust similarly. For example, does individuals' positive experience with the health care system reduce the competence distrust but not value distrust? Future studies should have more nuanced investigation of how these two dimensions differ.

There are several limitations to our study. The findings above were drawn from the Census tract level data. Several scholars have noted that using different geographic scales in health research may lead to inconsistent conclusions (Mobley, Kuo, & Andrews, 2008). To address this issue, this study also conducted the multiple comparisons with ZIP code level data as a sensitivity test. The results (not shown but available upon request) supported our previous conclusions, and therefore the findings of this study are fairly robust and reliable. Beyond this sensitivity test, however, several limitations of this study should be noted. First, the causal relationships between distrust and living arrangement are tentative due to use of cross-sectional data. An intervention study like Moving to Opportunity (Leventhal & Brooks-Gunn, 2003) should help researchers to clarify whether high distrust is a consequence of poor perceptions of living environment. Second, researchers and policy makers should be cautious when generalizing the findings to other regions of the United States as the PHMC survey was very specific to the population in the southeastern region of Pennsylvania, rather than a nationally representative data set. Third, while the distrust scale in this study is the most recently developed with an emphasis on health care system (Armstrong et al., 2008), using a distrust scale with a different focus (e.g., physicians or health insurance company) may yield different findings. Finally, our examination of the institute performance model mainly depends on the ACS data, which may not fully capture one's perception of the environment.

Despite these limitations, the results from this study have important implications for public policy and suggestions for future research. In sum, this study explicitly examined whether the dual-dimensional distrust fits the institutional performance model with MLCA and multiple comparison tests. While this study does not endeavor to investigate the causes per se of the soaring distrust since 1960s, our findings suggested that individuals reporting high distrust tend to be exposed to poor social and living neighborhood environments, which bears implications for future research and policies that aim to facilitate health behaviors and population health. Our finding also suggested that decreasing competence distrust may be a mechanism to encourage the use of preventive health care, though the overall distrust remains high.

ACKNOWLEDGMENTS

We acknowledge the support from the Center for Social and Demographic Analysis at the University at Albany, which receives core funding from the NICHD (R24-HD04494309). We would also like to acknowledge the help from Family Demography Training (T-32HD007514) from NICHD.

REFERENCES

Armstrong, K., McMurphy, S., Dean, L. T., Micco, E., Putt, M., Halbert, C. H., ... Shea, J. A. (2008). Differences in the patterns of health care system distrust between blacks and whites. *Journal of General Internal Medicine*, *23*(6), 827–833. doi:10.1007/s11606-008-0561-9

Armstrong, K., Rose, A., Peters, N., Long, J. A., McMurphy, S., & Shea, J. A. (2006). Distrust of the health care system and self-reported health in the United States. *Journal of General Internal Medicine*, *21*(4), 292–297. doi:10.1111/j.1525-1497.2006.00396.x

Asparouhov, T., & Muthén, B. (2008). Multilevel mixture models. In G. Hancock & K. Samuelsen (Eds.), *Advances in latent variable mixture models* (pp. 27–51). Charlotte, NC: Information Age Publishing, Inc.

Blendon, R. J. (2007). Why Americans don't trust the government and don't trust healthcare. In D. A. Shore (Ed.), *The trust crisis in healthcare: Causes, consequences, and cures* (pp. 21–31). New York, NY: Oxford University Press.

Clogg, C. C. (1988). Latent class models for measuring. In R. Langeheine & J. Ros (Eds.), *Latent trait and latent class models* (pp. 173–205). New York, NY: Plenum Press.

Consedine, N. S., Christie, M. A., & Neugut, A. I. (2009). Physician, affective, and cognitive variables differentially predict initiation versus maintenance PSA screening profiles in diverse groups of men. *British Journal of Health Psychology*, *14*(2), 303–322.

Corbie-Smith, G., & Ford, C. L. (2006). Distrust and poor self-reported health – Canaries in the coal mine? *Journal of General Internal Medicine*, *21*(4), 395–397.

Corbie-Smith, G., Thomas, S. B., & St George, D. M. M. (2002). Distrust, race, and research. *Archives of Internal Medicine*, *162*(21), 2458–2463.

Cunningham, C. O., Sohler, N. L., Korin, L., Gao, W., & Anastos, K. (2007). HIV status, trust in health care providers, and distrust in the health care system among Bronx women. *Aids Care-Psychological and Socio-Medical Aspects of Aids/HIV*, *19*(2), 226–234. doi:10.1080/09540120600774263

Hall, M. A., Dugan, E., Zheng, B. Y., & Mishra, A. K. (2001). Trust in physicians and medical institutions: What is it, can it be measured, and does it matter? *Milbank Quarterly*, *79*(4), 613–639.

Harris Interactive Polls. (2012). *Confidence in congress stays at lowest point in almost fifty years*. Retrieved from http://www.harrisinteractive.com/vault/Harris%20Poll%2044%20-%20Confidence%20Index_5%2021%2012.pdf. Accessed on January 20, 2013.

Henry, K. L., & Muthén, B. (2010). Multilevel latent class analysis: An application of adolescent smoking typologies with individual and contextual predictors. *Structural Equation Modeling: A Multidisciplinary Journal*, *17*(2), 193–215.

LaVeist, T. A., Isaac, L. A., & Williams, K. P. (2009). Mistrust of health care organizations is associated with underutilization of health services. *Health Services Research*, *44*(6), 2093–2105.

Lazarsfeld, P. F., & Henry, N. W. (1968). *Latent structure analysis*. New York, NY: Houghton Mifflin.

Leventhal, T., & Brooks-Gunn, J. (2003). Moving to opportunity: An experimental study of neighborhood effects on mental health. *Journal Information*, *93*(9), 1576–1582.

Matthews, S. A., & Yang, T.-C. (2010). Exploring the role of the built and social neighborhood environment in moderating stress and health. *Annual of Behavioral Medicine*, *39*(2), 170–183.

Mobley, L. R., Kuo, T. M. M., & Andrews, L. (2008). How sensitive are multilevel regression findings to defined area of context? A case study of mammography use in California. *Medical Care Research and Review*, *65*(3), 315–337.

Montgomery, D. C. (2008). *Design and analysis of experiments*. New York, NY: John Wiley & Sons.

Musa, D., Schulz, R., Harris, R., Silverman, M., & Thomas, S. B. (2009). Trust in the health care system and the use of preventive health services by older black and white adults. *American Journal of Public Health*, *99*(7), 1293–1299. doi:10.2105/ajph.2007.123927

Norris, P. (2007). Skeptical patients: Performance, social capital, and culture. In D. A. Shore (Ed.), *The trust crisis in healthcare: Causes, consequences, and cures* (pp. 32–46). New York, NY: Oxford University Press.

PHMC. (2008). The 2008 household health survey. Philadelphia, PA: Public Health Management Corporation.

Putnam, R. D. (2001). *Bowling alone: The collapse and revival of American community*. New York, NY: Simon & Schuster.

Rose, A., Peters, N., Shea, J. A., & Armstrong, K. (2004). Development and testing of the health care system distrust scale. *Journal of General Internal Medicine*, *19*(1), 57–63.

Sampson, R. J., Raudenbush, S. W., & Earls, F. (1997). Neighborhoods and violent crime: A multilevel study of collective efficacy. *Science*, *277*(5328), 918–924.

Shea, J. A., Micco, E., Dean, L. T., McMurphy, S., Schwartz, J. S., & Armstrong, K. (2008). Development of a revised health care system distrust scale. *Journal of General Internal Medicine*, *23*(6), 727–732.

Shoff, C., & Yang, T. C. (2012). Untangling the associations among distrust, race, and neighborhood social environment: A social disorganization perspective. *Social Science & Medicine*, *74*(9), 1342–1352.

Snijders, T. A. B., & Bosker, R. (2001). *Multilevel analysis: An introduction to basic and advanced multilevel modeling*. Thousand Oaks, CA: Sage.

US Census Burean. (2011). 2006–2010 American Community Survey from US Census Burean's American Community Survey Office.

Vermunt, J. K. (2003). Multilevel latent class models. *Sociological Methodology*, *33*(1), 213–239.

Vermunt, J. K. (2008). Latent class and finite mixture models for multilevel data sets. *Statistical Methods in Medical Research*, *17*(1), 33–51. doi:10.1177/0962280207081238

Wight, R. G., Aneshensel, C. S., Barrett, C., Ko, M., Chodosh, J., & Karlamangla, A. S. (2013). Urban neighbourhood unemployment history and depressive symptoms over time among late middle age and older adults. *Journal of Epidemiology and Community Health*, *67*(2), 153–158.

Yang, T. C., Matthews, S. A., & Hillemeier, M. M. (2011). Effect of health care system distrust on breast and cervical cancer screening in Philadelphia, Pennsylvania. *American Journal of Public Health*, *101*(7), 1297–1305.

Yang, T. C., Matthews, S. A., & Shoff, C. (2011). Individual health care system distrust and neighborhood social environment: How are they jointly associated with self-rated health? *Journal of Urban Health*, *88*(5), 945–958.

PART III
EDUCATION

IDENTIFYING AND MAPPING "HOT SPOTS" OF LOW HEALTH LITERACY: A POTENTIAL TOOL TO GUIDE INTERVENTION☆

Laurie T. Martin, Teague Ruder, José J. Escarce, Bonnie Ghosh-Dastidar, Daniel Sherman, Marc N. Elliott, Chloe E. Bird, Allen Fremont, Charles Gasper, Arthur Culbert and Nicole Lurie

ABSTRACT

Purpose – *Low health literacy is a hidden epidemic. Identifying individuals with low health literacy is a formidable barrier to eliminating disparities and improving health care quality and health outcomes. However, screening individual patients for low health literacy can be prohibitively expensive, time consuming, and inefficient. Focusing on communities, rather than individuals, provides opportunities for action.*

☆Disclaimer: The views expressed are solely those of the authors and do not necessarily reflect those of The Department of Health and Human Services.

Education, Social Factors, and Health Beliefs in Health and Health Care Services
Research in the Sociology of Health Care, Volume 33, 69–84

ISSN: 0275-4959/doi:10.1108/S0275-495920150000033026

Identifying geographic areas with large numbers of individuals with low health literacy can enable stakeholders to focus interventions in areas of greatest need. Creating such a measure also sheds light on health literacy as a community or neighborhood-level resource that contributes to health disparities and can inform health interventions.

Methodology – *We applied regression coefficients from a predictive model of health literacy to US Census data to estimate health literacy scores for census geographic areas in Missouri. We then created maps displaying the variability in health literacy levels. Finally, we compared areas identified by the predictive model to those identified on the basis of educational attainment alone.*

Findings – *Areas identified by the predictive model as having the lowest health literacy were substantially different from those identified using educational attainment alone, suggesting that a multivariate approach using a limited set of widely available predictors is considerably more accurate.*

Practical implications – *This study demonstrates a cost-effective and feasible method for estimating and mapping community-level health literacy. Predicting and mapping areas of low health literacy is relatively straightforward and inexpensive and makes complex data readily accessible to many stakeholders. Such maps can also identify and prioritize geographic areas for intervention by health care and public health providers. Moreover, this focus on community-level health literacy may help foster stakeholder collaboration, leading to efficient resource use that is targeted effectively and resulting in a positive return on investment for stakeholders.*

Keywords: Communication; social inequalities; health policy; small area studies; public health epidemiology

INTRODUCTION

Over the last decade, providers and policymakers have recognized the need to shift from only documenting the existence of gaps in quality of care and health outcomes to doing something about them. Health literacy has emerged as a potentially critical pathway through which education, income, and other fundamental determinants affect health care quality and disparities. Health literacy is "the degree to which individuals have the capacity to obtain, process, and understand basic health information and services needed to make appropriate health decisions" (Ratzan & Parker, 2000). One-third of the adult US population have health literacy skills that can be classified as basic or below basic (National Center for Education Statistics, 2006), yet low health literacy (LHL) remains a hidden epidemic costing the nation an estimated $106 billion to $236 billion annually (Vernon, Trujillo, Rosenbaum, & DeBuono, 2007).

Finding ways to support individuals and communities with low health literacy could substantially improve quality and outcomes and reduce disparities. While efforts to do this generally focus on identifying and intervening with individuals with low health literacy, health literacy is also a public health issue requiring a population approach. From a constrained-choice perspective (Bird & Rieker, 2008), individuals are affected or constrained not only by the upper limits of their own health literacy but also by their community's level of health literacy. For example, an individual with LHL who lives in an area with relatively high health literacy may benefit from the knowledge and abilities of his friends and neighbors to process health and health care information. In contrast, an individual with low health literacy who lives in a community where LHL is prevalent may actually receive counterproductive information from friends and neighbors who themselves may be less informed on current health practices and have limited abilities to obtain and assess new information on health and health care. Moreover, friends and neighbors with low health literacy may, in turn, share opinions and strategies aimed at minimizing health care costs without a clear understanding of the health consequences.

The feasibility of a population-based approach to improving care quality and reducing disparities due to LHL relies, in part, on the ability to identify geographic areas where large numbers of "at risk" people live and to determine optimal locations for interventions. It also requires tools to make complex data readily accessible and actionable to a range of stakeholders. For example, knowing that many of its clients live in areas characterized by low health literacy, some pharmacies may choose to implement health literacy interventions including special efforts to explain to patients how best to take their medicines or how to prepare pill cards. Health care providers could use such information to provide additional guidance to patients regarding how best to prepare for laboratory test, recognizing that written instructions are unlikely to be effective in helping patients arrive properly prepared (e.g., having fasted or having taken specific medications as precise intervals prior to the test). Similarly, public health departments implementing diabetes control programs, for example, may find it efficient to deploy their limited supply of community health workers to educate people in such neighborhoods or help patients from those neighborhoods better navigate the health care system.

To date, however, there has been no easy and cost-effective mechanism to estimate community-level health literacy. While individual-level health literacy assessments are available, including the Rapid Estimate of Adult Literacy in Medicine (REALM) (Murphy, Davis, Long, Jackson, & Decker, 1993), the Short Test of Functional Health Literacy in Adults (S-TOFHLA) (Parker, Baker, Williams, & Nurss, 1995), and the Newest Vital Sign (Osborn et al., 2007), they can be time consuming and resource-intensive to administer. While in isolated cases these assessments are being used to assess community-level literacy, these are massive undertakings, requiring significant resources to conduct in-person health literacy assessments of a large portion of the community, and a sophisticated sampling plan and weighting methodology for estimates to represent the broader community of interest. Such efforts are not feasible for the majority of communities hoping to address health disparities or poor health related to LHL.

Absent a way of identifying how individuals with various levels of health literacy may cluster, some have used area-level income or educational attainment as proxies. Several studies have indicated, however, that a multivariate predictive model of health literacy provides substantially more information about who is at risk for low health literacy (Gazmararian et al., 1999; Hanchate, Ash, Gazmararian, Wolf, & Paasche-Orlow, 2008; Martin et al., 2009) than any single proxy variable. Further, as Martin et al. have demonstrated, single-variable approaches can be insufficiently precise for optimal allocation of resources (Martin et al., 2009).

When census data are applied to coefficients of the predictive model, small area estimates of health literacy can be generated and subsequently mapped. Maps of community-level health literacy, particularly when coupled with more widely available maps of health outcomes, may help foster stakeholder collaboration around a shared goal, help stakeholders target population-focused interventions in communities of greatest need (Lalonde, 1974), and support the development of tailored approaches to improving health among vulnerable populations (Frolich & Potvin, 2008). Using the latter approach, stakeholders can work to change social and environmental conditions that cause people in these communities to be at higher risk of risks for poor health such as health literacy (CSDH, 2008), thereby decreasing health inequalities (Frolich & Potvin, 2008).

Therefore, we have developed such an approach using a predictive model which we previously published (Martin et al., 2009). Although we demonstrate the utility and feasibility of this approach for Missouri Public Use Microdata Areas (PUMAs) specifically, the same approach and technique can be used to estimate health literacy for any geographic area (e.g., counties, census tracts) for which demographic data are available. Finally, to further highlight the utility of the maps for health care decision-making, we compared the identification of areas of low health literacy derived from the multivariable predictive model with those identified using either educational attainment or poverty as a single-variable proxy for health literacy.

METHODS

Health Literacy

We used data from the 2003 National Assessment of Adult Literacy (NAAL) household sample, an in-person assessment of literacy among a nationally-representative sample community-dwelling US adults (National Center for Education Statistics, 2003) to create the predictive model of health literacy (Martin et al., 2009). Health literacy was measured on a 0–500 scale, with a national mean of 245 and a standard deviation of 55. While we utilize the continuous scores in the development of the maps, the National Research Council also classified these continuous scores into four ordinal performance categories: *below basic, basic, intermediate*, and *proficient* (National Center for Education Statistics, 2006). About 14% of the population had below basic health literacy skills (score of 0–184), indicating the ability only to perform tasks such as circling the date on an appointment slip. About 22% of individuals had basic health literacy skills (score of 185–225), indicating, for example, the ability to give two reasons why a person should be tested for a specific disease, based on information provided in a clearly written pamphlet. About 53% of the population had intermediate health literacy skills (score of 226–309); such individuals can perform moderately challenging health literacy activities, including determining at what time a person can take a prescription medication, using information on the prescription drug label. Only about 12% of the population had proficient health literacy (score of 310–500), indicative of the skills necessary to perform more complex and challenging literacy activities, such as calculating one's personal share of employer health costs using a table (National Center for Education Statistics, 2006). More information about the NAAL, its multi-stage sampling design, and scoring procedures is available in the 2006 National Center for Education Statistics report (National Center for Education Statistics, 2006).

Predictive Model of Health Literacy

We analyzed data from the 2003 National Assessment of Adult Literacy (NAAL), using linear regression to predict mean health literacy scores. Predictors included gender, age, race/ethnicity, educational attainment, poverty status, marital status, language spoken in the home, metropolitan statistical area (MSA), and length of time in United States. Although we present results from the model here to facilitate an understanding of how the maps were produced (see Table 1), detailed methods and results of how the predictive model was generated, along with a second model that used probit regression to predict the probability of an individual having "above basic" proficiency, can be found in Martin et al. (2009).

Socio-Demographic Characteristics

The American Community Survey (ACS) (U.S. Census Bureau, 2008) conducted by the US Census Bureau was initiated in 2005 to phase out the decennial census long form survey. It uses a series of monthly samples to produce annually updated data, and samples about 1 in 1,000 individuals within households. Because our predictive model is developed using individual-level observations, we use the ACS Public Use Microdata Sample (PUMS) from 2007. The main limitation of the ACS-PUMS is that in order to maintain confidentiality of the sample, the smallest unit of geography used is the PUMA. A PUMA has a population of approximately 100,000, with large urban counties typically subdivided into multiple PUMAs, while less populated rural areas PUMAs typically comprise smaller (population-wise) contiguous counties (Missouri Census Data Center, 2009).

Socio-demographic characteristics from the ACS applied to the predictive model include age, race/ethnicity, education, gender, marital status, poverty status, living in a metropolitan statistical area (MSA), language spoken in home, and years residing in the United States (parameterized categorically as shown in Table 1). We used information on income and household size to generate categories representing income relative to the

Table 1. Demographic Distributions of the Missouri 2007 ACS-PUMS and Multivariable Predictive Model of Health Literacy.

Characteristic	2007 ACS-PUMS $n = 46{,}090$	Predicting Mean Health Literacy Score β (SE)
Constant		290.0
Age		
18–24	12.9	Reference
25–39	25.6	7.9
40–49	19.6	−2.4
50–64	24.2	−7.8
65–74	9.0	−28.7**
75+	8.6	−39.1*
Education		
Still in HS	1.6	−44.2**
<HS	13.5	−40.7**
HS/GED	32.9	−32.1**
Some college	29.2	−12.4**
College degree or more	22.8	Reference
Sex		
Male	48.0	−7.7**
Female	52.0	Reference
Language spoken at home		
English	94.6	Reference
Other language	5.4	1.8
Marital status		
Married, living together	54.4	Reference
Never married	24.3	−4.0*
Divorced, separated, widowed	21.3	−3.3*
Metropolitan statistical area		
MSA	68.2	Reference
Non-MSA	31.8	−0.02
Income		
No income data	3.6	−6.8**
<100% FPL	8.4	−13.7**
100–200% FPL	16.1	−8.3**
200–300% FPL	16.5	−6.1**
≥300% FPL	55.4	Reference
Race/ethnicity		
White	84.4	Reference
Black	10.2	−33.1**
Hispanic	2.5	−33.3**
Asian/Pacific Islander	1.5	−18.3**
American Indian	0.3	−21.0
Multiracial	1.1	−21.9**

Table 1. *(Continued)*

Characteristic	2007 ACS-PUMS $n = 46{,}090$	Predicting Mean Health Literacy Score β (SE)
Time in the United States		
<5 years	1.0	−20.4**
6–10 years	0.9	−19.0**
>10 years	2.7	−14.2**
Born in the United States	95.4	Reference

*$p < 0.05$, **$p < 0.01$.

federal poverty limit (FPL), as defined by Health and Human Services (Assistant Secretary for Planning and Evaluation, 2006).

Development of Maps

To generate an estimate of health literacy for a given geographic area, we applied coefficients from our regression-based predictive model of health literacy (Martin et al., 2009) to information about the demographic makeup of each PUMA (e.g., 47.3% female) obtained from the ACS. Given that the ACS utilized individual-level data, and to account for the complex sample design of the ACS, we used replicate weights to generate point estimates and standard errors representative of the population in each PUMA (U.S. Census Bureau, 2007). Area-level estimates of health literacy were then mapped using ESRI ArcMap 9.3. Maps can be generated for any geographic region for which census-like data are available. Here, we present maps of PUMAs, but similar maps could be generated for counties or census tracts. This study was reviewed and approved by RAND Corporation's Institutional Review Board.

RESULTS

Mean Predicted Health Literacy Levels

The mean predicted mean health literacy scores for PUMAs are presented in Fig. 1. We used five categories of health literacy, each with a 15-point (0.27 standard deviation) range. Areas shown in white or shaded light gray have a mean health literacy score above the national average of 245.

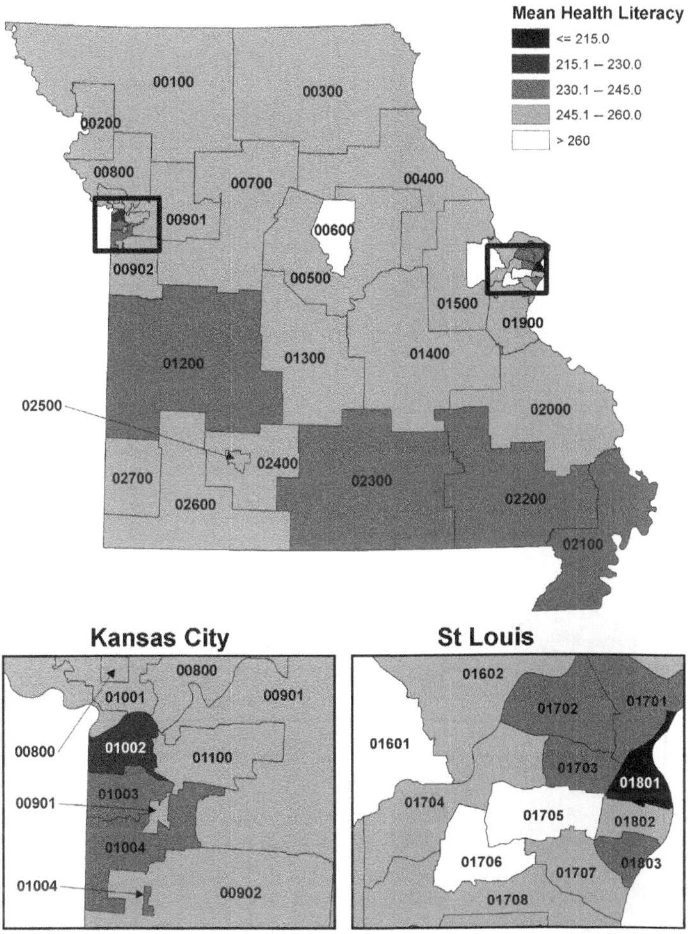

Fig. 1. Mean Health Literacy Levels for Population within PUMAs.

Fig. 1 suggests that the areas with the lowest average health literacy are clustered in Kansas City and north-eastern St. Louis. Fig. 2 provides a graphical representation of the 95% confidence intervals around the estimates and the distribution of health literacy scores overall and within PUMAs in Missouri. The columns correspond to the map shading in Fig. 1. For example, the regions shaded black represent communities with a mean estimated health literacy of 215.0 or less.

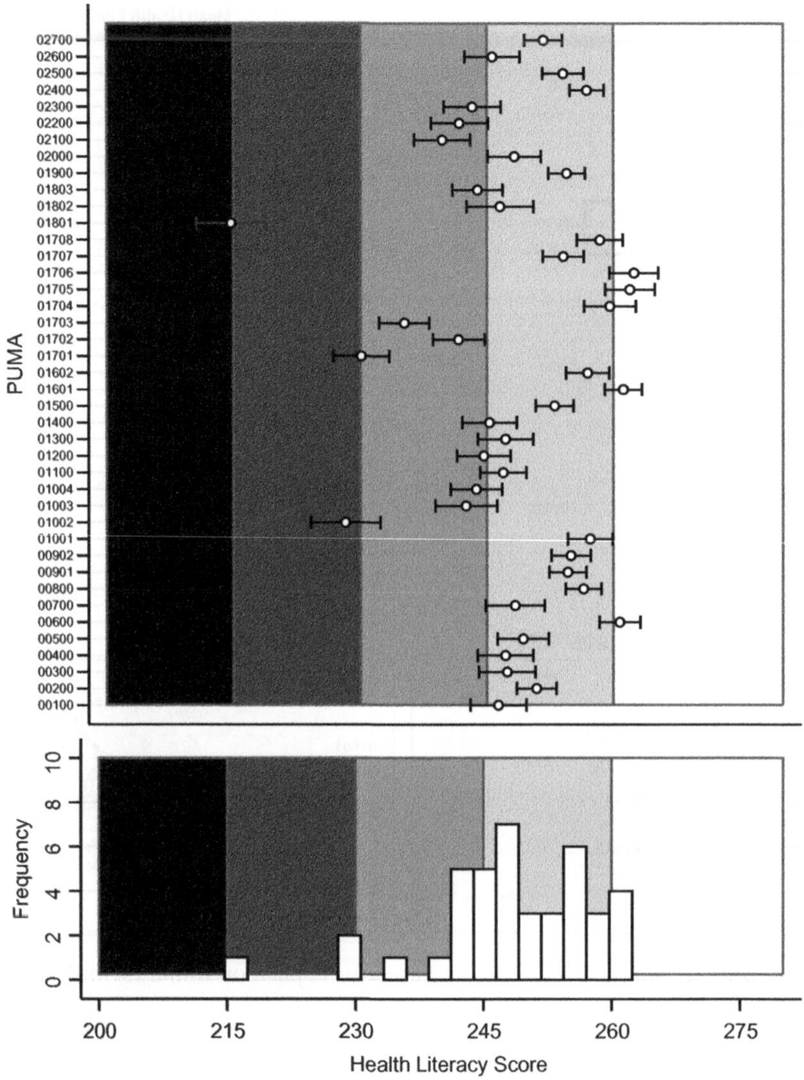

Fig. 2. Mean Health Literacy Score and 95% Confidence Intervals by PUMA. *Notes*: Numbers on *y*-axis correspond to PUMA identifiers.

Differences between the Multivariate Model and Single Predictors of Health Literacy

Fig. 3 presents a map of the percentage of individuals without a high school diploma. The areas shaded dark gray in Fig. 3 indicate that between 17% and 22% of the population has less than a high school diploma and black shaded areas indicate that between 22% and 31% of the population has

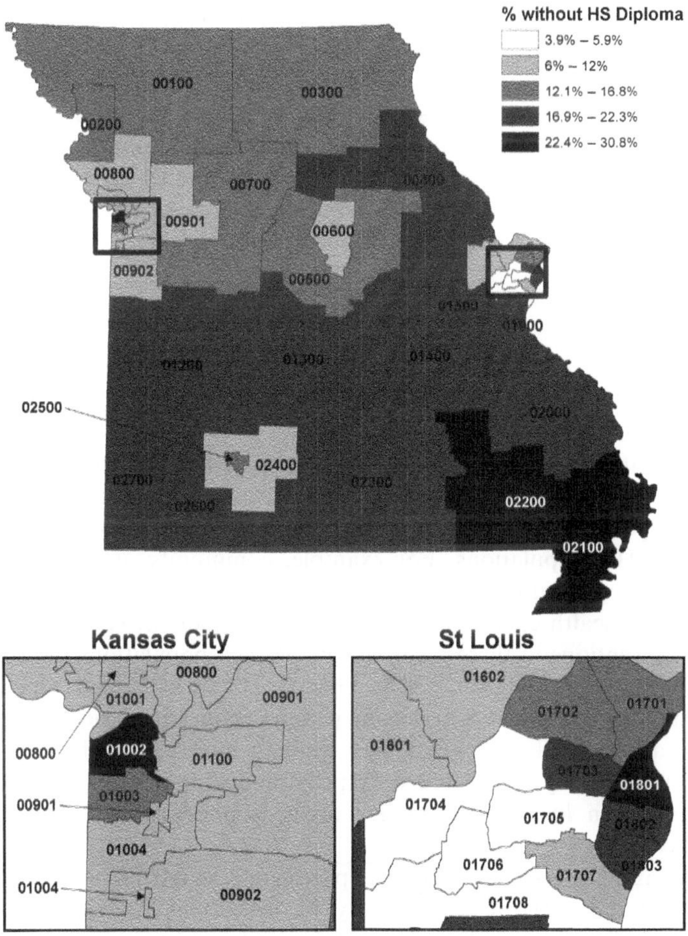

Fig. 3. Percent with Less Than a High School Education within PUMAs.

less than a high school diploma. Using education as a proxy for health literacy, both maps suggest that parts of St. Louis and Kansas City are "hot spots" with lower mean health literacy and lower educational attainment. However, the map of educational attainment might lead one to conclude that there was also a large concentration of low health literacy in the southeastern part of the state. Yet Fig. 1 indicates that, with the exception of a very small area, the average health literacy score of individuals in this region is at or just below the national average. Although individuals in the southeast may benefit from health literacy interventions, such interventions may yield a bigger return on investment when implemented in communities with lower average health literacy.

Similar patterns are seen when mapping other demographic characteristics such as poverty (results not shown) and indicators of lower educational attainment, such as the proportion who have not completed a 9th grade education. Thus, not only is the multivariate model of health literacy considerably more accurate than common single-variable proxies but it also produces substantially different geographic patterning than a single-variable proxy.

DISCUSSION

By pinpointing geographic areas in which estimated levels of health literacy are low, the maps identify populations at particular risk of the consequences of LHL and can help to efficiently focus interventions that can help LHL populations. For example, community organizations may wish to focus programs aimed at helping people with chronic diseases navigate the health care system in these low literacy areas or may wish to tailor interventions in these areas to low literacy populations. Drawing on the Ashville model (Eckel, 1988; Garrett, 1988) in which pharmacists were paid an increment to educate people about their medications and how to take them, health plans may want to intervene in the community rather than the physicians' office by providing support for pharmacists to act similarly in low health literacy areas, supporting better medication adherence.

Mapping may also help health departments, health plans and provider groups use resources more efficiently by identifying priority regions for other types of public health interventions. While producing health materials in plain language that everyone can read, understand, and act upon is a good universal precaution that should be widely promoted, newer technologies, such as computer-based education in physician waiting rooms tailored to individual patients, hold promise for improving the delivery of health messages but are not feasible to implement everywhere. As such, health literacy maps may help pinpoint geographic areas where such technologies may be particularly beneficial.

The maps also demonstrate that relying on a single-variable proxy for health literacy, such as area-level educational attainment or poverty status may lead one to substantial errors in identifying the population at risk in various regions, and that a multivariate approach using a limited set of widely available predictors is considerably more accurate. Using low education or income as an indicator of low health literacy is likely to identify areas in which individuals may not benefit as much, on average, as those living in areas identified through the multivariable model of health literacy. In other words, the return on investment from a given intervention has the potential to be significantly higher if implemented in a region with low health literacy specifically.

The maps of Missouri demonstrate that some areas of the state have low health literacy, while in other areas the average health literacy of residents is high. What is unknown is whether there is threshold at which "community health literacy" is achieved. For example, if over 40% of community residents have low health literacy, do adverse effects of low health literacy "spill over" to the rest of the population? Or is there a threshold of community health literacy sufficient to protect individuals living within that region, including those who have lower health literacy? Regardless, since so much health information is shared through social networks within a community, better understanding the health literacy of communities that are experiencing low quality care or poor health outcomes could be instructive in designing intervention efforts.

Several limitations to this study are noteworthy and should be the subject of further work. First, the predictive model used data from the National Assessment of Adult Literacy (NAAL), which assessed health literacy using only printed materials. As a result, the maps do not capture community estimates of other literacy skills including oral language (speaking) or aural language (listening) skills, both of which have been cited as important components of health literacy (Berkman et al., 2004; Institute of Medicine, 2004). Second, the NAAL only measured health literacy among English-speaking adults and we do not know how well these area-level estimates perform in communities that are primarily non-English speaking or that are new-immigrant destinations.

This approach to identify areas with varying levels of health literacy has also not yet been validated. Such validation will be challenging, as it would involve screening large numbers in a population for health literacy, well above what has been done in the NAAL and other studies. However, it may be possible to draw inferences about the validity of this approach by examining phenomena thought to be related to health literacy, such as medication adherence in populations with below basic as opposed to intermediate and proficient levels of health literacy. Finally, while mapping makes complex data readily accessible to many stakeholders, we do not yet know whether stakeholders will use the maps to implement appropriate and effectively targeted interventions to address low health literacy or its health impacts within their communities.

The analyses presented here have formed the basis for further work to examine the contribution of health literacy, among other factors, to quality of care. Several health plans have already made strides in mapping the quality of diabetes care (Lurie et al., 2008), for example, and by overlaying maps of poor quality of care and low health literacy, they can start to identify where, both geographically and within the health care delivery system, health literacy interventions might be implemented to improve quality. Then, moving from areas of lowest health literacy toward areas of proficiency, they can determine, on the basis of resource availability and return on investment, how far across the spectrum they want their interventions to reach.

To facilitate stakeholder decision-making and implementation of interventions, we developed a prototype interactive web-based mapping tool to help health care decision makers in Missouri identify community-level hot spots of suboptimal health or health care that may be due to LHL (Martin et al., 2010). The tool generates customizable color-coded maps of user-selected regions to help stakeholders quickly visualize hot spots of LHL and poor quality care and overlay information about neighborhood sociodemographic characteristics and access to health services in their communities. Feedback we receive from users of this tool will help to inform the refinement of such maps and tools to better facilitate stakeholder collaboration and action to improve care quality and reduce disparities in their communities.

ACKNOWLEDGMENT

This work was supported by the Missouri Foundation for Health.

REFERENCES

Assistant Secretary for Planning and Evaluation. (2006). *The 2007 HHS Poverty Guidelines.* Washington, DC: DHHS.

Berkman, N. D., DeWalt, D. A., Pignone, M. P., Sheridan, S., Lohr, K. N., Lux, L., ... Bonito, A. J. (2004). Literacy and Health Outcomes. Evidence Report/Technology Assessment No. 87. Agency for Healthcare Research and Quality, Rockville, MD.

Bird, C. E., & Rieker, P. P. (2008). *Gender and health: The effects of constrained choices and social policies.* New York, NY: Cambridge University Press.

CSDH. (2008). *Closing the gap in a generation: Health equity through action on the social determants of health.* Final report of the Commission on Social Determinants of Health. Geneva: World Health Organization.

Eckel, F. (Oct 2, 1988). The Asheville project – One year later. *Pharmacy Times Supplement*, pp. 6–8.

Frolich, K. L., & Potvin, L. (2008). The inequality paradox: The population approach and vulnerable populations. *American Journal of Public Health, 98*, 216–221.

Garrett, D. G. (Oct 14, 1988). The answer to how is when: The genesis of the Asheville project. *Pharmacy Times Supplement*, pp. 4–5.

Gazmararian, J. A., Baker, D. W., Williams, M. V., Parker, R., Scott, T. L., Green, D. C., ... Koplan, J. (1999). Health literacy among medicare enrollees in a managed care organization. *Journal of the American Medical Association, 281*, 545–551.

Hanchate, A. D., Ash, A., Gazmararian, J. A., Wolf, M. S., & Paasche-Orlow, M. K. (2008). The Demographic Assessment for Health Literacy (DAHL): A new tool for estimating associations between health literacy and outcomes in national surveys. *Journal of General Internal Medicine, 6.*

Institute of Medicine. (2004). Health literacy: A prescription to *end* confusion. In L. Nielsen-Bohlman, A. Panzer, & D. Kindig (Eds.). Washington, DC: National Academies Press.

Lalonde, M. (1974). A new perspective on the health of Canadians. Ottawa, ON: Ministry of Supply and Services Canada.

Lurie, N., Fremont, A., Somers, S., Coltin, K., Gelzer, A., Johnson, R. C., ... Zimmerman, D. (2008). The national health plan collaborative to reduce disparities and improve quality. *The Joint Commission Journal on Quality and Safety, 34*, 256–265.

Martin, L., Fremont, A., Felton, A., Ruder, T., Bird, C. E., Miyashiro, L., ... Lurie, N. (2010). *A prototype interactive mapping tool to target low health literacy in Missouri.* Santa Monica, CA: RAND Corporation.

Martin, L. T., Ruder, T., Escarce, J. J., Ghosh-Dastidar, B., Sherman, D., Elliott, M., ... Lurie, N. (2009). Developing predictive models of health literacy. *Journal of General Internal Medicine, 24*, 1211–1216.

Missouri Census Data Center. (2009). *Public Use Microdata Areas (PUMAs).* Jefferson City, MO: Office of the Missouri Secretary of State.

Murphy, P. W., Davis, T. C., Long, S. W., Jackson, R. H., & Decker, B. C. (1993). Rapid Estimate of Adult Literacy in Medicine (REALM): A quick reading test for patients. *Journal of Reading, 37*, 124–130.

National Center for Education Statistics. (2003). National Assessment of Adult Literacy (NAAL). Washington, DC: U.S. Department of Education.

National Center for Education Statistics. (2006). *The health literacy of America's adults: Results from the 2003 national assessment of adult literacy.* Washington, DC: U.S. Department of Education.

Osborn, C. Y., Weiss, B. D., Davis, T. C., Skripkauskas, S., Rodrigue, C., Bass, P. F., & Wolf, M. S. (2007). Measuring adult literacy in health care: Performance of the newest vital sign. *American Journal of Health Behavior*, *31*, S36–S46.

Parker, R., Baker, D. W., Williams, M. V., & Nurss, J. R. (1995). The test of functional health literacy in adults: A new instrument for measuring patients' literacy skills. *Journal of General Internal Medicine*, *10*, 537–541.

Ratzan, S. C., & Parker, R. (2000). Introduction. In C. Selden, M. Zorn, S. Ratzan, & R. Parker (Eds.), *National library of medicine current bibliographies in medicine: Health literacy*. Bethesda, MD: National Institutes of Health, U.S. Department of Health and Human Services.

U.S. Census Bureau. (2007). *PUMS accuracy of the data* (pp. 123). Edited by U. S. C. Bureau. Washington, DC: U.S. Department of Commerce.

U.S. Census Bureau. (2008). *American community survey*. Washington, DC: U.S. Department of Commerce.

Vernon, J. A., Trujillo, A., Rosenbaum, S., & DeBuono, B. (2007). *Low health literacy: Implications for national health policy*. University of Connecticut, Storrs, CT: National Bureau of Economic Research.

EDUCATION AND SELF-AWARENESS OF HEALTH: TOWARD A BETTER UNDERSTANDING OF SELF-RATED HEALTH

Heeju Sohn

ABSTRACT

Purpose – *To evaluate the extent to which a person's educational attainment moderates the relationship between his or her objective markers of health and self-rated health (SRH).*

Methodology/approach – *I use 10 years' worth of data from the National Health and Nutrition Examination Survey (NHANES 1999–2009;* N = *30,823) to examine how diagnosed medical conditions, health behaviors, and biomarkers are differentially associated with SRH by educational attainment. I use regression analysis to evaluate these relationships.*

Findings – *Results show that while medical conditions are negatively associated with SRH equally across education levels, behaviors and*

Education, Social Factors, and Health Beliefs in Health and Health Care Services
Research in the Sociology of Health Care, Volume 33, 85–103

ISSN: 0275-4959/doi:10.1108/S0275-495920150000033004

biomarkers have stronger association with SRH among individuals with greater education. Those with more education are more likely to have had their blood pressure and cholesterol checked in recent months. They are also more likely to correctly identify themselves as overweight when their body mass index exceeds 25.

Research implications – *The chapter's findings indicate that education may play a role in how people interpret and evaluate their own health. Real differences in how people evaluate their health can impact the conclusions that researchers can draw when comparing SRH between education groups. In addition these results can motivate further research in the causes of health disparities. Self-evaluation of health can potentially influence how people monitor and manage their health. Differences in self-evaluation between levels of educational attainment could contribute to disparities in health and mortality.*

Originality/value – *This chapter examines the relationship between self-rated health, objective markers of health, and education in a novel framework.*

Keywords: Self-rated health; education; biomarkers

Self-rated health is a widely used measure of general health. The question, most often structured to be answered with a five-point Likert scale, is easy to include in surveys and is considered to capture a sense of global health that individual health conditions cannot (Idler & Benyamini, 1997). Often, the respondent him or herself is most knowledgeable about conditions, behaviors, and family health history. Self-rated health is said to incorporate these factors in a holistic manner. Numerous studies have examined the predictive power of self-rated health. Idler and Benyamini (1997) and Benyamini and Idler (1999)'s review of the literature identifies a combined total of 46 studies prior to 1999 that examines self-rated health as a predictor of mortality. An overwhelming majority (42 out of 46) shows evidence of a significant negative relationship between self-rated health and mortality even after controlling for observed health conditions. The strong associations between self-rated health and mortality on the population-level face little debate. The contention enters as scholars present evidence supporting or challenging the notion that self-rated health is a reliable measure for differences in health between population sub-groups. If the determinants or the predictive power of self-rated health differ between the very groups that the researcher wishes to compare, the analyses may be vulnerable to biases. Thus, understanding this commonly used measure is crucial to designing and interpreting analyses that attempt to study health disparities within populations. This chapter focuses on how the determinants of self-rated health change with the respondent's educational attainment – a social strata that is of keen interest among scholars of health inequality.

BACKGROUND

Thomas and Frankenberg (2002) presents a model that decomposes self-rated health into four components: "true" health, individual idiosyncratic component, component specific to health indicators, and an individual health factor interaction component. According to this model, the degree of deviation between self-rated health and true health is partly determined by the person's individual characteristics. The person's age, gender, or education can modify the effect of health indicators as well as having an independent effect on self-rated health itself. Suffering from emphysema may have greater impact on self-rated health than a disease with less obvious symptoms such as hypertension. The person's education can change how much they factor in these health indicators in their self-rated health.

Researchers have empirically examined whether education play a significant role in moderating the relationship between actual and self-rated health. Most of these studies use mortality as a measure of "true health" and compare the predictive power of self-rated health between people of different educational backgrounds. The literature tests the effect of education on the predictive power of self-rated health on populations in Western Europe and North America. The common question that these researchers ask is, "Is self-rated health a better predictor of mortality among people with more education?" Studies that examine populations with larger heterogeneity in educational attainment tend to conclude that a person's education contribute to the predictive power of his or her self-rated health. Regidor and coauthors (2010) found that self-rated health predicted mortality better among Spanish men and women with secondary or higher education relative to those who are illiterate or did not complete primary school. Dowd and Zajacova (2007) also find strong educational gradients in the predictive power of self-rated health between those who did not graduate from high school and those who pursued a college degree in the United States. Both these studies use nationally representative samples of their respective countries and include people from a wide range of educational backgrounds. On the other hand, studies that use homogeneous populations to answer their research question produce results that point toward the answer, "No, education does not matter." Dalen, Huijts, Krokstad, and Eikemo (2012)'s study of adults from a rural county in Norway and McFadden et al. (2009)'s study of workers from the small region of Norfolk, UK showed no evidence supporting the notion that educated individuals have self-rated health measures that are better predictors of mortality. Similarly, Huisman, van Lenthe, and Mackenbach (2007) also find weak evidence of significant differences between education groups among Dutch adults residing in the southern part of the Netherlands. Larger differences between people in education groups lead to greater gradients in the association between self-rated health and mortality if education plays a non-insignificant role. The debate should move away from determining whether education moderates the predictive ability of self-rated health and toward asking how education shapes a person's self-assessment of health and why one person's self-rated health can be a better indicator than another's.

Jylha (2009) presents a conceptual model of a person's health evaluation process. She describes the process in three stages all formed under the influence of contextual factors such as culture and environment. While Jylha does not highlight education as a contextual factor, her model can easily explain how education can play a salient role in the person's evaluation process. First, the individual considers the factors that constitute "health" and compares his or her own status against these factors. Conceptions of "health" vary by the person's education as he or she may be aware of more diseases or conditions that determine a person's health. Education may also determine the awareness of the individual's own health status. Educational attainment could be correlated with the types of health signals – diagnoses, bodily sensations, genetics, and behavior – that he or she takes into consideration. Krause and Jay (1994)'s qualitative study based on 158 interviews tentatively finds that the specific health referents respondents consider when assessing general health differ by education. Schnittker (2009) tests education's moderating influence on the pathway linking disability and functional limitations to self-rated poor health using a much larger, nationally representative sample (US NHIS 1972–1996). The author finds statistically significant education interaction terms and highlights education's integral role in shaping the meaning of health.

This first stage can be summarized as "information collection." The second stage involves the interpretation and internalization of the information that the person gathered. Again, the respondent's education can influence how the information is translated into their own perception of health. Education can determine the reference group that the individual is comparing him or herself against. Persons with greater educational attainment would be evaluating their health against others similar to themselves rather than against those with less education and poorer health (Elo, 2009). Dowd and Zajacova (2010) find respondents with greater education had healthier biological indicators of health (blood pressure and cholesterol among others) for the same level of self-rated health. Education can also determine how a person evaluates their past health conditions and expected health developments. Past bouts of serious illnesses and bad health habits may signal deviation from optimal health even though the person is not currently sick (Agnew & Loving, 1998; Kirby & Petry, 2004; Reynolds, Richards, Horn, & Karraker, 2004).

This chapter focuses on how education can influence a person's health evaluation process. I ask if education is associated with the knowledge and internalization of health information that people consider when assessing their own health.

HYPOTHESIS

I directly test the moderating effects of education on the determinants of self-rated health: medical diagnosis, health behaviors, and biomarkers. I expect to find some evidence of disparate relationships between these health factors and self-rated health between education groups. My analysis data represents a heterogeneous US population incorporating persons who did not complete high school to those with post-secondary degrees. I also expect education's moderating effects to be stronger for health behaviors and biomarkers than medical diagnoses. Being told by a medical professional that one has a disease provides external confirmation by a health "expert." Such affirmation of sickness along with having experienced the symptoms of the illness would likely exert similar influence on self-rated health regardless of one's educational background. The relationship between health behaviors to self-assessment of health is less direct. Establishing the connection requires the respondent to have knowledge of which behaviors pose health risks and then to factor them into future expected health outcomes. Thus, individuals with greater education may discount their self-rated health in anticipation of future morbidity factoring in current unhealthy behaviors.

Indeed, education has been linked to healthy behaviors that prolong life expectancy. Cutler and Lleras-Muney (2008) observed very strong gradients where the better educated practiced healthier behaviors. With increasing education, people were less likely to smoke, drink a lot, to be overweight or obese, use illegal drugs, and to obtain preventive care. A similar study among British civil servants (Marmot, 1994) also found that individuals with greater educational attainment exhibited behaviors that promoted health. Both studies conclude that differences in these health behaviors can account for approximately 30% of the mortality differential between education groups. Persons with more education have greater knowledge of, and better means to engage in practices that lead to longevity and lower rates of lifestyle-related health problems.

Likewise, the process through which biological indicators of health can influence self-rated health is not straightforward. These biomarkers of health may or may not have physical manifestations and the knowledge of some of these measurements is dependent on access to medical care. Education is also correlated to access to care as individuals with higher educational attainment have greater earnings and better insurance coverage. Differential access to health care and income however, is not the sole source of this gradient. Cutler and Lleras-Muney (2008) and Lahelma, Martikainen, Laaksonen, and Aittomki (2004) find that income and access to health care could not account for more than 30% of the differences in health behaviors. Education may also play a role in people acquiring and internalizing new health information. De Walque (2004) find that people with greater education were faster to stop smoking after the 1964 Surgeon General Report publicizing the dangers of smoking.

Based on this discussion, I test the following.

1. The relationship between medical diagnoses and self-rated health does not depend on the respondent's educational attainment.
2. The association between self-rated health and health behaviors and biomarkers, however, is stronger among respondents with greater education.
3. Respondents with greater education are more likely to have better knowledge of their biological indicators of health.

4. Conditional on knowing their objective health measurements, persons with greater education are more likely to accurately assess their own health status.

DATA

I examine adults aged 25 and over living in the United States represented in the National Health and Nutrition Survey (NHANES 1999–2009). NHANES collected interviews, conducted clinical examinations, and recorded laboratory components in six cross-sectional waves between 1999 and 2010. The survey is designed to represent the U.S. population and over-samples African Americans, Asians, Hispanics, and persons aged 60 and older. Applying listwise deletion to observations without complete demographic variables results in an analysis sample size of 30,823 adults. Table 1 shows the descriptive characteristics of the sample.

Self-Rated Health

The NHANES asks respondents' self-rated health on two separate occasions – once before the physical examination in the home (HUQ010) and once during the examination at the Mobile Examination Center (HSD010). The question is identical but some participants gave different responses. I use the response that participants gave in their home (HUQ010) before they were subject to clinical examinations to avoid possible influence of the examination experience on their evaluations of their own health. Participants select a value between "Excellent" and "Poor" in response to the question, "In general, would you say your health is ...". I assign a numeric value to each of the five responses, 1 being "poor" and 5 being "excellent," and treat it as a continuous variable in all my analyses.

Socio-Demographic Variables

The key factor of interest in this chapter is the level of educational attainment. I categorize the sample into four education groups: did not graduate from high school, high school graduate or GED equivalent, some college

Table 1. Sample Characteristics; Adults Aged 25 and Over, NHANES 1999–2009.

	Mean	Std. Dev.
Self-rated health (1 poor – 5 excellent)	3.25	1.10
Age	52.98	16.97
Poverty ratio	2.62	1.61
	Count	**(%)**
Education		
Less than high school graduate	9,313	30.2
High school graduate	7,156	23.2
Some college/AS degree	7,982	25.9
4 yr college degree and above	6,372	20.7
Gender		
Male	14,996	48.7
Female	15,827	51.3
Marital status		
Never married	3,423	11.1
Currently married	17,752	57.6
Divorce/separated	4,532	14.7
Living with partner	1,794	5.8
Widowed	3,322	10.8
Race		
Non-Hispanic White	15,814	51.3
African American	5,923	19.2
Hispanic	7,776	25.2
Other	1,310	4.3
Total	30,823	100.0

or AA degree, and college graduate or above. In all my models, I include age, age-squared, gender, race, marital status, and logged ratio of family income to poverty threshold – factors that prior research shows relationships to self-rated health independent of observed health conditions (Schnittker, 2009).

Diagnosed Medical Conditions

The NHANES questionnaire asks respondents if they have ever been diagnosed with a particular medical condition by a physician. I examine whether education moderates the negative effects of ever having heart failure, diabetes, chronic obstructive pulmonary disease (COPD), liver condition, heart disease, heart attack, angina, and stroke on self-rated health. I also look at the relationship between taking medication for hypertension or high blood pressure and self-rated health.

Health Behaviors

I study three health behaviors that are repeatedly linked to health outcomes and mortality in this analysis. I use a dichotomous variable identifying current smokers and individuals who had a history of excessive alcohol consumption (ever drank five or more alcoholic drinks almost every day). I create a variable measuring the current level of recreational physical activity (0 none to 2 vigorous).

Biological Indicators

The NHANES conducts clinical examinations and laboratory blood testing for a wide range of biomarkers. I study the association between seven biological indicators of health and the participant's self-rated health: HDL cholesterol, hemoglobin level, C-reactive protein, resting heart rate, body mass index, waist-to-height ratio, and history of Hepatitis B infections. These biomarkers have been previously identified as health risk factors (PRB, 2008).

One of the nice features of the NHANES is that it asks participants to self-report their height, weight, and whether they consider themselves to be overweight before taking their measurements at the Mobile Examination Center. In the second part of my analysis, I estimate the likelihood of a respondent considering themselves overweight based on their actual Body Mass Index and educational attainment. In addition, the questionnaire asks respondents when they last had a health care provider check their blood pressure and their cholesterol levels. I use this information to observe differences in the likelihood of checking one's biomarkers by education.

ANALYSIS

The analysis is divided into two parts. The first demonstrates disparity in the associations between 10 health factors (diagnosed medical conditions, health behaviors, and biological indicators) and self-rated health between individuals of different educational attainment. The second part attempts to shed light onto how this may be the case.

A total of 10 (one for each health factor) OLS models estimate self-rated health (SRH) as a function of each health factor and its interaction with education. Significant health factor coefficients imply an association between the health factor and self-rated health independent of other socioeconomic variables. Interaction terms between health factors and education capture heterogeneity in the relationship between health factors and self-rated health across education levels. Health factors whose education interaction terms are significantly different from zero would be considered to have a different effect on a respondent's self-rated health depending on their educational attainment. All of these models include terms for education, gender, race, marital status, age, age-squared, and logged poverty ratio.

The second component of this chapter presents support for education's link to both greater knowledge of one's own health indicators and a better understanding of those measurements. I estimate the likelihood of an individual having his or her blood pressure or cholesterol checked by a health care provider in the past year. I then estimate the probability of respondents with BMI greater than 25 considering themselves overweight. I compare these odds between education groups while controlling for other relevant variables.

Due to the oversampling of persons above the age of 60, the distribution of self-rated health in the NHANES is not heavily skewed toward "Very Good" and "Excellent" as in many other large-scale surveys. The mean self-rated health is at 3.25 ("Good") with a standard deviation of 1.10. With the exception of coronary heart disease, the presence of medical conditions and bad health behaviors are correlated with lower self-rated health. Table 2 shows the unadjusted self-rated health of individuals reporting selected health factors relative to the overall sample. In concordance with previous findings, the prevalence of bad health behaviors, biological indicators of poor health and medical conditions is higher among individuals with less education. Table 3 shows college graduates as a healthier population than those without a high school degree on all indicators of health.

We now turn to the main results. Table 4 reports the coefficients and for each of the 20 health factors and their interaction terms with educational attainment. The top panel reports the 10 medical diagnoses and the bottom panel reports 10 health behaviors and biomarkers. Having been diagnosed

Table 2. Adverse Health Conditions and Behaviors Are Negatively Associated with Self-Rated Health. Mean Self-Rated Health (SRH) Are Not Adjusted for Socio-Demographic Factors.

Health Factor	Mean SRH	SD from Overall Mean
Smoker	3.07	−0.16
History of excessive drinking	2.98	−0.25
History of heart failure	2.23	−0.93
Ever had liver condition	2.68	−0.52
History of diabetes	2.48	−0.70
Ever had heart disease	3.47	0.20
Ever had heart attack	2.50	−0.68
Ever had angina	2.38	−0.79
History of COPD	2.60	−0.59
Ever had stroke	2.41	−0.76
Taking meds for hypertension	2.84	−0.37
Taking meds for high blood pressure	2.84	−0.373
Overall average self-rated health	3.25	

Table 3. Prevalence of Medical Conditions, Health Behaviors, and Average Biological Measurements by Educational Attainment.

	Less Than HS Graduate	HS Graduate	Some College	College Degree +
History of heart failure (%)	5.25	3.77	3.22	1.79
History of diabetes (%)	17.39	11.42	10.92	6.56
History of COPD (%)	8.57	7.95	7.96	5.17
Ever had liver condition (%)	3.65	3.33	3.71	2.91
Ever had heart disease (%)	6.10	4.82	4.10	4.06
Ever had heart attack (%)	6.58	5.44	4.37	3.30
Ever had angina (%)	4.26	3.86	3.55	2.28
Ever had stroke (%)	6.01	4.48	3.75	2.45
Taking meds for hypertension (%)	36.5	34.7	30.6	24.4
Taking meds for high blood pressure (%)	34.2	32.9	28.6	23.0
Smoker (%)	25.9	26.0	21.0	9.0
History of excess alcohol consumption (%)	22.0	17.1	14.1	8.2
Recreational activity level (0 low – 2 high)	0.40	0.63	0.79	1.11
HDL cholesterol (mg/dL)	50.3	51.0	52.7	54.0
Hemoglobin level (mg/dL)	14.1	14.3	14.2	14.2
C-Reactive protein (mg/dL)	0.52	0.47	0.48	0.37
Resting heart rate (pulse/60 sec)	72.4	72.9	73.0	71.2
BMI (kg/m^2)	29.2	29.2	29.6	27.8
Waist to height ratio	0.61	0.60	0.59	0.57
Past/current Hepatitis B infection (%)	9.75	7.08	6.17	5.43
Percentage of total sample (%)	30.21	23.22	25.9	20.67

Table 4. Moderating Effects of Education on the Association between Health Factors and Self-Rated Health (1 Poor – 5 Excellent).

Medical Diagnoses	Ever Had Heart Failure	Ever Had Diabetes	Ever Had COPD	Ever Had Liver Condition	Ever Had Heart Disease	Ever Had Heart Attack	Ever Had Angina	Ever Had Stroke	Taking Meds for Hypertension	Taking Meds for High Blood Pressure
Condition	−0.688***	−0.575***	−0.611***	−0.522***	−0.618***	−0.603***	−0.664***	−0.551***	−0.465***	−0.465***
Condition-education interaction terms										
Condition × less than HS	*(reference)*									
Condition × HS grad	−0.116	−0.0119	0.0205	0.0482	0.0347	0.022	−0.0529	−0.165*	0.0353	0.0533
Condition × some college/2 yr	−0.305***	−0.118**	0.0778	0.103	0.0144	0.0209	−0.135	−0.13	−0.0162	−0.0126
Condition × 4 yr college degree +	−0.338**	−0.162**	0.0268	0.0432	−0.136	−0.0717	−0.12	−0.146	0.0183	0.00108
R-squared	0.199	0.213	0.199	0.186	0.193	0.194	0.194	0.194	0.211	0.21

Table 4. *(Continued)*

Health Behaviors and Biomarkers	Smoker	History of Excess Alcohol Consumption	Recreational Activity Level	Logged HDL Cholesterol (mg/dL)	Logged Hemoglobin Level (mg/dL)	Logged C-Reactive Protein (mg/dL)	Logged Resting Heart Rate (Pulse/60 sec)	Logged BMI (kg/m^2)	Logged Waist to Height Ratio	Past/Current Hepatitis B Infection
	Lower values indicate health	Lower values indicate health	Higher values indicate health	Higher values indicate health	Higher values indicate health	Lower values indicate health	Lower values indicate health	Lower values indicate health	Lower values indicate health	Lower values indicate health
Condition or measurement	−0.0597*	−0.143***	0.178***	0.327***	0.538***	−0.0878***	−0.415***	−0.447***	−1.014***	0.0712
Condition-education interaction terms										
Condition × less than HS	*(reference)*									
Condition × HS grad	−0.111**	−0.0679	0.0720***	0.0369	0.128	−0.0141	−0.126	−0.309***	−0.195	−0.111
Condition × some college/2 yr	−0.120***	−0.0205	0.0376	0.134*	0.252	−0.0171	−0.0343	−0.444***	−0.369***	−0.146*
Condition × 4 yr college degree +	−0.170***	−0.151**	0.107***	0.247***	0.341*	−0.0543***	−0.266**	−0.544***	−0.417***	−0.162*
R-squared	0.183	0.186	0.204	0.194	0.185	0.196	0.19	0.203	0.211	0.182

Note: All models include controls for gender, race, marital status, age, age-squared, and logged poverty ratio.
***$p < 0.001$, **$p < 0.01$, *$p < 0.05$.

with a medical condition diminishes one's perception of general health. And, for the most part, an illness influences self-rated health equally across education groups. That is, persons with or without a high school degree will consider themselves equally less healthy if they have been diagnosed with a serious medical condition. Interestingly, I find that history of heart failure or diabetes is associated with lower self-rated health with increasing education. The reason for this distinction deserves further study; I conjecture that these two diseases require vigilant management of the patient's health measurements and behaviors. Indeed, when health behaviors – smoking, activity level, and history of excess alcohol consumption – are controlled for, the education interaction terms of diabetes and heart failure diminishes.

Current health behaviors have a stronger association with self-rated health among individuals with higher educational attainment as displayed in the bottom panel of Table 4. The statistically significant interaction terms of these health behaviors indicate that self-rated health is more responsive to smoking, drinking history, and exercise level among individuals with greater educational attainment. The sizes of these interaction terms are quite large, even exceeding the main effects by two to three times in the case for smokers.

Similarly to health behaviors, self-rated health has a stronger relationship with biological indicators of health. The effects of high HDL cholesterol and hemoglobin levels (associated with better health) are most salient among highest education category (college graduate and above). Likewise, C-reactive protein and resting heart rate have stronger association with lower self-rated health among the college graduates. Measures of obesity – body mass index and waist-to-height ratio – display a gradient with their relationship to self-rated health increasing with greater educational attainment. Indicators of past or current Hepatitis B infection (a risk factor for diseases of the liver) is related to self-rated health only among those with a college education (with or without a four-year degree). These results points toward a conclusion supporting heterogeneity in the association between health behaviors and biomarkers, and self-rated health. Medical diagnoses, on the other hand, show little educational gradient on their influence on self-rated health.

The second component of this study attempts to offer some explanations to the processes that lead to these educational gradients in the determinants of self-rated health. I show in Fig. 1 that education increases the likelihood of having a medical professional check one's blood pressure and cholesterol in the past 12 months controlling for gender, age, income, and marital

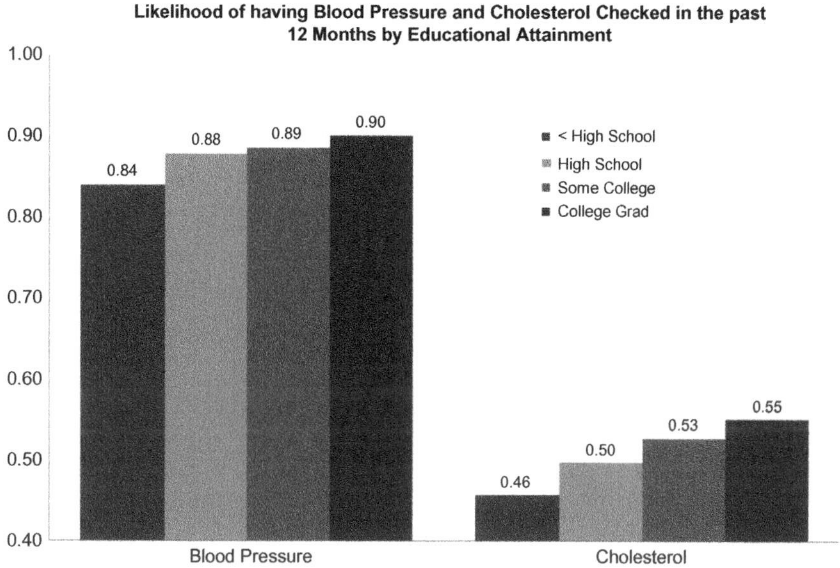

Fig. 1. Individuals with Higher Educational Attainment Are More Likely to Have Had Their Blood Pressure and Cholesterol Checked within the Past 12 Months. Probabilities Are Adjusted for Socio-Demographic Variables. *Note*: Odds are net of gender, race, marital status, age, age-squared, and logged poverty ratio.

status. Individuals with a college degree or higher are 7% more likely to have had their blood pressure checked and 20% more likely to have had their cholesterol measured in the past year. The NHANES records both the self-reported and measured blood pressure for persons self-identified as diabetic. Individuals living with diabetes are more likely to be aware of and to closely monitor their health than the average person. Even within this select group, those with high educational attainment report blood pressure levels that are closer to their actual levels. Table 5 shows the correlation coefficients between reported and measured (NHANES has physician examiners take up to four separate blood pressures readings from their participants. I take the average of the measurements) diastolic and systolic blood pressure. The correlation coefficient among those with a college degree is 2.5 times that of people without a high school degree for diastolic and 1.6 times for systolic blood pressure.

I then show that education is not only related to knowing one's biological health indicators but is also associated with how well the person can

Table 5. Correlation Coefficient between Reported and Measured Blood Pressure among Diabetic Persons.

	Diastolic	Systolic
Less than high school graduate	0.134	0.251
High school graduate	0.168	0.354
Some college or AS degree	0.373	0.302
College degree and above	0.342	0.404
Total observations	643	662

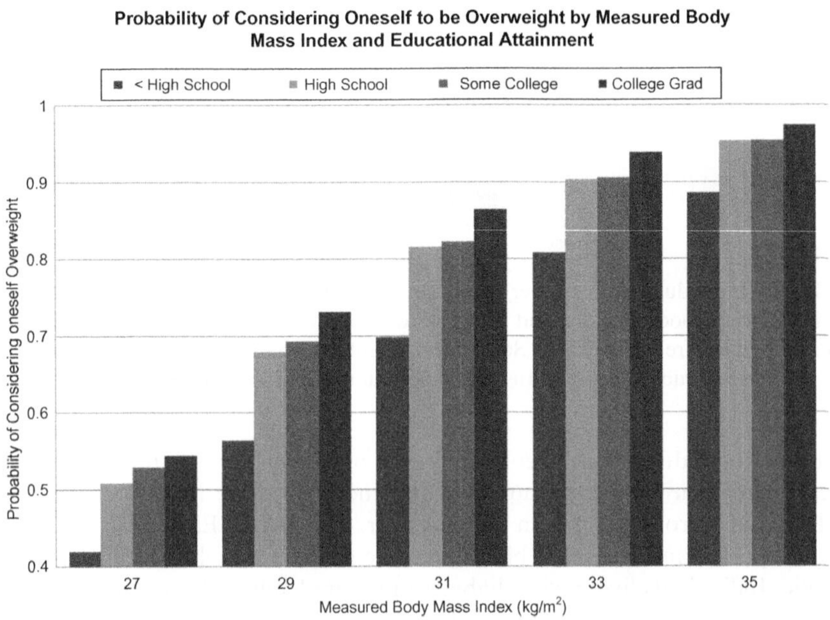

Fig. 2. Education Is Linked to a More Accurate Assessment of the Healthiness of One's Weight. Probabilities Are Adjusted for Socio-Demographic Variables. *Note*: Odds are net of gender, race, marital status, age, age-squared, and logged poverty ratio.

evaluate and internalize that measurement. Fig. 2 shows the probability that the respondent reports him or herself to be overweight given that they are actually clinically overweight (BMI greater than or equal to 25) or obese (BMI greater than or equal to 30). Education, again, is closely related to the likelihood that the respondent correctly assesses him or herself as overweight even when other socio-demographic factors are accounted for. The proportion of overweight or obese people recognizing that they exceed their healthy weight increases with educational attainment. Thirty percent of obese individuals with BMI of 31 without a high school degree do not recognize themselves to be overweight. Less than 14% of equivalent individuals with a college degree report that they are not overweight.

CONCLUSION

This chapter contributes to this growing literature through systematic examination of a wide range of health factors that has been previously linked to mortality and morbidity. I examine the three most salient health behaviors, seven biomarkers associated with current and future health risks, and 10 prevalent medical conditions. The rich health variables in the NHANES dataset allows for analysis incorporating a wider variety of health factors than prior studies.

These results show that the relationship between medical diagnoses and self-rated health does not change much by the respondents' education. Individuals can only report diagnoses when they have been informed by a medical professional and usually have experienced the illness. On the other hand, the relationships between self-rated health, and health behaviors and biomarkers are moderated by education. This distinction in health factors' correlations with self-rated health can help explain why some studies show evidence for educational gradients in the predictive power of self-rated health while others do not. Populations with greater disparity in access to care and health knowledge between people of different educational attainment would be more likely to display variability in the self-rated health-mortality relationship. Educational differences in the association between behaviors and biomarkers on self-rated health lead us to ask why these health factors operate differently from diagnosed medical conditions. I show that educational attainment is associated with having better awareness of biological indicators of health. Such differences in knowledge can affect their self-assessment of general health. The disparity is not limited to differences in the types and accuracy of information that people acquire. Individuals with greater education are not only more likely to be more knowledgeable about their own biological indicators of health but they are also more likely to understand and internalize these measurements. These findings draw attention to systematic biases that self-rated health may bring to the future analyses. Researchers of health inequalities along socioeco nomic boundaries, in particular, should be aware of the incongruity in the factors that shape self-rated measures of overall health.

REFERENCES

Agnew, C., & Loving, T. (1998). Future time orientation and condom use attitudes, intentions, and behavior. *Journal of Social Behavior and Personality, 13*(4), 755–764.

Benyamini, Y., & Idler, E. L. (1999). Community studies reporting association between self-rated health and mortality: Additional studies 1995–1998. *Research on Aging, 21*, 392–401.

Cutler, D., & Lleras-Muney, A. (2008). *Education and health: Evaluating theories and evidence*. New York, NY: Russell Sage Foundation.

Dalen, J. D., Huijts, T., Krokstad, S., & Eikemo, T. A. (2012). Are there educational differences in the association between self-rated health and mortality in Norway? The hunt study. *Scandinavian Journal of Public Health, 40*(7), 641–647.

De Walque, D. (2004). *Education, information, and smoking decisions: Evidence from smoking histories, 1940–2000*. Policy Research Working Paper Series No. 3362. The World Bank.

Dowd, J. B., & Zajacova, A. (2007). Does the predictive power of self-rated health for subsequent mortality risk vary by socioeconomic status in the US? *International Journal of Epidemiology, 36*(6), 1214–1221.

Dowd, J. B., & Zajacova, A. (2010). Does self-rated health mean the same thing across socioeconomic groups? Evidence from biomarker data. *Annals of Epidemiology, 20*(10), 743–749.

Elo, I. T. (2009). Social class differentials in health and mortality: Patterns and explanations in comparative perspective. *Annual Review of Sociology, 35*, 553–572.

Huisman, M., van Lenthe, F., & Mackenbach, J. (2007). The predictive ability of self-assessed health for mortality in different educational groups. *International Journal of Epidemiology, 36*(6), 1207–1213.

Idler, E., & Benyamini, Y. (1997). Self-rated health and mortality: A review of twenty-seven community studies. *Journal of Health and Social Behavior, 38*, 21–37.

Jylha, M. (2009). What is self-rated health and why does it predict mortality? Towards a united conceptual model. *Social Science & Medicine, 69*(3), 307–316.

Kirby, K., & Petry, N. (2004). Heroin and cocaine abusers have higher discount rates for delayed rewards than alcoholics or non-drug-using controls. *Addiction, 99*(4), 461–471.

Krause, N. M., & Jay, G. M. (1994). What do global self-rated health items measure? *Medical Care, 32*(9), 930–942.

Lahelma, E., Martikainen, P., Laaksonen, M., & Aittomki, A. (2004). Pathways between socioeconomic determinants of health. *Journal of Epidemiology and Community Health, 58*(4), 327–332.

Marmot, M. G. (1994). Social differentials in health within and between populations. *Daedalus, 123*(4), 197–216.

McFadden, E., Luben, R., Bingham, S., Wareham, N., Kinmonth, A.-L., & Khaw, K.-T. (2009). Does the association between self-rated health and mortality vary by social class? *Social Science & Medicine*, *68*(2), 275–280.

PRB. (2008). *Use of biomarkers in predicting health and mortality*. Technical report. Today's Research on Aging, Populations Reference Bureau.

Regidor, E., Guallar-Castilln, P., Gutirrez-Fisac, J. L., Banegas, J. R., & Rodrguez-Artalejo, F. (2010). Socioeconomic variation in the magnitude of the association between self-rated health and mortality. *Annals of Epidemiology*, *20*(5), 395–400.

Reynolds, B., Richards, J. B., Horn, K., & Karraker, K. (2004). Delay discounting and probability discounting as related to cigarette smoking status in adults. *Behavioral Processes*, *65*, 35–42.

Schnittker, J. (2009). Mirage of health in the era of biomedicalization: Evaluating change in the threshold of illness, 1972–1996. *Social Forces*, *87*, 2155–2182.

Thomas, D., & Frankenberg, E. (2002). The measurement and interpretation of health in social surveys. In C. J. L. Murray (Ed.), *Summary measures of population health: Concepts, ethics, measurement and applications, chapter the measurement and interpretation of health in social surveys* (pp. 387–420). Geneva: World Health Organization.

PART IV
MENTAL HEALTH

PSYCHOLOGICAL DISTRESS, NATIVITY, AND HELP-SEEKING AMONG FILIPINO AMERICANS

Ethel G. Nicdao, Aileen A. Duldulao and David T. Takeuchi

ABSTRACT

Purpose – *This study examines Filipino Americans with high levels of psychological distress. We report on whether ethnic identity, discrimination, and nativity are predictors for help-seeking from a medical professional.*

Methodology – *We derived our data from the Filipino American Community Epidemiological Study which surveyed Filipino adults living in the United States (*N = *2,285). We used OLS regression to examine the association between psychological distress and help-seeking among US-born Filipinos and immigrants.*

Findings – *The majority of US-born and foreign-born Filipinos sought help for psychological distress from a lay person. Years spent in the United States, ethnic identity, and discrimination were strong predictors for help-seeking. US-born Filipinos were more likely to seek help. Those*

Education, Social Factors, and Health Beliefs in Health and Health Care Services
Research in the Sociology of Health Care, Volume 33, 107–120

ISSN: 0275-4959/doi:10.1108/S0275-495920150000033005

with low ethnic identity and experienced medium to high discrimination were less likely to seek help.

Conclusions – *Our findings suggest that years in United States, ethnic identity and discrimination are associated with help-seeking. Future research should consider factors such as social support and acculturation to examine whether these contribute to psychological distress and help-seeking.*

Keywords: Filipino; psychological distress; help-seeking; ethnic identity; discrimination

PSYCHOLOGICAL DISTRESS AND SOCIAL FACTORS INFLUENCING HELP-SEEKING FOR ASIAN AMERICANS

Research studies investigating the association between psychological distress and a combination of factors including race, age, socioeconomic status (SES), ethnic identity, acculturation, nativity, and help-seeking behavior of ethnic minorities have produced varied results (Jarvis, Kirmayer, Weinfeld, & Lasry, 2005; Kirmayer et al., 2007; Mak & Zane, 2004; Shim & Schwartz, 2008). Elevated psychological distress is attributed to a combination of factors. In a study comparing older Korean immigrants and non-Hispanic Whites, race and SES were associated with psychological distress. Compared to their White counterparts, older Korean immigrants reported higher levels of distress. Additionally, Korean immigrants with increased levels of social support significantly reduced their psychological distress (Min, Moon, & Lubben, 2005). And for Filipino immigrants, attendance at religious services was associated with lower levels of psychological distress (Jarvis et al., 2005), yet rates of help-seeking for mental health services remains low for Asian Americans (David, 2010; Kirmayer et al., 2007).

In a critical review of the relationship between acculturation and health, increased levels of acculturation predicted increased help-seeking and utilizing medical professional services (Salant & Lauderdale, 2003). Another study reported that highly acculturated adults predicted lower levels of depression (Suinn, 2010). And Asian Americans who were more acculturated were likely to be more receptive to seeking professional psychological services than those less acculturated to US culture (Kim, 2007). Furthermore, Kim (2007) found an inverse relationship between enculturation to Asian cultural norms and seeking professional psychological help. In other words, the attitudes of Asian Americans towards help-seeking were associated with loss of traditional Asian cultural norms. Conversely, individuals who are less acculturated, adhere more strongly to Asian values, and live in the United States for a shorter period of time predicted increased levels of psychological distress (Shim & Schwartz, 2008). Interestingly, another study presented evidence that for immigrant Chinese Americans, acculturation and length of stay in the United States was not related to somatization, but psychological distress provided possible explanations for somatization tendencies (Mak & Zane, 2004).

Psychological distress has also been linked to discrimination and ethnic identity. In a nationally representative study of Asian Americans, researchers found that discrimination was a strong predictor of mental disorders, even when controlling for other characteristics such as acculturative stress and family cohesion. Among the ethnic subgroups in the sample, Filipinos had the highest levels of self-reported discrimination (Gee, Spencer, Chen, Yip, & Takeuchi, 2007). Additionally, ethnic identity was shown to buffer and exacerbate discrimination and psychological distress, dependent on the age of Asian adults. Specifically, Filipinos who reported more discrimination had more distress, and those with stronger ethnic identity were likely to have less distress (Yip, Gee, & Takeuchi, 2008). While some studies indicate that ethnic identity serves to protect against ethnic discrimination (Mossakowski, 2003), other studies report that ethnic identity does not moderate the effects of discrimination. According to Yoo and Lee (2005), ethnic identity only serves as a protective factor for effects of discrimination when the discrimination is not severe. While these studies provide evidence that distinct Asian ethnic groups experience psychological distress in different ways, and offer explanations on the many social factors that contribute to distress and help-seeking, few studies have examined the association between psychological distress, nativity, discrimination, and ethnic identity among Filipino Americans.

MENTAL HEALTH AND HELP-SEEKING AMONG FILIPINO AMERICANS

The help-seeking process of Filipino Americans with mental health problems can be understood by considering the role of culture and acculturation in their health and illness beliefs, and as a consequence, their health behaviors. In particular, Anderson (1983) noted that among less acculturated Filipino immigrants, psychopathology was largely explained as having hereditary tendencies. Together with the stigma attached to mental illness, the desire to protect a positive self-image and avoid embarrassment, the sociocultural practice of maintaining balance to achieve good health, and perceptions of mental health attributed to religion, social support systems, and coping styles (Anderson, 1983; Nadal, 2000; Sanchez & Gaw, 2007), Filipinos are hindered from seeking mental health care services, and more likely to seek help from religious leaders (Kirmayer et al., 2007).

Drawing from the body of work indicating that ethnic identity serves to buffer against the deleterious effects of discrimination (Mossakowski, 2003), we use data from the Filipino American Community Epidemiological Study (FACES) to elucidate on the mental health of Filipinos. Research based on the FACES data have already resulted in some key findings, namely the association between higher levels of psychological distress and job dissatisfaction (de Castro, Gee, & Takeuchi, 2008), differences in nativity showing that foreign-born Filipinos compared to US-born Filipinos have significantly lower levels of depressive symptoms (Mossakowski, 2007), the likelihood that Filipino Americans use the lay system as their usual source of care compared to professional or folk systems (Gong, Gage, & Tacata, 2003), the risk and protective factors for alcohol use disorders for Filipinos living in different sociocultural environments (Kim, Kim, & Nochajski, 2010), and that highly religious Filipino Americans were more likely to seek help from religious clergy, while those who were highly spiritual were less likely to seek help for mental health issues (Abe-Kim, Gong, & Takeuchi, 2004). Our study aims to examine whether the previously mentioned associations between psychological distress, years in United States, nativity, ethnic identity, and discrimination hold true for Filipino Americans. We hypothesize that Filipinos that have spent more years living in the United States, are US-born, have strong ethnic identity and experience high levels of discrimination are more likely to seek help. In contrast, those who have spent less years living in the United States, are foreign-born, have low ethnic identity and low levels of experiencing discrimination are less likely to seek help.

METHODS

We derived our data from the Filipino American Community Epidemiological Study. The study was conducted between 1998 and 1999 and surveyed Filipino American adults 18 years of age and older living in and around Honolulu, Hawai'i, and San Francisco, California on a variety of health issues. Participants were given the option of having the survey administered in Tagalog or Ilocano as well as English. A total of 2,285 interviews were completed with a response rate of 78%. Due to missing data, this study uses 1987 observations. Detailed sampling procedures have been documented in previous literature (Gong et al., 2003; Mossakowski, 2003).

Measures

Sociodemographic variables included sex (1 = female, 0 = male), marital status (1 = married, 0 = not married), county of residence (1 = Honolulu, HI, 0 = San Francisco, CA), and education (continuous variable measuring number of years of education). The number of years in the United States was measured using the variable "Years in the US" which consisted of five categories. Respondents who were recent immigrants (in the United States 5 years or less) were coded as "1," with categories for respondents who had been in the United States for longer periods of time (2 = 6–10 years in the United States, 3 = 11–20 years in the United States, 4 = 20 years or more in the United States). Respondents born in the United States were coded as "5."

Ethnic identity was measured using 12 items using a Likert scale (1 = strongly disagree, 4 = strongly agree). For this study, the Cronbach's alpha for this scale is 0.78. Items assessed the level that respondents identified with being Filipino and included items such as "I have a clear sense of my Filipino background and what it means to me," "I have spent time trying to learn more about Filipino history, traditions, and cultures," and "I am happy that I am Filipino." Scores for each item were summed to create an aggregate score for each respondent. Each score was categorized into "High," "Medium," and "Low" based on the aggregate score.

Everyday discrimination was measured using nine items from the Detroit Area Study and in this study the Cronbach's alpha is 0.87. Respondents were asked to rate the frequency of their experiences with discrimination in the past month using a Likert scale (1 = never, 5 = very often). A categorical variable was created based on the sum of responses to the scale questions and divided into the categories "High," "Medium," and "Low." Items asked if respondents had been treated with less "respect" or with less "courtesy" as well as if the respondents had been "called names or insulted" and "threatened or harassed." These experiences could be attributed to race, ethnicity, or other characteristics.

Help-seeking was measured using a dichotomous variable (1 = yes, 0 = no) and represents whether or not respondents had ever sought help from a health service provider in the past 12 months. Options for help-seeking were based on three possible sources: general medical care (e.g., general practitioner or physician), mental health specialist (e.g., psychiatrist, psychologist, or other mental health worker), and other care (e.g., religious clergy, counselor, folk healer, etc.).

Psychological distress is based on 21 items from the Symptom Checklist-90-Revised (Derogatis, 1994). The minimum score on this scale is zero with a maximum score of 120, with higher scores indicating higher levels of psychological distress.

Analyses

This study used multivariate logistic regression in three models to explore the relationship between help-seeking and the dependent variables. Data was weighted to account for the different probabilities of selection between the two counties of residence. The first model examines the likelihood of help-seeking by sociodemographic variables. The second model examines the likelihood of help-seeking according to the number of years in the United States, ethnic identity and discrimination, controlling for psychological distress. The third model examines help-seeking in the context of all of the dependent variables, controlling for psychological distress.

RESULTS

Descriptive statistics are shown in Table 1. Analyses for missing data yielded an overall sample size of 1987 respondents. The majority of foreign-born respondents ($N = 1{,}681$) were male (50.3%) and married (65.8%) and had a mean age of 43 years old (SE = 0.32). In contrast, the US-born respondents ($N = 403$) were mostly female (53.23%) and unmarried (36%). Additionally, US-born respondents were generally younger than foreign-born respondents with a mean age of 35.8 years old (SE = 0.68). The majority of respondents in both groups resided in Honolulu. Among foreign-born Filipino Americans, approximately one-third of the sample (32%) had been living in the United States for over 20 years and one-fifth (20.7%) were recent immigrants who had been living in the United States for 5 years or less.

Table 1. Descriptive Statistics by Nativity for Whole Sample ($N = 1,987$).

	Foreign-Born $N = 1,579$ Mean (SE) or %	Psychological Distress Mean (SE)	US-Born $N = 408$ Mean (SE) or %	Psychological Distress Mean (SE)	Entire Sample $N =$ 1,987 Mean (SE) or %
Overall	100	6.98 (0.23)	100	9.71 (0.58)	7.54 (0.22)
Sex					
Male	50.29	8.29	46.77	12.22	49.57
Female	49.71	5.65	53.23	7.52	50.43
Marital status					
Married	65.78	6.45	64.05	6.79	59.65
Unmarried	34.22	7.99	35.95	11.36	40.35
County of residence					
Honolulu	57.1	3.96	62.19	7.66	58.14
San Francisco	42.9	11	37.81	13.1	41.86
Education, years	11.50 (0.12)	–	11.58 (0.23)	–	11.51 (0.11)
Age	43 (0.32)	–	35.8 (0.68)	–	41.54 (0.30)
Years in the United States					
0–5 years	20.74	6.10	–	–	16.48
6–10 years	18.11	6.01	–	–	14.39
11–20 years	29.19	7.61	–	–	23.19
Over 20 years	31.95	7.52	–	–	25.39
Ethnic identity					
Low	22.67	7.44	17.77	8.12	21.66
Medium	52.06	6.53	46.63	8.47	50.94
High	25.27	7.47	35.61	12.15	27.40
Discrimination					
Low	53.98	3.96	44.96	5.76	52.12
Medium	26.04	8.20	28.96	12.10	26.64
High	19.99	13.53	35.61	13.89	21.24
Help-seeking					
Yes	21.08	5.83	36.24	6.07	24.20
No	78.92	11.29	63.76	16.14	75.80

Most foreign-born and US-born respondents were categorized as having "medium" ethnic identity (52.1% and 46.6%, respectively). More US-born respondents (35.6%) expressed having "high" ethnic identity compared to foreign-born respondents (25.3%). Additionally, more US-born respondents (35.6%) were categorized as having experienced high levels of discrimination compared to foreign-born respondents (20%), although among both groups the majority of respondents expressed that they had experienced low levels of discrimination. There were also differences in mean scores on psychological distress, with US-born respondents having a higher mean score (9.71, SE = 0.58) than foreign-born respondents (6.98, SE = 0.23).

Descriptive statistics for those individuals who expressed high levels of psychological distress symptoms are shown in Table 2. Only people over one standard deviation from the mean for psychological distress were included. Analyses for missing data yielded an overall sample size of 274 respondents with high levels of psychological distress. The majority of respondents ($N = 274$) were male (74%), unmarried (54%) and resided in San Francisco (72%). Respondents had a mean age of 38 years old (SE = 0.82), and only 28% were US-born Filipino Americans. Approximately one-fourth of the sample (24%) had been living in the United States for

Table 2. Descriptive Statistics for Filipinos with High Psychological Distress ($N = 274$).

	Mean (SE) or %
Sex	
Male	73.72
Female	26.28
Marital status	
Married	46.35
Unmarried	53.65
County of residence	
Honolulu	28.47
San Francisco	71.53
Education, years	12.88 (0.25)
Age	38.28 (0.82)
Years in the United States	
0–5 years	12.77
6–10 years	12.41
11–20 years	22.99
Over 20 years	23.72
US-born	28.10
Ethnic identity	
Low	19.71
Medium	48.54
High	31.75
Discrimination	
Low	21.17
Medium	28.83
High	50
Help-seeking	
Yes	47.08
No	52.92

over 20 years and nearly one-fourth (23%) had been living in the United States 11–20 years.

Most respondents were categorized as having "medium" ethnic identity (48.54%). Additionally, half of the respondents (50%) were categorized as having experienced high levels of discrimination. Lastly, the majority of respondents reported not seeking help (53%).

Table 3 provides the results of the weighted multivariate logistic regression models. Model 1 examined the relationship between help-seeking and several demographic variables. Significant differences in the likelihood of help-seeking were found when examining marital status. Married Filipino Americans were more likely (OR = 3.05, 95% CI = 1.76, 5.27) than unmarried Filipino Americans to seek help for psychological distress, controlling

Table 3. Multiple Logistic Regression Models Predicting Help-Seeking.

	Model 1		Model 2		Model 3	
	Odds ratio	95% CI	Odds ratio	95% CI	Odds ratio	95% CI
Sex						
Male[a]	–		–		–	
Female	1.43	0.79, 2.67			1.67	0.83, 3.68
Marital status						
Unmarried[a]	–		–		–	
Married	3.05**	1.76, 5.27			2.49*	1.22, 5.08
County of residence						
Honolulu[a]	–		–		–	
San Francisco	0.86	0.46, 1.63			0.61	0.27, 1.35
Years in the United States						
0–5 years	–		–		–	
6–10 years			1.44	0.46, 4.53	1.49	0.43, 5.12
11–20 years			1.58	0.57, 4.35	3.91*	1.22, 12.55
Over 20 years			1.58	0.57, 4.35	2.82	0.87, 9.15
US-born			7.34**	2.56, 21.11	8.98**	2.64, 30.57
Ethnic identity						
High[a]	–		–		–	
Medium			0.87	0.45, 1.70	0.98	0.49, 1.97
Low			0.58	0.27, 1.26	0.80	0.34, 1.90
Discrimination						
Low[a]	–		–		–	
Medium			0.6	0.30, 1.19	0.62	0.30, 1.26
High			0.30*	0.15, 0.60	0.36*	0.15, 0.74

All models control for psychological distress.

[a]Referent category.

*$p \leq 0.05$; **$p \leq 0.001$.

for all other variables. There were no significant differences by sex and county.

Model 2 examined the relationship between help-seeking and the number of years in the United States, ethnic identity, and discrimination, while controlling for psychological distress. US-born Filipinos (OR = 7.34, 95% CI = 2.56, 21.11) were over seven times as likely to seek help than recent immigrants controlling for other variables. There were no differences in help-seeking between recent immigrants (in the United States 5 years or less) and immigrants who had been in the United States 11 years or more. Additionally, Filipino Americans who experienced high levels of discrimination (OR = 0.30, 95% CI = 0.15, 0.60) were less likely to seek help compared to those who experienced low levels of discrimination, controlling for all other variables including psychological distress.

Model 3 examined help-seeking by sociodemographic variables, immigration and identity variables, and psychological distress. As in the first model, there were no significant differences by sex and county. Married Filipino Americans continued to be more likely (OR = 2.49, 95% CI = 1.22, 5.08) than those unmarried to seek help for psychological distress. Unlike Model 2, there were significant differences between recent immigrants in the United States 5 years or less and immigrants who had been in the United States 11 years or more. Filipino Americans living in the United States 11–20 years were more likely to seek help (OR = 3.91, 95% CI = 1.22, 12.55) than recent immigrants. Moreover, Filipino American immigrants who were born in the United States (OR = 8.98, 95% CI = 2.64, 30.57) were nearly nine times as likely to seek help for psychological distress than recent immigrants. Significant differences also remained between Filipino Americans who had experienced different levels of discrimination, with those experiencing high levels of discrimination (OR = 0.36, 95% CI = 0.15, 0.74) being less likely to seek help than those experiencing low levels of discrimination.

DISCUSSION

Our study examined the help-seeking behavior of foreign-born Filipinos and US-born Filipinos with psychological distress. Findings point to several factors like nativity, marital status, and discrimination as significant predictors for help-seeking. In two of our predictive models, marital status was a strong predictor for help-seeking. Marital status may serve as a protective factor for married Filipinos compared to those who are unmarried.

The higher likelihood of married Filipinos seeking help for psychological distress may be due to the support provided from one's spouse. Social support has been shown to "promote health" and serve as a buffer for life stressors (Thoits, 1982, 1986).

In our examination of the relationship between help-seeking and the number of years spent in the United States, level of ethnic identity, and experiences of discrimination, we found that US-born Filipinos were more likely to seek help for psychological distress than recent immigrants. This finding may represent different levels of acculturation for US-born versus immigrant Filipinos. A possible explanation could be that US-born Filipinos may not adhere strongly to Asian cultural norms and their increased level of acculturation may lead them to consider seeking psychiatric and mental health services (Kim, 2007; Salant & Lauderdale, 2003). In contrast, length of time spent in residence in the United States has resulted in a decline of health status for immigrants (Frisbie, Cho, & Hummer, 2001). Additionally, those who experienced high levels of discrimination were less likely to seek help. We postulate that Filipinos experiencing high levels of discrimination based on phenotype or skin color (Kiang & Takeuchi, 2009; Rondilla & Spickard, 2007) may be less likely to seek help out of fear that they might experience discrimination in the health care setting.

Our results revealed that low ethnic identity does not correlate with discrimination and seem to suggest that Filipino Americans can possess low ethnic identity and experience high levels of discrimination, which may lead them to avoid seeking help for psychological distress. In contrast, a study by Richman, Kohn-Wood, and Williams (2007) determined that Black Americans with high racial identity who also experienced discrimination predicted a lower likelihood of utilizing mental health services compared to those with low racial identity (Richman et al., 2007). Indeed, ethnic identity for minority groups is complex and can manifest differently when considering sociocultural factors. As Tuason et al. (2007) noted in their findings, the Filipino American identity is dependent on numerous characteristics including being US- or Philippine-born, religion, sense of belonging, identifying with Filipino cultural values, and American values.

CONCLUSION

Our study has several limitations. The data used is cross-sectional and only reflects the behaviors, beliefs, and mental health status of respondents at one point in time. This may be problematic since behaviors and beliefs critical to this study such as ethnic identity, discrimination, and psychological distress change over time. A longitudinal study would better capture the changes over time as well as the complex relationship between help-seeking and its covariates. Additionally, variation in the levels of psychological distress and help-seeking behaviors of US-born and foreign-born Filipinos could be the result of other factors not considered in this study such as social support and acculturation levels. We did not have an actual measurement for acculturation in our model. We used years in the United States as a proxy measurement, but this did not include acculturative stress. Lastly, our measure of discrimination only included racial and ethnic discrimination, and did not consider other types of discrimination, which may or may not have contributed to under- or over-reporting of experiences of discrimination.

Despite our limitations, our study has potential to expand the direction of future research on examining the associations between ethnic identity, discrimination, and acculturation. In particular, our focus on Filipinos emphasizes the fact that not all Asian American groups are the same and, especially in the case of Filipinos who were colonized by the West, have very distinct immigration and sociocultural histories that impact their interactions with different institutions. The ethnic identity of Filipinos is complex and warrants further investigation. A qualitative study could help explain how ethnic identity and discrimination are related. Specifically, we assume that individuals experience discrimination in their host country, but for Filipino immigrants, discrimination based on phenotype and skin color begins in their home country. Measures must take into consideration the sociohistorical context of Filipinos, namely the history of colonization and immigration, and how these elements relate to their experiences of discrimination, levels of psychological distress, and help-seeking.

ACKNOWLEDGMENT

The Filipino American Community Epidemiological Study was supported by the National Institute on Alcohol Abuse and Alcoholism (grant 098633 to David T. Takeuchi).

REFERENCES

Abe-Kim, J., Gong, F., & Takeuchi, D. T. (2004). Religiosity, spirituality, and help-seeking among Filipino Americans: Religious clergy or mental health professionals? *Journal of Community Psychology*, *32*(6), 675–689.

Anderson, J. N. (1983). Health and illness in Pilipino immigrants. *Western Journal of Medicine*, *139*(6), 811–819.

David, E. J. R. (2010). Cultural mistrust and mental health help-seeking attitudes among Filipino Americans. *Asian American Journal of Psychology*, *1*(1), 57–66.

de Castro, A. B., Gee, G. C., & Takeuchi, D. T. (2008). Relationship between job dissatisfaction and physical and psychological health among Filipino immigrants. *AAOHN Journal*, *56*(1), 33–40.

Derogatis, L. R. (1994). *Symptom checklist-90-R (SCL-90-R): Administration, scoring and procedures manual* (3rd ed.). Minneapolis, MN: NCS Pearsons, Inc.

Frisbie, W. P., Cho, Y., & Hummer, R. A. (2001). Immigration and the health of Asian and pacific islander adults in the United States. *American Journal of Epidemiology*, *153*(4), 372–380.

Gee, G. C., Spencer, M., Chen, J., Yip, T., & Takeuchi, D. (2007). The association between self-reported racial discrimination and 12-month DSM-IV mental disorders among Asian Americans nationwide. *Social Science & Medicine*, *64*(10), 1984–1996.

Gong, F., Gage, S.-Je L., & Tacata, L. A. Jr. (2003). Helpseeking behavior among Filipino Americans: A cultural analysis of face and language. *Journal of Community Psychology*, *31*(5), 469–488.

Jarvis, G. E., Kirmayer, L. J., Weinfeld, M., & Lasry, J.-C. (2005). Religious practice and psychological distress: The importance of gender, ethnicity and immigrant status. *Transcultural Psychiatry*, *42*(4), 657–675.

Kiang, L., & Takeuchi, D. T. (2009). Phenotypic bias and ethnic identity in Filipino Americans. *Social Science Quarterly*, *90*(2), 428–445.

Kim, B. S. (2007). Adherence to Asian and European American cultural values and attitudes toward seeking professional psychological help among Asian American college students. *Journal of Counseling Psychology*, *54*(4), 474–480.

Kim, W., Kim, I., & Nochajski, T. H. (2010). Risk and protective factors of alcohol use disorders among Filipino Americans: Location of residence matters. *American Journal of Drug and Alcohol Abuse*, *36*, 214–219.

Kirmayer, L. J., Weinfeld, M., Burgos, G., Du Fort, G. G., Lasry, J.-C., & Young, A. (2007). Use of health care services for psychological distress by immigrants in an Urban multicultural milieu. *Canadian Journal of Psychiatry*, *52*(5), 295–304.

Mak, W. W. S., & Zane, N. (2004). The phenomenon of somatization among community Chinese Americans. *Social Psychiatry & Psychiatric Epidemiology*, *39*(12), 967–974.

Min, J. W., Moon, A., & Lubben, J. E. (2005). Determinants of psychological distress over time among older Korean immigrants and non-Hispanic white elders: Evidence from a two-wave panel study. *Aging & Mental Health*, *9*(3), 210–222.

Mossakowski, K. N. (2003). Coping with perceived discrimination: Does ethnic identity protect mental health? *Journal of Health and Social Behavior*, *44*(3), 318–331.

Mossakowski, K. N. (2007). Are immigrants healthier? The case of depression among Filipino Americans. *Social Psychology Quarterly*, *70*(3), 290–304.

Nadal, K. L. (2000). F/Pilipino American substance abuse: Sociocultural factors and methods of treatment. *Journal of Alcohol & Drug Education*, *46*(2), 26–36.

Richman, L. S., Kohn-Wood, L. P., & Williams, D. R. (2007). The role of discrimination and racial identity for mental health service utilization. *Journal of Social and Clinical Psychology*, *26*(8), 960–981.

Rondilla, J. L., & Spickard, P. (2007). *Is lighter better? Skin-tone discrimination among Asian Americans*. Lanham, MD: Rowman & Littlefield.

Salant, T., & Lauderdale, D. S. (2003). Measuring culture: A critical review of acculturation and health in Asian immigrant populations. *Social Science & Medicine*, *57*(1), 71–90.

Sanchez, F., & Gaw, A. (2007). Mental health care of Filipino Americans. *Psychiatric Services*, *58*(6), 810–815.

Shim, Y. R., & Schwartz, R. C. (2008). Degree of acculturation and adherence to Asian values as correlates of psychological distress among Korean immigrants. *Journal of Mental Health*, *17*(6), 607–617.

Suinn, R. M. (2010). Reviewing Acculturation and Asian Americans: How acculturation affects health, adjustment, school achievement, and counseling. *Asian American Journal of Psychology*, *1*(1), 5–17.

Thoits, P. A. (1982). Conceptual, methodological, and theoretical problems in studying social support as a buffer against life stress. *Journal of Health and Social Behavior*, *23*(2), 145–159.

Thoits, P. A. (1986). Social support as coping assistance. *Journal of Consulting and Clinical Psychology*, *54*(4), 416–423.

Tuason, M., Teresa, G., Taylor, A. R., Rollings, L., Harris, T., & Martin, C. (2007). On both sides of the hyphen: Exploring the Filipino-American identity. *Journal of Counseling Psychology*, *54*(4), 362–372.

Yip, T., Gee, G. C., & Takeuchi, D. T. (2008). Racial discrimination and psychological distress: The impact of ethnic identity and age among immigrant and United States-Born Asian adults. *Developmental Psychology*, *44*(3), 787–800.

Yoo, H. C., & Lee, R. M. (2005). Ethnic identity and approach-type coping as moderators of the racial discrimination/well-being relation in Asian Americans. *Journal of Counseling Psychology*, *52*(4), 497–506.

CONNECTIONS AND TRANSITIONS IN MENTAL HEALTH CARE ORGANIZATIONS AND SYSTEMS

Michael Polgar

ABSTRACT

Purpose – *Sociology promotes and describes public health, helping to explain macro-social dynamics of mental health care through studies of organizations, networks, and systems of care.*

Methodology/approach – *This chapter summarizes sociological research on mental health care organizations and systems, illustrating a macro-social perspective by examining the problem of transitions in care for young adults. Summary findings from a regional mental health services research project describe a system of care that includes 100 organizations. This system helps young adults with mental health needs.*

Findings – *The scope and management of care involves a focus on modes of treatment supported by research evidence and delivered effectively by people with cultural competencies. Care and continuity of care are delivered through coordinated systems of inter-organizational networks, linking organizations and providers. Active inter-organizational*

Education, Social Factors, and Health Beliefs in Health and Health Care Services
Research in the Sociology of Health Care, Volume 33, 121–138

ISSN: 0275-4959/doi:10.1108/S0275-495920150000033006

linkages are needed to support mental health for young adults during challenging and sometimes difficult transitions.

Originality/value – *This research summarizes original and regional data on mental health care organizations within a regional system of care. Practical implications include support for the importance of coordination, transition planning, and cultural competence within and among organizations. Sociological and original research on organizations and systems should continue to elaborate the needs and values of mental health services for regional planning and public health.*

Keywords: Mental health; mental health care; organizations; systems

INTRODUCTION

This chapter will summarize sociological research that examines organizations and systems, illustrating the importance of this macro-social perspective by applying it to the problem of transitions in care for youth (Costello, He, Sampson, Kessler, & Merikangas, 2014) and young adults (Clark, Koroloff, Geller, & Sondheimer, 2008; Davis & Vander Stoep, 1997). Mental health and mental health care, like all types of health and care, are related to social context (Horwitz, 2013). Problems of health and care are understood and addressed concurrently through biological, psychological, and socio-cultural frameworks (Kendler, 2008). There is a growing research base that provides evidence for the effectiveness and importance of a variety of types of mental health care services (Dougherty et al., 2014). Mental health problems, including substance abuse disorders, are based on symptoms and diagnoses that range from mild to severe.

Mental health problems are studied first and foremost at an individual level of analysis, especially as mental disorders are objectively identified, classified, treated, and providers reimbursed through the categories of the Diagnostic Statistical Manual (DSM), now in its fifth version (American Psychiatric Association, 2013). Mental health problems across the lifespan are only sometimes identified and treated (Pottick, Bilder, Vander Stoep, Warner, & Alvarez, 2008), often through a medicalized process (Conrad & Leiter, 2004) that may include both pharmaceutical treatment and psychosocial interventions, often but not always including illness management and recovery (McGuire et al., 2014).

Like many social problems, mental health concerns are often first conceptualized as personal troubles which seem at first to mainly affect individual lives, problems that also need to be explained etiologically and epidemiologically. Sociologists have also helped to understand how these problems are part of public health and are also addressed through solutions that recognize both individual and social proximate causes (Horwitz, 2013). Mental health and care are thus concurrently individual and social conditions which reflect and complicate other social problems (such as poverty, violence, natural disasters, and crime). Therefore, mental health and mental health care are important and ongoing national public health concerns which help inform national health policies (Olin, 2000; U.S. Department of Health and Human Services, 1999a, 1999b).

The social and sociological nature and scope of mental health come into focus at those times when mental health problems are viewed in the context of pervasive and sometimes alarming or extreme problems, like those of sudden and decontextualized violence (McGinty, Webster, & Barry, 2014; Yang, Mulvey, Loughran, & Hanusa, 2012). Mental health problems also have an empirical relationship to strong emotions, including anger (Brown & Turner, 2012), but mental disorders are defined through symptoms beyond the usual scope of human emotion under adverse situations (Wakefield, 1999). In contrast, the process of recovery from mental illness, while an important and measurable outcome (Shanks et al., 2013) is more rarely at the center of research or public attention, resulting in more limited awareness of recovery and consequently fewer resources for research.

Furthermore, sociological research helps clarify the importance of understanding mental health as both individual and social conditions. Many strands of research indicate that mental problems and disorders have both social antecedents (like stress etiologies) and social consequences where disorders may cause stress for groups or institutions (Aneshensel & Phelan, 1999). Growing mental health care needs and uses across demographic groups generates ongoing and informative empirical statistics in psychiatric epidemiology, building upon population, community, and clinical studies of morbidity, symptomatology, and service use in the United States and around the world. However, some of the problems of psychiatric epidemiology, including etiologies, remain clouded in uncertainty related to debates over classification systems (Horwitz & Grob, 2011). As health patterns emerge and change in complex environments, including a growing focus on disabilities (Carmona & McCabe, 2005), systems of care may also improve through social services to social and support systems beyond the individuals with mental illness, including education and help for relatives and families (Dixon et al., 2011).

Sociology has a long and ongoing tradition of studying contextual factors related to the development and care of mental health problems, including social stress, coping (Thoits, 2011), and stigma (Pescosolido, 2013). Social epidemiology has described the distribution of disorders and treatments throughout communities and populations, searching for explanations for correlations between poverty and mental disorder through theories of social causation and social selection (Link & Phelan, 2000). Critical studies have examined the social history of mental health care, including the limits to a singularly medical model of mental illness (Horwitz, 2002).

Macro-social research first aggregates individuals into populations to describe both epidemiology and use of health care. At an organizational level, research on mental health care aggregates sets, populations, fields, and systems of organizations within changing environments (Scott & Davis, 2007). Sets and networks of mental health providers and organizations are linked into systems of care, which operate within organizational populations and fields (Evan, 1993; Morrissey et al., 1994). Organizations work together in systems and also may change in response to institutional environments (Scott, 2003).

Mental health care systems are used by a variety of individuals experiencing illness trajectories and illness careers (Pescosolido, Boyer, & Medina, 2013). These individual, as well as caregivers, family members, and colleagues, are affected by the cultural contexts of both health and health care (Pescosolido, McLeod, & Avison, 2007). Inequalities and disparities in needs for and uses of mental health care are complex and dynamic; disparities can be related to social conditions including differential exposure to a stressors (Mezuk et al., 2013), including racism (Williams & Mohammed, 2009), perceived discrimination (Pascoe & Smart Richman, 2009), and other forms of discrimination (Miller, Rote, & Keith, 2013; Takeuchi & Williams, 2003). As sociologists often document, problems including stressors related to mental health increase where there are intersections between inequalities, such as race and poverty (Miller et al., 2013).

Organizations and Systems

There are many types of macro-social research and scholarship that describe organizations and systems of mental health care, particularly in light of ongoing health care financing trends and debates (Mark, Levit, Vandivort-Warren, Buck, & Coffey, 2011). Examining organizations and systems through the sociologies of medicine and mental health involves studies of health and care providers who work in organizations and networks of care (Polgar, 2010). This can mean reframing ("flipping" in the new pedagogical jargon) attention from the health care consumer (or patient or person with illness/disorder) back upon the provider organizations and workforce (Hoge et al., 2013) and away from the sometimes privileged or medical viewpoints which take individuals, illnesses and diseases as a primary and more objective subject of study. The frame of macro-social analysis, concurrent with health services research generally (Cook et al., 2014), involves working to explain patterns and behavior among providers, organizations, and systems that provide informal or formal treatment, support, and care, to complement the concurrent focus on variations in disease patterns, people with disorders, or trajectories in individual illness careers. The scope and management of health care, which is too often assessed primarily in terms of its economic value, involves a focus not just on people with or at risk of health problems but on the workings of social institutions and organizations.

People in organizations form systems of care that are designed for and using modes of treatment which are empirically supported by research evidence (Dougherty et al., 2014) and delivered effectively by people with cultural and professional competencies (Betancourt, Green, Carrillo, & Ananeh-Firempong, 2003). Looking through even wider "lenses," social network analyses of health care systems allow us to understand that care and its financing are delivered through inter-organizational systems, linking organizations and providers to gain economies of scale, standardize care, and better ensure both coordination and continuity of care. These systems are especially important for large-scale organizations and the expansion of managed care (Light, 2004; Mechanic, 1999; Mechanic, McAlpine, & Olfson, 1998; Mechanic, Schlesinger, & McAlpine, 1995). Organizational systems are also potentially helpful in ensuring that people in need of care are traverse difficult transitions at pivotal periods in the life course, such as during young adulthood or surrounding life-course transitions.

Mental health care organizations and systems, linked with medical and social institutions in both public and private sectors, help individuals and communities respond to mental health problems. The patterns in organization and distribution of mental health care vary across contexts and social structures, within dynamic systems of organizations and institutions (Scheid & Greenberg, 2007). Mental health care, like health care and caregiving more generally, is provided by a professional and allied workforce (Hoge et al., 2013) that includes providers in multiple professions and sometimes also volunteers in organizations. Caregiving is led by physicians and allied health professionals who are increasingly and technologically integrated with hospitals and health care systems (Rundall, Shortell, & Alexander, 2004) and complemented by growing ranks family and other supportive caregiving (Glenn, 2010). These systems of care are formally integrated and also socially interconnected by inter-organizational networks of increasingly dynamic complexity (Morrissey, Johnsen, & Calloway, 1997, 2005).

Mental health services and systems research produces a variety of indicators and information about the organization, distribution, and performance of mental health providers. While it has often been a challenge to comprehensively integrate macro- and micro-level perspectives, organizational and systemic data on mental health providers enhance sociological theory and research (Scott & Davis, 2007). Consumers, providers, and policy analysts may all seek out and benefit from this research literature, especially during periods of health care reform, as developments in treatments often change the structure and performance of mental health care services (Henggeler, Schoenwald, Pickrel, Rowland, & Santos, 1994).

For example, scholars estimate the need for mental health professionals in the United States (Hoge et al., 2013). This requires not just epidemiological information but also data on the nation's medical and mental health workforce to estimate the number and locations of mental health providers (prescribing and otherwise) required to treat the epidemiologically estimated populations of people with mental illness, adjusting for data on average duration of mental health service delivery and use (Linzer et al., 2002). Adjusting for need by county and the work of primary care physicians, this work can help direct mental health care to underserved areas and populations. Inter-organizational linkages between providers anchored in different systems, particularly through referral and information networks, can often provide continuity along avenues of care for people with mental health care needs.

In organizational studies, the degree to which populations use or administer mental health care services is measured within sets or types of organizations or population. More or less effective or efficient uses of services may be used as a performance indicator (Proctor, Rosen, & Staudt, 1999; Rosen, Proctor, & Staudt, 1999; Schoenwald & Hoagwood, 2001). Comparing treatment modalities, some treatments are hypothesized or found to be more effective for adults (Schoenwald & Hoagwood, 2001) and others for youth (Burns, Hoagwood, & Mrazek, 1999). Measures of health care quality, in mental health as in other forms of health care, are important but highly variable and sometimes contested (Cretin, Farley, Dolter, & Nicholas, 2001; Glisson & Hemmelgarn, 1998; Hermann & Palmer, 2002). Consumers, organizations, regulators, and accreditors variously use different types of quality measures for different purposes. Many studies examine the effects of policy changes on organizations and those staff who provide mental health care. For example, research often estimates effects of managed care on mental health care variables, such as provider job satisfaction (Morris & Bloom, 2002).

The most general macro-social level of abstraction, using an even wider scope for research and analysis, is called inter-organizational research on systems of mental health care. This research can consider the effects of system-level interventions on the structure and performance of mental health provider organizations within broad social networks. Generalizing across multiple organizations and sometimes regions, entire local, state, or national systems of care for people with mental health problems are examined empirically. Sets and networks of organizations within regions are compared both with each other and with other sets of organizations or regions. For example, in evaluating federal support for people with mental illness who became homeless, researchers showed that grantee organizations improved inter-organizational relationships (project-centered integration) in 18 sites in 15 cities across the nation, although the overall degree of system integration was not significantly greater when additional funds were provided to encourage systems change (Morrissey, Calloway, Johnsen, & Ullman, 1997). In addition, housing outcomes were progressively better when networks of organizations were became more integrated (Rosenheck et al., 1998). However the integration of service systems did not itself produce significantly better (or direct) mental health outcomes for clients of mental health services (Goldman, Morrissey, & Ridgely, 1994).

Research methods that study inter-organizational systems start by identifying a group of provider organizations, health and human service agencies that work within a region, described as organizational sets (Evan, 1993). Then researchers gather data from surveys of each organization, focusing on the presence and strength of a myriad of organizational relationships (Van De Ven & Astley, 1981; Van De Ven & Ferry, 1980). Inter-organizational research examines the dynamic and complex structures of mental health service systems. Inter-organizational structures and changes in these structures can have consequences for organizational performance and on outcomes (Morrissey et al., 1994). Mental health care systems research examines providers of services for children (Morrissey et al., 2005) and adults (Morrissey et al., 1997). The extent or degree of communication and exchange within a network of mental health provider organizations helps describe systems of care; empirically these inter-organizational systems are variably operational as social networks. The form and the performance of a system may be affected by changes in social network variables such as density, centralization, and fragmentation. Social network analyses require researchers to study how and why these variables may compare across different service systems, using matrix-based analyses and measures of social structural variables that identify group forms and structures, not only attributes of individual units of analysis (Wasserman & Faust, 1994).

Mental Health Systems during Young Adult Transitions

Young people are putting increasing demands on multiple social institutions; growing up now involves passage through an increasingly long and complex life stage that sociologists and demographers are describing as young or early adulthood. This stage expands over time, concurrent with increases in national average ages at first marriage and having a first child (Furstenberg, Kennedy, McLoyd, Rumbaut, & Settersten, 2004). Concurrently, epidemiologists document that modern service use for mental health problems is far below measures of need and incidence in the United States population, usually around 40% (Wang et al., 2005). For youth, nationally representative epidemiological sample surveys estimate similar "utilization" rates, indicating that more than only between 36% and 45% of adolescents with mental disorders received services for their illness, more often in school or specialty mental health settings (Costello et al., 2014; Merikangas et al., 2011). Thus, from a life-course perspective, people in modern cohorts of young adults emerge as independent health consumers with high rates of unmet need for mental health care, need that includes populations already underserved even before a transition (growing up) into legal independence in early adulthood.

Concurrently, limitations exist on both demand- and supply-sides of mental health care. The rates of insurance coverage and the acceptance of underinsured or uninsured patients in psychiatry are indeed limited, partial, and incomplete (Bishop, Press, Keyhani, & Pincus, 2014). While the affordable care act (ACA) has important consequences in this area, expanding for young adult health insurance options and provider requirements, and while the ACA may help expand coverage for mental health and specifically promote (but not guarantee) presence and sometimes continuity of insurance coverage for young adults up through age 26 (Mechanic, 2012), young adults health service use may still and always be discontinued when young people grow into adulthood. This discontinuity in care may be due to cost and related insurance limitations, among other factors (Pottick et al., 2008). Initial research shows some limited effects of the ACA on the use of care by young adults, but still significant gaps remain (Meara et al., 2014). At the same time, families matter for all type of health including mental health, providing informal care in many ways and across generations. For example, family caregivers help informally (Glenn, 2010) and parents of young adults receive mental health benefits from helping their adult children (Bangerter, Kim, Zarit, Birditt, & Fingerman, 2014).

Public services, consumer payers, and other supporters of health care organizations fund a variety of help and health systems for youth and young adults with or at risk of mental health problems (Heflinger & Hoffman, 2008). Research shows that systems of care for youth and young adults depend, among other things, upon the relationships among service providers in systems of care (Stiffman et al., 2000). Many youth come to mental health care through social networks that become established as pathways and gateways (Stiffman, Pescosolido, & Cabassa, 2004). These begin with and include educational systems in particular (Farmer, Burns, Phillips, Angold, & Costello, 2003). Findings show that systems need specifically to improve access to services for older youth during transitional ages and to customize services to the needs of different age cohorts and groups (Manteuffel, Stephens, Sondheimer, & Fisher, 2008). Transition support programs for youth can improve outcomes in a variety of areas, including employment, education, criminal justice, mental health (including substance abuse) (Haber, Karpur, Deschênes, & Clark, 2008). Without support for health in general and mental health in particular, young people may experience discontinuities in insurance coverage and also (subsequently) health care just at the time of independence when a variety of life circumstances are becoming more challenging and costly. This transition is especially difficult for higher-risk populations, such as youth in foster care (Cabrera, Auslander, & Polgar, 2009; Harman, Childs, & Kelleher, 2000; McMillen, Auslander, Elze, et al., 2003).

Young adults with mental health problems can thus confront both developmental and institutional transitions as they become more independent, moving from secondary school and into adulthood. Optimal systems of health care for youth coordinate transitions from youth services into adult services (Davis & Vander Stoep, 1997; Vander Stoep,

Davis, & Collins, 2000). Research on service transitions for young adults measures and examine these transition points and structural links that serve as bridges from youth to young adulthood. Inter-organizational bridges at service transition points are important components of mental health service delivery in the United States (Clark & Davis, 2000).

Research Findings for Young Adults

Researchers fielded a survey of organizational representatives to examine 100 regional organizations, a nearly full set of those actively serving youth with mental health needs in a large Midwestern metropolitan area (including two counties, urban and suburban). The object of research is the organizational transition structures between child and adult systems of care, thereby illuminating the pathways for young people at risk of exiting from care when they are epidemiologically most at risk of major mental disorder (Polgar & Cabassa, 2007). In this region and across the United States, not all providers of care are similar; there are multiple and systemic variations in the service sectors, organizational locations, and systemic interconnections of those organizations providing services to youth and young adults who need mental health care. Key informants within provider organizations shared information about these providers, including organizational information, inter-organizational network relationships, and descriptive organizational performance data.

There are many ways to understand and measure structural features in this or any system or network of organizations which indicate both coordination and also potentials for discontinuities between youth and adult mental health services. In this research, data include both aggregated attributes of the full set of organizations in the region and relational data on coordination and structural linkages in this system of care. Case management, transition planning, and referral networks indicate the mechanisms and extent of pathways from youth to adult service systems. Organizational variation in the use of these bridging mechanisms at service transition points is an important subject of analysis (Polgar & Cabassa, 2007).

Survey methods integrate two types of mental health service system evaluation data (Morrissey et al., 2005). First, survey and sample use a key-informant approach to assess service system performance. This approach summarizes expert opinions from organizational leaders, using multidimensional scaling. Second, survey and sample examine social network relationships in an organizational set, assessing agencies which help young adults with mental health problems. This approach allows analysts to calculate peer-ratings of organizations and to measure the range and average strength of inter-organizational relationships. Research methods and measures are more fully described in previous publications (Polgar & Cabassa, 2007).

First, about half (53%) of regional organizations who provided services to people with mental health needs during the transition to young adulthood provided services to both youth and adults. Some in the educational sector (secondary schools) served only youth while some other organizations served only adults. Some specialized in mental health care (the majority of organizational respondents) or substance abuse treatment, while others focused on more general services in health or education. As a result of respondent selection criteria, all organizations provided help or care for fairly sizable numbers of youth with mental health care needs. The care was usually of significant duration; median number of sessions provided for mental health service clients was 11 annually. Most provided the recommended methods (Oliver, Nims, Hughey, & Somers, 1998; Pescosolido, Wright, & Sullivan, 1995) to increase success after difficult transitions: these include case management (63%), transition planning (81%) follow-up on client referrals (71%), and les often long-term planning (55%) to help clients continue to get help subsequent to care within their organization.

Summary statistics indicate that organizations offering a greater variety of services, particularly medical care, offered a significantly rosier view of the system of care. Organizations which emphasized cultural competence or helped young people with transitional services also had a brighter view of the system. Among mental health specialty organizations there was a significant correlation between organizational peer-performance ratings and the degree to which an organization was integrated through inter-organizational linkages. This suggests that those mental health providers who were more respected by their peers were also more connected with other organizations that helped young people with mental problems. In other words, positive peer-evaluation is related to inter-organizational relationships only within the mental health sector.

In addition, organizational practices that promoted continuity of care correlate significantly with several organizational variables, including total staff size ($r = .27$, $p = .01$), client-provider ratio ($r = -.25$, $p = .01$), greater variety of services ($r = .72$, $p = .00$), cultural competence in principle ($r = .28$, $p = .00$), and culturally competent practices in particular

($r = .38$, $p = .00$). Organizations which monitor their caseloads to ensure proportional racial and ethnic representation scored higher on the continuity of care index ($r = .32$, $p = .00$). Inter-organizational collaboration through referral networks and other social linkages was more abundant in larger organizations ($r = .43$, $p = .00$) and organizations offering greater service variety ($r = .31$, $p = .00$).

CONCLUSION

Sociology helps public health through working to understand and sometimes to explain the macro-social dynamics of mental health and its care through studies of organizations, networks, and systems of care. We can understand some of the challenges for systems of care by exploring and researching the problem of transitions in mental health and care for young adults. Summary findings from an original regional mental health services research project describe a system of care that helps facilitate transitions through planning, referral, and case management. The scope and management of care involves a focus on using modes of treatment supported by research evidence and delivered effectively by people with cultural competencies. Care and continuity of care are also delivered through systems of inter-organizational networks, linking organizations and providers to better ensure both coordination and continuity, which may be more challenging during difficult transitions.

This research describes only one system in one region at one point in time and therefore has limited scope and generalizability. It also focuses on organizations and systems without complementary data on the outcomes of mental health service use. Therefore future research, in combination with findings across social and medical sciences, should continue to explore both opportunities and limitations in health care and social services for young people with mental health service needs. Research in this area supports intersecting values of coordination, transition planning, and cultural competence within and among organizations. Policies and practices can extend and improve the use, quality, scope, and duration of care for people in need of help due to mental health problems. Original and creative research on organizations and systems should continue, linking sociological understanding to managerial concerns with health care treatment methods and financing, and also increasing the value of mental health services research for regional planning and public health.

ACKNOWLEDGMENTS

This research was supported by the National Institutes of Health (NIH), NIMH grant #R03MH59108.

REFERENCES

American Psychiatric Association. (2013). *Diagnostic and statistical manual of mental disorders: DSM-5*. Washington, DC: American Psychiatric Association.

Aneshensel, C., & Phelan, J. C. (Eds.). (1999). *Handbook of the sociology of mental health*. New York, NY: Plenum Press.

Bangerter, L. R., Kim, K., Zarit, S. H., Birditt, K. S., & Fingerman, K. L. (2014). Perceptions of giving support and depressive symptoms in late life. *The Gerontologist*, *54*, 1–10.

Betancourt, J., Green, A., Carrillo, E. E., & Ananeh-Firempong, O. (2003). Defining cultural competence. *Public Health Reports*, *118*(4), 293–302.

Bishop, T. F., Press, M. J., Keyhani, S., & Pincus, H. (2014). Acceptance of insurance by psychiatrists and the implications for access to mental health care. *JAMA Psychiatry*, *71*(2), 176–181.

Brown, R. L., & Turner, R. J. (2012). Physical limitation and anger: Stress exposure and assessing the role of psychosocial resources. *Society and Mental Health*, *2*(2), 69–84.

Burns, B. J., Farmer, E. M. Z., Angold, A., Costello, E. J., & Behar, L. (1996). A randomized trial of case management for youths with serious emotional disturbance. *Journal of Clinical Child Psychology*, *25*(4), 476–486.

Burns, B. J., Hoagwood, K., & Mrazek, P. J. (1999). Effective treatment for mental disorders in children and adolescents. *Clinical Child and Family Psychology Review*, *2*(4), 199–253.

Cabrera, P., Auslander, W., & Polgar, M. (2009). Future orientation of adolescents in foster care: Relationship to trauma, mental health, and HIV risk behaviors. *Journal of Child & Adolescent Trauma*, *2*(4), 271–286.

Carmona, R. H., & McCabe, J. (2005). Improving the health and wellness of persons with disabilities: A call to action. *American Journal of Public Health*, *95*(11), 1883–1884.

Clark, H., & Davis, M. (2000). *Transition to adulthood: A resource for assisting young people with emotional or behavioral difficulties*. Baltimore, MD: Paul Brookes.

Clark, H., Koroloff, N., Geller, J., & Sondheimer, D. (2008). Research on transition to adulthood: Building the evidence base to inform services and supports for youth and young adults with serious mental health disorders. *The Journal of Behavioral Health Services and Research*, *35*(4), 365–372.

Conrad, P., & Leiter, V. (2004). Medicalization, markets and consumers. *Journal of Health and Social Behavior*, *45*(Special Issue), 158–176.

Cook, B. L., Zuvekas, S. H., Carson, N., Wayne, G. F., Vesper, A., & McGuire, T. G. (2014). Assessing racial/ethnic disparities in treatment across episodes of mental health care. *Health Services Research*, *49*(1), 206–229.

Costello, E. J., He, J.-p., Sampson, N. A., Kessler, R. C., & Merikangas, K. R. (2014). Services for adolescents with psychiatric disorders: 12-month data from the national comorbidity survey-adolescent. *Psychiatric Services*, *65*(3), 359–366.

Cretin, S., Farley, D. O., Dolter, K. J., & Nicholas, W. (2001). Evaluating an integrated approach to clinical quality improvement: Clinical guidelines, quality measurement, and supportive system design. *Medical Care, 39*(8), 70–84.

Davis, M., & Vander Stoep, A. (1997). The transition to adulthood for youth who have serious emotional disturbance: Developmental transition and young adult outcomes. *Journal of Mental Health Administration, 24*(4), 400–427.

Dixon, L. B., Lucksted, A., Medoff, D. R., Burland, J., Stewart, B., Lehman, A. F., & Murray-Swank, A. (2011). Outcomes of a randomized study of a peer-taught family-to-family education program for mental illness. *Psychiatric Services, 62*(6), 591–597.

Dougherty, R. H., Lyman, D. R., George, P., Ghose, S. S., Daniels, A. S., & Delphin-Rittmon, M. E. (2014). Assessing the evidence base for behavioral health services: Introduction to the series. *Psychiatric Services, 65*(1), 11–15.

Evan, W. M. (1993). *Organization theory: Research and design*. New York, NY: Macmillan.

Farmer, E. M. Z., Burns, B. J., Phillips, S. D., Angold, A., & Costello, E. J. (2003). Pathways into and through mental health services for children and adolescents. *Psychiatric Services, 54*(1), 60–66.

Furstenberg, F. F., Kennedy, S., McLoyd, V. C., Rumbaut, R. G., & Settersten, R. A. (2004). Growing up is Harder to do. *Contexts, 3*(3), 33–41.

Glenn, E. N. (2010). *Forced to care: Coercion and caregiving in America*. Cambridge, MA: Harvard University Press.

Glisson, C., & Hemmelgarn, A. (1998). The effects of organizational climate and interorganizational coordination on the quality and outcomes of children's service systems. *Child Abuse & Neglect, 22*(5), 401–421.

Goldman, H. H., Morrissey, J. P., & Ridgely, M. S. (1994). Evaluating the Robert Wood Johnson foundation program on chronic mental illness. *Milbank Quarterly, 72*, 37–47.

Haber, M., Karpur, A., Deschênes, N., & Clark, H. (2008). Predicting improvement of transitioning young people in the partnerships for youth transition initiative: Findings from a multisite demonstration. *The Journal of Behavioral Health Services & Research, 35*(4), 488–513.

Harman, J. S., Childs, G. E., & Kelleher, K. J. (2000). Mental health care utilization and expenditures by children in foster care. *Archives of Pediatrics & Adolescent Medicine, 154*(11), 1114–1117.

Heflinger, C., & Hoffman, C. (2008). Transition age youth in publicly funded systems: Identifying high-risk youth for policy planning and improved service delivery. *The Journal of Behavioral Health Services & Research, 35*(4), 390–401.

Henggeler, S. W., Schoenwald, S. K., Pickrel, S. G., Rowland, M. D., & Santos, A. B. (1994). The contribution of treatment outcome research to the reform of children's mental health services: Multisystemic therapy as an example. Special section: Mental health services for children, youth, and families. *Journal of Mental Health Administration, 21*(3), 229–239.

Hermann, R. C., & Palmer, R. H. (2002). Common ground: A framework for selecting core quality measures for mental health and substance abuse care. *Psychiatric Services, 53*(3), 281–287.

Hoge, M. A., Stuart, G. W., Morris, J., Flaherty, M. T., Paris, M., & Goplerud, E. (2013). Mental health and addiction workforce development: Federal leadership is needed to address the growing crisis. *Health Affairs, 32*(11), 2005–2012.

Horwitz, A. V. (2002). *Creating mental illness*. Chicago, IL: University of Chicago Press.

Horwitz, A. V. (2013). The sociological study of mental illness: A critique and synthesis of four perspectives. In C. Aneshensel, J. Phelan, & A. Bierman (Eds.), *Handbook of the sociology of mental health* (pp. 95–112). Dordrecht, The Netherlands: Springer.

Horwitz, A. V., & Grob, G. N. (2011). The checkered history of American psychiatric epidemiology. *Milbank Quarterly*, *89*(4), 628–657.

Kendler, K. S. (2008). Explanatory models for psychiatric illness. *The American Journal of Psychiatry*, *165*(6), 695–702.

Light, D. W. (2004). Ironies of success: A new history of the American health care "System." *Journal of Health and Social Behavior*, *45*(Special Issue), 1–24.

Link, B. G., & Phelan, J. C. (2000). Evaluating the fundamental cause explanation for social disparities in health. In C. Bird, P. Conrad, & A. Freemont (Eds.), *Handbook of medical sociology* (5th ed., pp. 37–59). Upper Saddle River, NJ: Prentice Hall.

Linzer, M., Gerrity, M., Douglas, J. A., McMurray, J. E., Williams, E. S., & Konrad, T. R. (2002). Physician stress: Results from the physician worklife study. *Stress and Health*, *18*(1), 37–42.

Manteuffel, B., Stephens, R., Sondheimer, D., & Fisher, S. (2008). Characteristics, service experiences, and outcomes of transition-aged youth in systems of care: Programmatic and policy implications. *The Journal of Behavioral Health Services & Research*, *35*(4), 469–487.

Mark, T. L., Levit, K. R., Vandivort-Warren, R., Buck, J. A., & Coffey, R. M. (2011). Changes in US spending on mental health and substance abuse treatment, 1986–2005, and implications for policy. *Health Affairs*, *30*(2), 284–292.

McGinty, E. E., Webster, D. W., & Barry, C. L. (2014). Gun policy and serious mental illness: Priorities for future research and policy. *Psychiatric Services*, *65*(1), 50–58.

McGuire, A. B., Kukla, M., Green, A., Gilbride, D., Mueser, K. T., & Salyers, M. P. (2014). Illness management and recovery: A review of the literature. *Psychiatric Services*, *65*(2), 171–179.

McMillen, C., Auslander, W., Elze, D., White, T., & Thompson, R. (2003). Educational experiences and aspirations of older youth in foster care. *Child Welfare*, *82*(4), 475–495.

Meara, E., Golberstein, E., Zaha, R., Greenfield, S. F., Beardslee, W. R., & Busch, S. H. (2014). Use of hospital-based services among young adults with behavioral health diagnoses before and after health insurance expansions. *JAMA Psychiatry*, *71*(4), 404–411.

Mechanic, D. (1999). *Mental health and social policy: The emergence of managed care* (4th ed.). Needham Heights, MA: Allyn & Bacon.

Mechanic, D. (2012). Seizing opportunities under the affordable care act for transforming the mental and behavioral health system. *Health Affairs*, *31*(2), 376–382.

Mechanic, D., McAlpine, D., & Olfson, M. (1998). Changing patterns of psychiatric inpatient care in the United States, 1988–1994. *Archives of General Psychiatry*, *55*(9), 785–791.

Mechanic, D., Schlesinger, M., & McAlpine, D. (1995). Management of mental health and substance abuse services: State of the art and early results. *The Milbank Quarterly*, *73*(1), 19–55.

Merikangas, K. R., He, J.-P., Burstein, M., Swendsen, J., Avenevoli, S., Case, B., ... Olfson, M. (2011). Service utilization for lifetime mental disorders in U.S. adolescents: Results of the national comorbidity survey-adolescent supplement (NCS-A) [journal]. *Journal of the American Academy of Child & Adolescent Psychiatry*, *50*(1), 32–45.

Mezuk, B., Abdou, C. M., Hudson, D., Kershaw, K. N., Rafferty, J. A., Lee, H., & Jackson, J. S. (2013). "White Box" epidemiology and the social neuroscience of health behaviors: The environmental affordances model. *Society and Mental Health, 3*(2), 79–95.

Miller, B., Rote, S. M., & Keith, V. M. (2013). Coping with racial discrimination: Assessing the vulnerability of African Americans and the mediated moderation of psychosocial resources. *Society and Mental Health, 3*(2), 133–150.

Morris, A., & Bloom, J. R. (2002). Contextual factors affecting job satisfaction and organizational commitment in community mental health centers undergoing system changes in the financing of care. *Mental Health Services Research, 4*(2), 71–83.

Morrissey, J. P., Calloway, M., Bartko, W. T., Ridgely, M. S., Goldman, H. H., & Paulson, R. I. (1994). Local mental health authorities and service system change: Evidence from the Robert Wood Johnson program on chronic mental illness. *Milbank Quarterly, 72*(1), 49–80.

Morrissey, J. P., Calloway, M. O., Johnsen, M. C., & Ullman, M. D. (1997). Service system performance and integration: A baseline profile of the ACCESS demonstration sites. *Psychiatric Services, 48*(3), 374–380.

Morrissey, J. P., Johnsen, M., & Calloway, M. (2005). Methods for system-level evaluations of child mental health service networks. In M. Epstein, K. Kutash, & A. Duchnowski (Eds.), *Outcomes for children and youth with emotional and behavioral disorders and their families: Programs and evaluations, best practices* (pp. 297–307). Austin, TX: Pro-Ed.

Morrissey, J. P., Johnsen, M. C., & Calloway, M. O. (1997). Evaluating performance and change in the mental health systems serving children and youth: An interorganizational network approach. *Journal of Mental Health Administration, 24*(1), 4–21.

Olin, S. S. (2000). *U.S. public health service, report of the surgeon general's conference on children's mental health: A national action agenda* (pp. 1–56). Washington, DC: Department of Health and Human Services.

Oliver, R. D., Nims, D. R., Hughey, A. W., & Somers, J. R. (1998). Case management wraparound expenses: Five-year study. *Administration and Policy in Mental Health, 25*(5), 477–491.

Pascoe, E. A., & Smart Richman, L. (2009). Perceived discrimination and health: A meta-analytic review. *Psychological Bulletin, 135*(4), 531–554.

Pescosolido, B. (2013). The public stigma of mental illness: What do we think; what do we know: What can we prove? *Journal of Health and Social Behavior, 54*(1), 1–21.

Pescosolido, B., Boyer, C., & Medina, T. (2013). The social dynamics of responding to mental health problems. In C. Aneshensel, J. Phelan, & A. Bierman (Eds.), *Handbook of the sociology of mental health* (pp. 505–524). Dordrecht, The Netherlands: Springer.

Pescosolido, B., McLeod, J. D., & Avison, W. R. (2007). Reflections through the sociological looking glass. In W. R. Avison, J. D. McLeod, & B. A. Pescosolido (Eds.), *Mental health, social mirror* (pp. 3–32). New York, NY: Springer Science.

Pescosolido, B., Wright, E. R., & Sullivan, W. P. (1995). Communities of care: A theoretical perspective on case management models in mental health. *Advances in Medical Sociology, 6*, 37–79.

Polgar, M. (2010). Mental health care in organizations and systems. In T. L. Scheid & T. N. Brown (Eds.), *A handbook for the study of mental health* (2nd ed., pp. 499–509). New York, NY: Cambridge University Press.

Polgar, M., & Cabassa, L. (2007). Helping young adults with mental health problems: Providers evaluate a regional system of care. *Sociological Viewpoints, 83*(Fall), 85–100.

Pottick, K., Bilder, S., Vander Stoep, A., Warner, L., & Alvarez, M. (2008). US patterns of mental health service utilization for transition-age youth and young adults. *The Journal of Behavioral Health Services and Research*, *35*(4), 373–389.

Proctor, E. K., Rosen, A., & Staudt, M. M. (1999). Social work research and the quest for effective practice. *Social Work Research*, *23*(1), 4–14.

Rosen, A., Proctor, E., & Staudt, M. (1999). Social work research and the quest for effective practice. *Social Work Research*, *23*, 4–14.

Rosenheck, R., Morrissey, J. P., Lam, J., Calloway, M., Johnsen, M., Goldman, H., ... Teague, G. (1998). Service system integration, access to services, and housing outcomes in a program for homeless persons with severe mental illness. *American Journal of Public Health*, *88*(11), 1610–1615.

Rundall, T. G., Shortell, S. M., & Alexander, J. A. (2004). A theory of physician-hospital integration: Contending institutional and market logics in the health care field. *Journal of Health and Social Behavior*, *45*(Extra Issue), 102–117.

Scheid, T. L., & Greenberg, G. (2007). An organizational analysis of mental health care. In W. R. Avison, J. D. McLeod, & B. A. Pescosolido (Eds.), *Mental health, social mirror* (pp. 379–406). New York, NY: Springer Science.

Schoenwald, S. K., & Hoagwood, K. (2001). Effectiveness, transportability, and dissemination of interventions: What matters when? *Psychiatric Services*, *52*(9), 1190–1197.

Scott, W. R. (2003). The old order changeth: The evolving world of health care organizations. In S. S. Mick (Ed.), *Advances in health care organization theory* (pp. 23–43). New York, NY: Jossey-Bass.

Scott, W. R., & Davis, G. (2007). *Organizations and organizing: Rational, natural, and open systems perspectives*. Upper Saddle River, NJ: Pearson Prentice Hall.

Shanks, V., Williams, J., Leamy, M., Bird, V. J., Le Boutillier, C., & Slade, M. (2013). Measures of personal recovery: A systematic review. *Psychiatric Services*, *64*(10), 974–980.

Stiffman, A., Hadley-Ives, E., Dore, P., Polgar, M., Horvath, V., Striley, C., & Elze, D. (2000). Youths' access to mental health services: The role of providers' training, resource connectivity, and assessment of need. *Mental Health Services Research*, *2*(3), 141–154.

Stiffman, A., Pescosolido, B., & Cabassa, L. J. (2004). Building a model to understand youth service access: The gateway provider model. *Mental Health Services Research*, *6*(4), 189–198.

Takeuchi, D. T., & Williams, D. R. (2003). Race, ethnicity and mental health: Introduction to the special issue. *Journal of Health and Social Behavior*, *44*(3), 233–236.

Thoits, P. A. (2011). Mechanisms linking social ties and support to physical and mental health. *Journal of Health and Social Behavior*, *52*(2), 145–161.

U.S. Department of Health and Human Services. (1999a). *Mental health: A report of the surgeon general*. Rockville, MD: U.S. Department of Health and Human Services, Substance Abuse and Mental Services Administration, Center for Mental Health Services, National Institutes of Health, National Institute of Mental Health.

U.S. Department of Health and Human Services. (1999b). *Mental health: A report of the surgeon general–executive summary* (p. xxi). Rockville, MD: U.S. Department of Health and Human Services, Substance Abuse and Mental Services Administration, Center for Mental Health Services, National Institutes of Health, National Institute of Mental Health.

Van De Ven, A., & Astley, W. G. (1981). Mapping the field to create a dynamic perspective on organizational design and behavior. In A. H. V. D. Ven & W. F. Joyce (Eds.), *Perspectives on organization design and behavior* (pp. 427–468). New York, NY: Wiley.

Van De Ven, A., & Ferry, D. (1980). *Measuring and assessing organizations*. New York, NY: Wiley.

Vander Stoep, A., Davis, M., & Collins, D. (2000). Transition: A time of developmental and institutional clashes. In B. H. Clark & M. Davis (Eds.), *Transition to adulthood* (pp. 2–28). Baltimore, MD: Paul Brookes.

Wakefield, J. C. (1999). The measurement of mental disorder. In A. V. Horwitz & T. L. Scheid (Eds.), *A handbook for the sociology of mental health* (pp. 29–57). New York, NY: Cambridge University Press.

Wang, P. S., Lane, M., Olfson, M., Pincus, H. A., Wells, K. B., & Kessler, R. C. (2005). Twelve-month use of mental health services in the United States: Results from the national comorbidity survey replication. *Archives of General Psychiatry*, *62*(6), 629–640.

Wasserman, S., & Faust, K. (1994). *Social network analysis*. New York, NY: Cambridge University Press.

Williams, D., & Mohammed, S. (2009). Discrimination and racial disparities in health: Evidence and needed research. *Journal of Behavioral Medicine*, *32*(1), 20–47.

Yang, S., Mulvey, E. P., Loughran, T. A., & Hanusa, B. H. (2012). Psychiatric symptoms and alcohol use in community violence by persons with a psychotic disorder or depression. *Psychiatric Services*, *63*(3), 262–269.

PERSONAL RELIGIOSITY AND MENTAL HEALTH CARE UTILIZATION AMONG ADOLESCENTS

Thomas Christian Quinn and Rebecca L. Utz

ABSTRACT

Purpose – *This study set out to examine whether personal religiosity was in any way associated with adolescents' propensity to seek out formal mental health care.*

Methodology/approach – *Using the National Longitudinal Study of Adolescent Health (Add Health), this study uses logistic regression models to test for an association between personal religiosity and mental health services use net of depressive symptomology and demographic controls.*

Findings – *Results showed a negative, statistically significant relationship between personal religiosity and mental health services use. Highly religious adolescents had lower odds of having seen a mental health professional compared to their less religious counterparts even after controlling for depressive symptomology.*

Education, Social Factors, and Health Beliefs in Health and Health Care Services
Research in the Sociology of Health Care, Volume 33, 139–159

ISSN: 0275-4959/doi:10.1108/S0275-495920150000033007

Research limitations/implications – *Data restrictions required that we limit our analysis to one specific form of mental health services: talk therapy. Nevertheless, this study suggests that religiosity represents a potentially important consideration in addressing the mental health needs of adolescents.*

Originality/value – *To our knowledge, this is the first study in which a nationally representative sample of adolescents is used to examine the relationship between personal religiosity and mental health services use.*

Keywords: Religion; mental health; adolescence

INTRODUCTION

The effect of religiosity on mental illness and the factors that cause an adolescent to seek out or forgo professional help have thus far been treated as entirely unrelated matters. Indeed, psychologists have written prolifically on treating religious patients, yet have not addressed the question of how religion might affect the decision to seek out such services (Harris, Edlund, & Larson, 2006). Likewise, there is a growing consensus that religious activity may have an effect on mental health outcomes (McCullough & Smith, 2003) as well as shaping one's belief systems and the social support networks used to cope with or understand life stressors (Maton, 1989), yet few models of health services use have included religion as a predictive variable. This study seeks to determine whether or not religiosity – measured as a combination of religious salience, frequency of church attendance, frequency of church-sponsored youth group attendance and frequency of prayer – has an association with the probability of one's having sought emotional or psychological counseling in the last year. This study focuses specifically on an adolescent population – defined as ages 11–18 – given the developmental characteristics of this life stage, as well as the unique mental health needs of this age group.

Mental Health among Adolescents

Until recently, relatively few studies have sought to examine the prevalence and incidence rates of mental illness among an adolescent population.

Although interest in adolescent mental health has increased in recent years, estimates of true prevalence rates are still somewhat tentative and tend to vary from one source to the next. Estimates of the prevalence of any type of psychiatric disorder, for example, range from a low of 8.2 percent to a high of 42 percent. Similarly, estimated prevalence rates for any type of depressive disorder range from a low of 0.2 percent to a high of 18.2 percent (Costello, Mustillo, Erkanli, Keeler, & Angold, 2003).

Recent research suggests that the majority of adolescents in need of mental health care do not receive it (Cummings, 2010; Munson, Floersch, & Townsend, 2009). For example, Samargia, Saewyc, and Elliott (2006) estimated that as many as 10 percent of adolescents suffer from a mental illness severe enough to cause of functional impairment, yet only a small minority of the aforementioned 10 percent actually receive treatment. With the exception of some childhood disorders such as ADHD, the propensity to utilize mental health care immediately following the initial onset of mental and/or emotional distress is extremely low among adolescents, though this propensity does increase with age (Wang, 2005). The reasons for this delay are not entirely known, but potential explanations include a belief that the problem will go away on its own, a lack of access to mental health care, concerns about confidentiality and problems communicating distress to parents, guardians or other adults (Elliott & Larson, 2004).

Providers of Adolescent Mental Health Care

To the extent that adolescents do seek mental health care, schools are the major providers (Rones & Hoagwood, 2000). Although providing mental health care is hardly the primary mandate of the public school system, public health officials view schools as being essential to in identifying and addressing the needs of adolescents who are in need of mental health care (Adelman & Taylor, 1998). Because school-based interventions are often able to incorporate teachers, peers and family members into a treatment plan, such interventions have the potential to be uniquely effective at eliminating behavioral problems and teaching social skills (Rones & Hoagwood, 2000). Furthermore, school-based interventions have the potential to eliminate barriers associated with cost and/or insurance status, since there is no out-of-pocket fee assessed when seeing guidance counselors or other such providers.

Schools, however, represent but one means whereby adolescent mental illness can be treated or even prevented. Churches or one's personal religiosity (defined as either personal conviction or affiliation with a specific tradition) could very well affect – either directly or indirectly – the probability of an adolescent's seeking mental health care. Potential causal mechanisms are at least twofold: first, religion is thought to act as a buffer to mental health, effectively insulating the devout from some of life's stressors, particularly in times of crisis (Maton, 1989). Regardless of whether such benefits are due to faith itself or due to the larger social support systems enjoyed by active members of religious congregations (Ellison & George, 1994), religion would indirectly affect the probability of utilizing mental health services by mediating the severity of mental illness or preventing it entirely. Secondly, religious individuals presumably have access to clergy, many of whom might facilitate religious coping behaviors or even play a role similar to that of a therapist or counselor. Research has shown that adults seek advice from clergy more often than any other type of counsel (Chalfant, Heller, Roberts, & Briones, 1990), and the same would likely hold true for adolescents. Furthermore, some faiths, such as Scientology, actively market their respective belief systems as alternatives to formal mental health services (Fink, 2000). Religion, therefore, may decrease one's need for or utilization of formal mental health care.

Religiosity and Mental Health among Adolescents

Generally speaking, religion plays a significant role in the lives of American youth. As many as 95 percent of adolescents believe in God (or some variation thereof), and all but 13 percent affiliate with some religious group or tradition (Cotton, Zebracki, Rosenthal, Tsevat, & Drotar, 2006; Smith, Denton, Faris, & Regnerus, 2002). Furthermore, approximately 50 percent regularly participate in religious organizations either by attending formal religious services or via participation in youth groups (Smith et al., 2002). Even as overall religiosity has declined in the general population – self reported religious involvement has declined over the last 40 years – today's youth remain relatively devout. In fact, rates of adolescent church attendance were slightly higher in 2000 than they were in 1971 (Bengtson, Copen, Putney, & Silverstein, 2009).

Adolescence is thought to be a phase of life during which individuals accrue the sort of life experience that can dramatically affect religious commitment both now and later in life (Eliassen et al., 2005). Unsurprisingly, there is considerable debate regarding the significance of religion during adolescence. Some researchers view adolescents' religious beliefs as mere reflections of or reactions to those espoused by parents or primary caretakers (Miller, 2001). Others, in contrast, argue that childhood religious socialization has very little effect on religious beliefs and/or attendance during adolescence (Arnett & Jensen, 2002). In fact, adolescence is the lifestage during which religious conversion is most likely to occur (Smith et al., 2002). This is likely attributable to the increased autonomy that accompanies adolescent maturation (Smith et al., 2002). Adolescence is typically thought of as a lifestage in which individuals establish their own identities and personal beliefs, including their personal religiosity (Regnerus, 2004).

A limited number of studies have sought to discover which elements of adolescent religiosity are associated with mental health outcomes. Among the specific aspects of religiosity that have been shown to have statistically as well as clinically significant effects on mental health within an adolescent population are frequency of prayer, religious affiliation, religious salience (the importance that a given individual places on his or her religion) and participation in formal religious activities (Harker, 2001; Miller & Gur, 2002; Mosher & Handal, 1997). While the effects of these components vary by both the context in which they are studied and the way in which they are conceptualized, they are each considered reliable indicators of religiosity and robust predictors of mental health status (Cotton, 2006). That is, higher religiosity among adolescents is associated with more favorable mental health outcomes. Part of this effect may be attributable to the fact that religion serves as a means by which teens can learn and practice the sort of coping skills that will help them deal with the typical turbulence of adolescence. For example, Smith (2003) found that religiously based activities such as prayer, meditation, confession and forgiveness can help youth address and process personal challenges. Similarly, the belief that a loving and omnipotent deity is in control of one's life can lend a sense of orderliness and predictability to the turbulence of adolescence (Ellison, 1991).

While no research has specifically examined the effect of religiosity on mental health service utilization in an adolescent population, there are reasons why faith may play a role in an adolescent's decision to seek or forgo therapy. Research has shown, for example, that adolescents are most likely to receive help if they have already established a trusted relationship with someone who can either provide help directly or supply a referral to a qualified professional (Rickwood, Deane, & Wilson, 2007). Having not yet developed the capacity for self-referral, young adolescents may depend on adults to recognize that a problem exists and identify potential sources of help (Rickwood et al., 2007). These adults are generally thought to include parents, friends, and school counselors, but some research

(Rumberger & Rogers, 1982) has shown that clergy can also fulfill such a role. Similarly, Harris et al. (2006) found a positive correlation between church attendance and mental health service utilization among young adults with severe mental illness, a fact that may point to the existence of referral processes within many religious organizations. In contrast, some research suggests that those who utilize clergy as their initial source of aid may be less likely to ultimately utilize formal mental health services. Meylink and Gorsuch (1988), for example, found that fewer than 10 percent of those coming to clergy for help with a mental health problem are ever referred to a psychiatrist or psychologist.

Variations in Adolescent Help-Seeking Behaviors

In addition to an individual's personal level of religiosity, there are several factors that ought to be considered when analyzing the help-seeking behavior of adolescents. Foremost among these factors are the demographic characteristics of the adolescent in question. Gender, for example, has proven to be a consistent predictor of mental health care utilization; girls tend to seek mental health care with greater frequency than boys (Saunders, Resnick, & Hoberman, 1994). Moreover, boys are generally thought to be more likely to forego mental health care based on the hope that the problem will go away on its own (Elliott & Larson, 2004). Equally salient in this discussion is the race of the adolescent, as Caucasians have been shown to utilize mental health services with greater frequency than other ethnicities (Wu et al., 2001).

An individual's insurance status has also been shown to affect mental health service utilization (Zwaanswijk, Van Der Ende, Verhaak, Bensing, & Verhulst, 2003). For most Americans, one's insurance status and financial situation represent the most significant barrier to health care access in general and mental health services in particular (Zwaanswijk et al., 2003). In situations where such services are widely available, however, insurance status and related socioeconomic variables lose their significance (Sourander et al., 2001). The provision of counselors within the school setting may decrease the importance of health insurance on adolescents' decision to seek mental health services.

Familial and parent characteristics may also influence adolescent help seeking behavior. While some research has shown that adolescents in single-parent households are more likely to need and subsequently utilize mental health care than their counterparts in two-parent households

(Zwaanswijk et al., 2003), single-parent households are often more likely to lack the economic resources or health insurance needed to seek mental health services (Saunders et al., 1994). The role of parental educational attainment is similarly unclear. Although individuals who utilize mental health services often come from educated backgrounds (Yu et al., 2008), the significance of parental education, like that of insurance status, tends to decline in situations where mental health care is widely available (Zwaanswijk et al., 2003). Finally, the quality of the parent-child relationship is thought to play a role in an adolescent's decision to seek formal mental health care (Sourander et al., 2001). As discussed in the previous section, adolescents who enjoy a close relationship with their parents are more likely to both seek and receive help (Rickwood et al., 2007). In contrast, those who have had experiences in which their needs were not met or their problems not taken seriously are more likely to express distrust in mental health professionals and subsequently forgo care (Rickwood et al., 2007).

The Current Study

The primary objective of this analysis is to explore a potential association between the religiosity and the help-seeking behaviors of adolescents. We have chosen to focus on adolescence not only because it is regarded as a unique stage in the life course where personal identities and autonomous decision making begin to emerge but also due to the tendency of adolescents to delay or forego treatment for mental health issues. We hypothesize that the use of mental health services will vary among adolescents, with those who report high levels of religiosity having lower levels of utilization. This comprehensive analysis is able to control for factors that may also affect the differential utilization rates of mental health services, such as age, race, gender, insurance status, parental educational attainment, and parental involvement in the life of the adolescent.

METHODS

Data come from the first wave of the Add Health survey, which was carried out by the Carolina Population Center at the University of North Carolina from 1994 to 2008. The Add Health Study is a school-based project that selected a nationally representative sample of 7th–12th grade students from 132 middle and high schools.

Sample

The public access version of the ADD Health dataset contains 6,504 observations. The eligible sample for this study consisted of individuals who were between the ages of 12 and 18 and enrolled in school at the time of the first interview ($n = 6{,}454$) and those for whom parental data were available ($n = 5{,}627$). Admittedly, restricting the analysis to individuals who were enrolled in school runs the risk of biasing our sample by excluding early dropouts, a group that may include adolescents who are perhaps most likely to need mental health services and least likely to receive them. This issue is addressed in more detail in the Discussion section of this study. An additional 963 respondents were excluded due to missing data on one or more of the key variables, yielding a final analytic sample of 4,684 individuals or about three quarters of the full ADD Health sample.

Outcome Variable

Utilization of mental health services was determined by the respondents' answer to the question, "In the past year, have you received psychological or emotional counseling?" Individuals who answered, "yes" in Wave I were counted as having utilized mental health services, resulting in a dichotomous outcome. While it's true that some individuals receive treatment from sources other than counselors or therapists (e.g., primary care physicians prescribing antidepressants), this study attempted to focus on talk therapy, which is qualitatively different from the sort of care one would receive from other medical sources such as primary care physicians. Admittedly, the question itself is somewhat ambiguous as to the exact meaning of "psychological or emotional counseling," a fact that will be addressed in more detail in the discussion section.

Independent Variables

Religiosity

For the purposes of this project, a scale composed of four standardized religion variables – frequency of church attendance, frequency of participation in youth-oriented religious activities, frequency of prayer, and the importance of religion to the respondent – served as the primary independent variable of interest. All four items were measured on four-point Likert scales in which one represented either the highest frequency or greatest subjective importance and four represented the lowest or least. In constructing the index, all four items were reverse-coded so that higher numbers would correspond to greater religiosity and then added together, forming a religiosity score ranging from 4 (lowest) to 16 (highest). However, given skewness of responses, the variables were standardized prior to being combined into an index, and the resulting values, measured in standard deviation units, ranged from a minimum of −2.58 to a maximum of 1.33. The alpha coefficient for this computed variable is 0.87.

Worth noting is the fact that Add Health respondents who answered "no religious affiliation" on the first question of the religion section were not given the opportunity to answer the remaining religion-oriented questions. While some ADD Health users have circumvented this oversight by assigning those who were skipped the lowest possible value on all religion-oriented variables (i.e., Petts, 2008; Regnerus & Uecker, 2006), we instead opted to drop the 617 adolescents for whom there was no religious information. Supplementary analyses showed that this decision did not substantially affect our results or conclusions.

Depressive Symptomology

Depression was appraised with questions taken from the Center for Epidemiologic Studies Depression Scale (CES-D), a 20-item questionnaire developed to measure depressive symptomology in adolescents and adults (Nooney, 2005). The Add Health survey contains 19 of the 20 aforementioned questions. The alpha coefficient for these 19 items is 0.86. Like the variables having to do with religiosity, all measures of mental health status were standardized prior to their being combined into an index. The resulting scale, measured in standard deviation units, ranged from a minimum of −1.47 to a maximum of 5.59.

Demographic Characteristics

Demographic factors included age (measured continuously in years), race (white vs. nonwhite), and gender (male vs. female), all of which were measured at Wave I when the respondent was between ages 12 and 18. The Add Health survey required that respondents choose one racial/ethnic category from a list that included Hispanic, white, black, Native American, Asian/Pacific Islander, or other. Respondents were not permitted to choose more than one category.

Health Care Access

Access to mental health services was conceptualized as a function of insurance status and student status. Insurance status was measured dichotomously with a dummy variable indicating those individuals who had been continuously insured over the preceding year. Because schools provide an environment in which mental health services are available, school enrollment may be an additional proxy for mental health care access. Limiting the analytic sample to only those individuals who were enrolled in school eliminated the need for a variable indicating student status.

Parental Characteristics

Due to the extent to which parental traits are thought to influence adolescent development, a considerable number of the predictors described the resources of the parents or with the parent/child relationship. Such variables included socioeconomic indicators like the education level of the parent (operationalized here as having completed at least some college or not) who filled the questionnaire, the vast majority (93.4 percent) of whom were mothers. The parental survey also included marital status (married vs. unmarried) of the responding parent at the time of completion. Furthermore, the quality of the parent/child relationship was assessed via two standardized, 10-item scales designed to measure the extent to which mother and fathers are involved in the life of the adolescent. These scales included questions like "How close are you to your mom/dad?" and "How much would you say your mom/dad cares about you?" Indices were constructed separately for mothers and fathers, which boasted alpha coefficients of reliability of 0.97 and 0.81, respectively. Scores for the maternal involvement scale, expressed in standard deviation units, ranged from −3.07 to 1.88. Scores for the paternal involvement scale, similarly expressed, ranged from −1.37 to 2.01.

In order to avoid a significant decrease in sample size, the final analysis utilized a single parental involvement score for each individual. This consisted of the higher of the two parental scores for adolescents who had responses for both a mother and a father, or the only available score for those who only had one parent. The reasoning for adopting this measurement strategy is that a child may have different involvement levels from a mother versus a father, but only one involved parent is needed to help identify and address a child's mental health needs. Approximately one in three (33 percent) of respondents reported living in a single-parent household at the time of the survey.

Analytic Plan

This analysis used a series of five logistic regression model to assess a potential association between the aforementioned independent variables and one's having gone to therapy or counseling in the last year. AIC and BIC statistics are included for each model as an indicator of model fit.

Model 1 assesses only the association between religiosity and the dependent variable net of depressive symptomology. Model 2 incorporates the adolescents' demographic information, as rates of mental health service use have been shown to vary by age, race, and gender (Saunders et al., 1994; Wu et al., 2001). Model 3 considers the importance of health insurance status. Model 4 assesses the possible effects associated with parental traits and their potential to factor into the relationship between religiosity and mental health service utilization. Finally, Model 5 includes all aforementioned variables in order to evaluate what association, if any, religiosity has with mental health service utilization after having controlled for demographic, socioeconomic and familial traits. Due to the extremely complex relationship that exists between religion, race, gender and mental health service utilization, the final model also tested for potential interaction effects between race and religiosity (i.e. the possibility that religious involvement has a different effect for nonwhites than it does for whites), gender and religiosity (i.e., the possibility that religious involvement has a different effect on females than it does for males) and religiosity and depression (i.e., the possibility that the effect of one's religiosity is dependent on one's being depressed or vice versa). All analyses were performed using STATA (version 11).

RESULTS

Just over one in ten (12 percent) adolescents reported that they had received psychological or emotional counseling. As shown in Table 1, several noteworthy differences existed between the youth who have utilized mental health services and those who have not. Of particular interest are the differences in the mean depression and religiosity scores (as assessed by independent samples *t*-tests comparing those who did and did not see a therapist); those who have sought counseling appeared to be significantly more depressed and slightly less religious than their counterparts who had not sought counseling.

Table 1. Descriptive Statistics Comparing Respondents Based on Mental Health Service Utilization.

		Mean	Standard Deviation	Min	Max
Did not see a therapist	Religiosity score	0.03***	0.99	−2.58	1.33
($N = 4{,}139$)	Depression score	−0.07***	0.95	−1.47	5.55
	Parental involvement	0.19**	0.99	−2.19	3.49
	Age	15.91	1.72	12.00	18.00
Saw a therapist	Religiosity score	−0.23	0.97	−2.58	1.33
($N = 555$)	Depression score	0.52	1.17	−1.47	5.17
	Parental involvement	−0.14	1.03	−2.18	3.49
	Age	15.84	1.66	12.00	18.00

Note: Mean differences were assessed with independent samples *t*-tests.
$^{**}p < .01$; $^{***}p < .001$.

Table 2 summarizes the results of the five logistic regression models. Model 1 shows the effects of religiosity and depression on the probability of having received counseling or therapy in the past year. The odds ratios – 0.81 and 1.62, respectively – suggest substantial main effects for each, and both are highly statistically significant ($p < 0.001$). As expected, those with high depressive scores had higher odds of receiving counseling. Furthermore, as hypothesized, those who had higher levels of religiosity had lower odds of receiving counseling.

Model 2 incorporates the adolescents' demographic characteristics. Age proved to be statistically significant ($p < 0.05$), though its slight negative effect (odds ratio = 0.93) is contrary to what one might predict based on the literature. Similarly, the race variable is noteworthy for both its statistical significance and the size of its effect. Relative to whites, nonwhite adolescents are much less likely to have utilized mental health services (odds ratio = 0.65, $p < 0.001$). In contrast to the robust, statistically significant effect of race, the gender variable showed only borderline statistical significance ($p < 0.10$). While the associations of both religiosity and depression with the outcome variable are slightly diluted when demographic controls were included, they retain their statistical significance.

Model 3 considers the adolescents' access to health care. As was discussed previously, the entire analytic sample was enrolled in school at the time of the survey, which likely would have provided them access to some form of mental health services regardless of insurance status. As a result, the dummy variable for those respondents who had insurance is not

Table 2. Odds Ratios for Logistic Regressions Predicting Mental Health Services Use.

	Model 1	Model 2	Model 3	Model 4	Model 5
Religiosity	0.81***	0.83***	0.81***	0.80***	0.84**
	(0.04)	(0.04)	(0.04)	(0.04)	(0.04)
Depression	1.62***	1.66***	1.63***	1.62***	1.67***
	(0.07)	(0.07)	(0.07)	(0.07)	(0.07)
Demographic variables					
Nonwhite		0.65***			0.56***
		(0.07)			(0.07)
Female		1.18			1.20
		(0.12)			(0.11)
Age		0.93*			0.94
		(0.03)			(0.03)
Insured			1.26		01.12
			(0.19)		(0.18)
Parental variables					
No college education				0.67***	0.65***
				(0.07)	(0.07)
Married				0.56***	0.49***
				(0.06)	(0.05)
Parental involvement				1.01	0.97
				(0.05)	(0.03)
Interaction terms					
Nonwhite × religiosity					0.89
					(0.09)
Female × religiosity					0.93
					(0.06)
Depression × religiosity					1.00
					(0.05)
AIC	3653.26	3614.72	3630.06	3561.62	3479.73
BIC	3672.24	3652.68	3655.33	3605.84	3549.11

Note: Standard errors in parentheses.
$^{*}p < .05$; $^{**}p < .01$; $^{***}p < .001$; n.s. not significant.

statistically significant, though its positive association is in concordance with what one might expect. Again, both the religiosity and depression indices remain statistically significant in this model.

Model 4 examines the possible contributing effects of parental characteristics. Relative to those whose parents had at least some college education, adolescents whose parents who possessed only a high school diploma were considerably less likely to have participated in psychological or emotional counseling in the last year (odds ratio = 0.67, $p < 0.001$). Similarly, adolescents whose parents were married showed a lower probability of having sought counseling than adolescents whose parents were single, divorced, separated or widowed (odds ratio = 0.56, $p < 0.001$). Unlike the parental education and marital status, parental involvement in the life of the respondent had no association with the outcome variable. Although the association of religiosity is lessened somewhat by the inclusion of the parental variables, it remains statistically significant, as does depression.

Model 5 combines predictors from all four previous models. The respective effects and significance of the aforementioned predictors remain largely unchanged, though the religiosity association decreases somewhat when the other predictors are included in the same model.

Model 5 also reveals the results of the interaction effects that were explored. Neither one's race nor depressive symptoms nor gender modified the effect of religiosity on mental health care utilization.

Table 3 shows the results of an exploratory analysis, in which the four individual religious behaviors (i.e., church attendance, prayer, participation in youth activities, importance of religion in daily life) were correlated with the dependent variable to assess whether the effect of religiosity on mental health care utilization was driven primarily by one aspect of religious behavior versus the others. Although the effects of the individual items were in the same direction of the effect reported earlier in Table 2, none of the individual items were significantly related to the utilization of mental health services. Only the combined scale measuring one's overall level of religiosity was significantly correlated with utilization. This suggests that the effects reported herein are not driven by an isolated aspect of religious involvement or belief.

Table 3. Mean Religiosity Scores by Whether Mental Health Care Was Received.

	Saw a Therapist ($n = 555$)	Did Not See a Therapist ($n = 4139$)
Religiosity score (−2.58 to 1.33)	−0.18***	0.06
Religious attendance (1–4)	2.56***	2.82
Participation in youth activities (1–4)	1.92***	2.16
Frequency of prayer (1–4)	3.32***	3.62
Importance of religion (1–4)	2.83***	3.02

Note: Mean differences were assessed with independent samples t-tests.
***$p < .001$.

DISCUSSION

This study tested whether or not religiosity is associated with adolescents' probability of seeking emotional or psychological counseling. The findings discussed in the previous section suggest that adolescent religiosity has a negative and statistically significant effect on the probability of having sought therapy even after controlling for depression, demographic characteristics, insurance status and familial context. In other words, a high score on the religious index – which encompasses the importance of religion to the respondent, frequency of prayer, frequency of attendance and participation in non-service activities – is associated with a decreased likelihood of having received psychological or emotional counseling.

This negative relationship is not entirely unexpected. Although research examining the effect of religious involvement on mental health in an exclusively adolescent population is sparse, existing studies have generally pointed to religiosity as being protective against mental illness. Wright and Wisecarver (1993), for example, found that high levels of spirituality, defined as the importance of religion in defining the purpose of one's life, was directly associated with lower levels of depression among adolescents. Additional studies have found religiosity to be negatively correlated with depression (Petts, 2006), stress (Nooney, 2005) and suicidal ideation (Greening & Stoppelbein, 2002).

The current study builds on these findings by demonstrating that religiosity – either directly or indirectly – is also associated with a lower probability of an adolescent's having sought therapy. The causal mechanisms through which this effect might operate, however, are less clear. That the odds ratio associated with the CES-D scale is both statistically significant and greater than one, suggests that depression is (unsurprisingly) correlated with a greater likelihood of having sought mental health services. To the extent that religion acts as a prophylactic against the symptoms of depression – by teaching positive coping skills, promoting healthy interaction with parents and peers and providing a framework through which life's challenges can be understood – it could be seen in some cases as decreasing the need for psychological or emotional counseling.

The fact that religiosity remained statistically significant after controlling for mental health status suggests that religious participation and religious salience play a role above and beyond that of prevention. Considerable research on the subject of religion and mental health points to clergy as being among the first resources sought in times of emotional distress

(Chalfant, 1990; Ellison, 2002; Leavey, 2007). Although the Add Health data do not provide a measure of the extent to which adolescents utilize the resources provided by their respective religions as a form of coping behavior, the negative effect of religiosity on mental health service utilization is consistent with previous findings on the subject.

Furthermore, the supposition that religious youth turn to clergy rather than mental health professionals in times of stress has the potential to partially explain the difference in mental health services use among whites and minorities, as the latter are thought to rely on informal mental health services to a greater extent than their white counterparts. Blank et al. (2002), for example, found that predominantly black churches (urban and rural) play a significantly larger role in the prevention and treatment of mental illness than do their predominantly white equivalents. Additionally, the former tend to provide a much wider range of services than do the latter. It is not out of the realm of possibility, then, that a portion of the negative effect associated with minority status could be due to greater use of religion-centric coping resources. However, preliminary analyses found the interaction between race and religiousness to be statistically insignificant.

Another possible explanation for the negative association between religiosity and mental health services use has to do with the often-acrimonious relationship that exists between religion and psychology. Although considerable common ground has been found in the approximately 80 years since Sigmund Freud effectively threw down the gauntlet with the publication of *The Future of an Illusion*, there are circumstances in which religion and the mental health field remain uneasy bedfellows. As recently as 1995, for example, Pope John Paul II warned his followers that "a purely experimental psychology, unaided by metaphysics, and unenlightened by Christian moral teaching, would lead to a reductive concept of humans that would ultimately expose them to decidedly degrading treatment" (Address to the Tribunal of the Roman Rota, 1995). Similarly, some psychologists have speculated that to many religious individuals, "a challenge to the biblical concept of insanity seems to be a challenge to Christianity itself ... to abandon the idea that sin and the devil are the origin of most psychoses would be to deny the clearly stated views of Christ as reported in the New Testament" (Dain, 1992). To the extent that the Add Health Survey's respondents subscribe to the notion of mental illness as a spiritual matter, it stands to reason that such individuals would be unlikely to seek mental health services, either because they doubt the potential effectiveness of such care or because they fear the implications and/or stigma associated with mental illness as interpreted by their own theology.

In these data and in past literature, there is some debate regarding for whom and under what circumstances religiosity is associated with positive mental health outcomes. Among the factors thought to confound this relationship is gender. Petts (2006), for example, found that the effect of religious attendance on adolescent depression was strongly negative for boys but curvilinear and sometimes positive for girls, a finding that points to girls' possibly receiving fewer benefits from religious participation than boys. The interaction analyses, however, suggest that the effect of religiosity on the probability of utilizing mental health services is actually greater for girls than for boys.

Familial context also explained some of the variation in adolescents' mental health care utilization. As expected, those adolescents with married parents had significantly lower probabilities of seeking psychological or emotional counseling than those from single parent households. Because children in single parent households have in some cases been shown to be more likely to need and subsequently utilize mental health services, the negative effect associated with having married parents is not unexpected. The negative effect associated low parental education, in contrast, is not as easily explained and warrants further investigation.

These findings must be considered in the context of several limitations. The Add Health Study, because it sampled from schools, excluded youths who had dropped out of school or those who were being homeschooled. The youth comprising these two groups would likely face different barriers to treatment than would those included in the study. The analysis carried out in this study further constrained the sample by including only those who were enrolled in school. These findings, therefore, may only be applicable to this select group.

The measures of religiosity in the Add Health data are also somewhat limiting. Although the survey includes religious salience as well as frequency of prayer, attendance and participation in non-service activities, none of these items are directly related to religious coping behaviors, the subjective meaning of religion to a given adolescent or the nature of the relationship that exists between the respondent and his/her clergy. These problems are exacerbated by the skip pattern that resulted in no religion-centric data being collected for anyone who answered "no religious affiliation" to the first question. A more nuanced evaluation of adolescent religious beliefs and behaviors would thus allow for a more detailed analysis.

Finally, the dependent variable leaves something to be desired. We as researchers have no way of knowing how respondents interpreted the phrase "psychological or emotional counseling" in the question of interest, nor do we have any information about the type of counseling received. Furthermore, it is worth noting that parental characteristics may in many cases be the driving force behind adolescents' participation in both counseling and religious activities, though supplementary analyses showed no association between parental religiosity and adolescent depression, religiosity or participation in counseling.

In spite of these limitations, this project supports the somewhat contentious notion that clergy ought to be viewed as a potentially valuable resource in promoting community mental health. Insofar as the negative effect of religiosity on the propensity to seek mental health services is the result of better overall mental health among the devout, clergy should seen as allies of the mental health professionals. Because not all of the variance in mental health service utilization can be attributed to good mental health, however, clergy owe it to their respective congregations to recognize the limits of spiritual counseling and work with mental health professionals as the first step toward service use. Moreover, as trusted advisors of both parents and teens, clergy find themselves in a unique position to support parents, combat stigma, and promote understanding of mental illness in the community.

In summary, this study represents what may be the first attempt to use a nationally representative sample to tease out the relationship between religiosity and mental health service utilization among adolescents. This project demonstrated a negative, statistically significant relationship between high levels of religiosity and the probability of having seen a therapist or counselor even after controlling for mental health status, demographic variables, and familial context.

REFERENCES

Address to the Tribunal of the Roman Rota | John Paul II. (n.d.). Retrieved from http://w2.vatican.va/content/john-paul-ii/en/speeches/1995/february/documents/hf_jp-ii_spe_19950210_roman-rota.html. Accessed on August 5, 2014.

Adelman, H. S., & Taylor, L. (1998). Reframing mental health in schools and expanding school reform. *Educational Psychologist*, *33*, 135–152.

Arnett, J. J., & Jensen, L. A. (2002). A congregation of one: Individualized religious beliefs among emerging adults. *Journal of Adolescent Research*, *17*, 451–467.

Bengtson, V. L., Copen, C. E., Putney, N. M., & Silverstein, M. (2009). A longitudinal study of the intergenerational transmission of religion. *International Sociology*, *24*(3), 325–345.

Blank, M. B., Mahmood, M., Fox, J. C., & Guterbock, T. (2002). Alternative mental health services: The role of the black church in the South. *American Journal of Public Health, 92*(10), 1668–1672.

Chalfant, H. P., Heller, P. L., Roberts, A., & Briones, D. (1990). The clergy as a resource for those encountering psychological distress. *Review of Religious Research, 31*(3), 305–313.

Costello, E., Mustillo, S., Erkanli, A., Keeler, G., & Angold, A. (2003). Prevalence and development of psychiatric disorders in childhood and adolescence. *Archives of General Psychiatry, 60*(8), 837–844.

Cotton, S., Zebracki, K., Rosenthal, S. L., Tsevat, J., & Drotar, D. (2006). Religion/spirituality and adolescent health outcomes: A review. *Journal of Adolescent Health, 38*(4), 472–480.

Dain, N. (1992). Madness and the stigma of sin in American Christianity. In P. J. Fink & A. Tasman (Eds.), *Stigma and mental illness* (pp. 73–84). Arlington, VA: American Psychiatric Association.

Eliassen, H. A., & Taylor, J. (2005). Subjective religiosity and depression in the transition to adulthood. *Journal for the Scientific Study of Religion, 44*(2), 187–199.

Elliott, B. A., & Larson, J. T. (2004). Adolescents in mid-sized and rural communities: Foregone care, perceived barriers, and risk factors. *Journal of Adolescent Health, 35*, 303–309.

Ellison, C. G. (1991). Religious involvement and subjective well-being. *Journal of Health and Social Behavior, 32*(1), 80–99.

Ellison, C. G., & George, L. K. (1994). Religious involvement, social ties, and social support in a southeastern community. *Journal for the Scientific Study of Religion, 33*(1), 46–61.

Ellison, C. G., & Levin, J. S. (1998). The religion-health connection: Evidence, theory, and future directions. *Health Education and Behavior, 25*(6), 700–720.

Fink, M. (2000). Electroshock revisited. *American Scientist, 88*, 162–167.

Gorsuch, R. L. (1972). Single vs. multiple-item scales for measuring religious values. *Journal for the Scientific Study of Religion, 11*(1), 53–64.

Greening, L., & Stoppelbein, L. (2002). Religiosity, attributional style, and social support as psychosocial buffers for African American and white adolescents' perceived risk for suicide. *Suicide and Life-Threatening Behavior, 32*, 404–417.

Hall, D. E., Meador, K. G., & Koenig, H. G. (2008). Measuring religiousness in health research: Review and critique. *Journal of Religion and Health, 47*(2), 134–163.

Harker, K. (2001). Immigrant generation, assimilation, and adolescent psychological well-being. *Social Forces, 79*(3), 969–1004.

Harris, K. M., Edlund, M. J., & Larson, S. L. (2006). Religious involvement and the use of mental health care. *Health Services Research, 41*(2), 395–410.

Krause, N. (1995). Religiosity and self-esteem among older adults. *Journal of Gerontology: Psychological Sciences, 50*, 236–246.

Leavey, G., & King, M. (2007). The devil in the detail: Partnership between psychiatry and faith based organizations. *The British Journal of Psychiatry, 191*, 97–98.

Maton, K. I. (1989). The stress-buffering role of spiritual support: Cross-sectional and prospective investigations. *Journal for the Scientific Study of Religion, 28*(3), 310–323.

Meylink, W. D., & Gorsuch, R. (1988). New perspectives for clergy-psychologist referrals. *Journal of Psychology and Christianity, 5*, 62–70.

Miller, L. (2001). Religiosity, depression and physical maturation in adolescent girls. *Child and Adolescent Psychiatry*, *41*(2), 206–214.
Miller, L., & Gur, M. (2002). Sexual maturation, depression and religion in adolescent girls. *Journal of the American Academy of Child and Adolescent Psychiatry*, *41*(2), 206–214.
Mosher, J. P., & Handal, P. J. (1997). The relationship between religion and psychological distress in adolescents. *Journal of Psychology and Theology*, *25*, 449–457.
Munson, M. R., Floersch, J. E., & Townsend, L. (2009). Attitudes toward mental health services and illness perceptions among adolescents with mood disorders. *Child and Adolescent Social Work Journal*, *26*(5), 447–466.
Nooney, J. G. (2005). Religion, stress, and mental health in adolescence: Findings from add health. *Review of Religious Research*, *46*(4), 341–354.
Petts, R. J. (2008). Religion and adolescent depression: The impact of race and gender. *Review of Religious Research*, *49*(4), 395–414.
Poloma, M. M., & Pendleton, B. F. (1990). Religious domains and general well-being. *Social Indicators Research*, *22*(3), 255–276.
Regnerus, M. (2004). Social context in the development of adolescent religiosity. *Applied Developmental Science*, *8*(1), 27–38.
Rickwood, D., Deane, F., & Wilson, C. (2007). When and how do young people seek professional help for mental health problems? *Medical Journal of Australia*, *187*(7), S35–S39.
Rones, M., & Hoagwood, K. (2000). School-based mental health services: A research review. *Clinical Child and Family Psychology Review*, *3*(4), 223–241.
Rumberger, D. J., & Rogers, M. L. (1982). Pastoral openness to interaction with a private Christian counseling service. *Journal of Psychology and Theology*, *10*, 337–345.
Samargia, L. A., Saewyc, E. M., & Elliott, B. A. (2006). Foregone mental health care and self-reported access barriers among adolescents. *The Journal of School Nursing*, *22*(1), 17–24.
Saunders, S. M., Resnick, M. D., & Hoberman, H. M. (1994). Formal help-seeking behavior of adolescents identifying themselves as having mental health problems. *Journal of the American Academy of Child and Adolescent Psychiatry*, *33*(5), 718–728.
Smith, C., Denton, M. L., Faris, R., & Regnerus, M. (2002). Mapping American adolescent religious participation. *Journal for the Scientific Study of Religion*, *41*(4), 397–612.
Smith, T. B., McCullough, M. E., & Poll, J. (2003). Religiousness and depression: Evidence for a main effect and the moderating influence of stressful life events. *Psychological Bulletin*, *129*, 614–636.
Sourander, A., Helstelä, L., Ristkari, T., Ikäheimo, K., Helenius, H., & Piha, J. (2001). Child and adolescent mental health service use in Finland. *Social Psychiatry and Psychiatric Epidemiology*, *36*, 294–298.
Uecker, J. E., Regnerus, M., & Vaaler, M. L. (2007). Losing my religion: The social sources of religious decline in early adulthood. *Social Forces*, *85*(4), 1667–1692.
Wright, L., Frost, C., & Wisecarver, S. (1993). Church attendance, meaningfulness of religion, and depressive symptomatology among adolescents. *Journal of Youth and Adolescence*, *22*, 559–568.
Wu, P., Hoven, C., Liu, X., Morre, R. E., Tiet, Q., Okezie, N., ... Bird, H. R. (2001). Factors associated with use of mental health services for depression by children and adolescents. *Psychiatric Services*, *52*, 189–195.

Yu, W. J., Adams, S. H., Burns, J., Brindis, C. D., & Irwin, C. E. (2008). Use of mental health counseling as adolescents become young adults. *Journal of Adolescent Health, 43*(3), 268–276.

Zwaanswijk, M., Van Der Ende, J., Verhaak, P. F. M., Bensing, J. M., & Verhulst, F. C. (2003). Factors associated with adolescent mental health service need and utilization. *Journal of the American Academy of Child & Adolescent Psychiatry, 42*(6), 692–700.

PART V
OTHER SOCIAL FACTORS

RACIAL AND ETHNIC DIFFERENCES IN TRUST IN SOURCES OF HEALTH INFORMATION: A GENERALIZED DISTRUST IN PHYSICIANS

Celeste Campos-Castillo

ABSTRACT

Purpose – *A fairly consistent finding in research on trust in physicians is that racial and ethnic minorities cite lower levels than whites. This research typically samples only health care users, which limits our understanding of what underlies distrust. It remains unclear whether the distrust is generalized, which is distrust that is unrelated to using health care regularly or recently.*

Methodology/approach – *Using data from the Health Information National Trends Survey, multivariable logistic regressions assessed whether racial and ethnic differences in distrust (1) are equivalent among health care users and non-users; (2) regardless of respondents' health and socio-economic status; and (3) manifest in other health information sources.*

Education, Social Factors, and Health Beliefs in Health and Health Care Services
Research in the Sociology of Health Care, Volume 33, 163–186

ISSN: 0275-4959/doi:10.1108/S0275-495920150000033008

Findings – *Racial and ethnic minorities are less likely than whites to trust physicians as health information sources. These racial and ethnic differences are equivalent among health care users and non-users, regardless of respondents' health and socio-economic status. The racial and ethnic patterns do not manifest when predicting trust in other health information sources (Internet, family or friends, government health agencies, charitable organizations).*

Research limitations/implications – *Data are derived from a cross-sectional survey, which makes it difficult to account comprehensively for self-selection into being a health care user. Despite the limitations, this research suggests that racial and ethnic minorities possess a generalized distrust in physicians, necessitating interventions that move beyond improving health care experiences.*

Originality/value – *Many researchers have surmised that a generalized distrust in physicians exists among racial and ethnic minorities. This chapter is the first to explicitly examine the existence of such distrust.*

Keywords: Trust; race and ethnicity; health care use; health information sources

Despite rising use of the Internet to access health information, individuals still turn to physicians or other health care professionals as sources of health information. In particular, individuals seek a health care professional's guidance to help make sense of the information they find on the Internet (e.g., Kivits, 2006; Sommerhalder, Abraham, Zufferey, Barth, & Abel, 2009). Physicians remain central in the contemporary health information environment, yet trust in them as a health information source remains divided. A fairly consistent finding in the literature on trust in physicians is that racial and ethnic minorities tend to report lower levels than whites (Boulware, Cooper, Ratner, LaVeist, & Powe, 2003; Corbie-Smith, Thomas, & St George, 2002; Doescher, Saver, Franks, & Fiscella, 2000; Gordon, Street, Sharf, Kelly, & Souchek, 2006; Keating, Gandhi, Orav, Bates, & Ayanian, 2004; LaVeist, Nickerson, & Bowie, 2000; Saha et al., 2011; Schnittker, 2004). Trust in a physician is the expectation that the physician has our best interests in mind (Mechanic, 1996). It is positively associated with health and health care outcomes, such as coping with a disease or illness (Wileman, May, & Chew-Graham, 2002), treatment adherence (Piette, Heisler, Krein, & Kerr, 2005; Saha, Jacobs, Moore, & Beach, 2010), and utilization (LaVeist, Isaac, & Williams, 2009; O'Malley, Sheppard, Schwartz, & Mandelblatt, 2004; Whetten et al., 2006), leading to the conclusion that racial and ethnic differences in trust contribute to disparities. The conclusion has spurred efforts to increase trust in physicians among racial and ethnic minorities through improving health care experiences, particularly the patient-provider interaction (e.g., Fiscella et al., 2004; McCabe, 2004; Thom, 2001).

Unfortunately, much of the research in this area oftentimes samples only recent or regular users of the health care system, which leaves unanswered questions about what underlies these racial and ethnic differences. The convention in previous research on trust in physicians – both quantitative (e.g., Cooper et al., 2003; Doescher et al., 2000; LaVeist et al., 2000; Saha et al., 2011; Schnittker, 2004) and qualitative (e.g., Cooper-Patrick et al., 1997; Jacobs, Rolle, Ferrans, Whitaker, & Warnecke, 2006; Kroll, Richardson, Sharf, & Suarez-Almazor, 2007) – has been to sample respondents who were health care users, defined empirically as those who either (1) have a usual source of care or (2) made a visit within a recent timeframe. There are exceptions to this trend, where the study samples include both health care users and non-users, and such studies still find that racial and ethnic minorities report greater distrust in a physician or other health care provider (Boulware et al., 2003; Corbie-Smith et al., 2002; Halbert, Armstrong, Gandy, & Shaker, 2006; but for one exception, see Savage, 2011). This information alone, however, is insufficient for determining whether racial and ethnic minorities possess a generalized distrust in physicians, which is distrust unaffected by recent or regular experience with a physician because it generalizes across physicians (LaVeist & Nuru-Jeter, 2002; Malat, 2001; Stepanikova, Mollborn, Cook, Thom, & Kramer, 2006).

A generalized distrust in physicians among racial and ethnic minorities implies that the magnitude of racial and ethnic differences is similar among health care users and non-users. Its existence indicates the need to move beyond just improving the patient-provider interaction and other aspects of the health care experience, to improving wider perceptions of physicians among racial and ethnic minorities. I develop a model of what type of evidence is necessary for identifying the existence of generalized distrust and test it using a nationally representative sample of health care users and non-users to address the limitations in previous research.

THEORETICAL MODEL

There are substantive reasons to believe that generalized distrust does not exist. Many cite the actual encounter with a physician as a primary source of racial and ethnic disparities in health and health care (for one review, see Van Ryn & Pu, 2003). Indeed, reports of experiencing discrimination in health care are positively related to distrust in physicians (Doescher et al., 2000; Hammond, 2010; LaVeist et al., 2000; Schuster et al., 2005). Accordingly, one hypothesis is that racial and ethnic minority distrust in physicians may manifest only among health care users and not non-users, because the former group experienced inequality. An interesting corollary of this line of thought is that the existing research on distrust – where much of the research samples health care users – is actually overestimating the level of distrust in the broader population of racial and ethnic minorities.

H1a. Racial and ethnic minority distrust is greater among health care users than non-users.

As mentioned earlier, generalized distrust occurs when recent or regular experience with a physician is unrelated to the distrust. The physician role is highly symbolic in that many individuals possess a general understanding of its archetypal features (Parsons, 1951). Trust in a physician may therefore be highly generalized and stable (Hall et al., 2002), with only broader societal and cultural shifts affecting it (e.g., Pescosolido, Tuch, & Martin, 2001). Such a characterization of distrust in physicians among racial and ethnic minorities contrasts with the one that H1a summarizes. It suggests that existing research that documents greater distrust among racial and ethnic minorities than whites – where much of the research samples health care users – is indeed reflective of the level of distrust in the broader population of racial and ethnic minorities because it is capturing generalized distrust. Others have surmised that racial and ethnic patterns of distrust in physicians likely reflect a generalized distrust (e.g., LaVeist & Nuru-Jeter, 2002; Malat, 2001; Stepanikova et al., 2006), but to date no one has offered empirical support for such claims. Empirical support for the existence of a generalized distrust would be if racial and ethnic patterns of distrust were equivalent among health care users and non-users.

H1b. Racial and ethnic minority distrust is equivalent among health care users and non-users.

Because numerous background variables may account for differences in distrust among health care users and non-users, considering these is necessary to corroborate equivalence in racial and ethnic minority distrust between health care users and non-users. For example, socio-demographics – such as education and income – are correlated with health care usage and trust (e.g., LaVeist et al., 2009; Schnittker, 2004). Health status is also correlated with health care usage and trust (e.g., LaVeist et al., 2009; O'Malley et al., 2004; Whetten et al., 2006). If racial and ethnic minority distrust remains equivalent among health care users and non-users after accounting for these background variables, then it further corroborates an account that generalized distrust exists.

H2. Racial and ethnic distrust remains equivalent among health care users and non-users after adjusting for socio-demographics.

H3. Racial and ethnic distrust remains equivalent among health care users and non-users after adjusting for health status.

Finally, it is necessary to differentiate a generalized distrust in physicians from a generalized distrust in any other health information source. Much research documents racial and ethnic distrust in numerous domains, besides in accessing information from a health care professional. For example, racial and ethnic minorities often cite a lack of trust in a "generalized other," which shapes their lack of trust in institutions (McKnight, Cummings, & Chervany, 1998). Consequently, finding that racial and ethnic distrust is equivalent between health care users and non-users may simply indicate that racial and ethnic minorities distrust institutions and a "generalized other," a situation substantively different from a generalized distrust uniquely tied to physicians as health information sources. Accordingly, if racial and ethnic minorities cite distrust in physicians as sources of health information *and* not in any other source, then it supports the existence of a generalized distrust in physicians.

H4. Racial and ethnic minorities will cite distrust in physicians as sources of health information, but not in any other source of health information.

Together, these hypotheses delineate whether a generalized distrust in physicians exists among racial and ethnic minorities. If such a generalized distrust exists, then it fuels the need to develop community-level efforts that improve racial and ethnic minorities' perceptions of the health care system in order to address health and health care disparities comprehensively. Existing efforts to improve physician trust that focus on the patient-physician encounter (e.g., Fiscella et al., 2004; McCabe, 2004;

Thom, 2001) deserve merit in that they draw our attention to ways that reduce disparities, but the drawback of these efforts is that they are targeted toward those already interacting with health care. The presence of a generalized distrust among racial and ethnic minorities implies that we need to devote additional efforts that go beyond just the health care experience. The findings from an analysis of the 2007 Health Information National Trends Survey (HINTS) can inform research and practice regarding such efforts.

DATA AND METHODS

Data Source

I relied on the 2007 cross-section of the HINTS, which the National Cancer Institute developed to capture the experiences of U.S. adults with cancer-related information. More recent iterations of HINTS exist, but the 2007 data were collected using a dual survey mode design (telephone and mail). Because researchers have identified survey mode to influence responses to various health communication items (e.g., Nan, Zhao, & Briones, 2013; Wallace, Chisolm, Abdel-Rasoul, & DeVoe, 2013), it is crucial for this initial and novel assessment that I draw on the best data sources available to account for sources of bias comprehensively. Future research can determine whether patterns continue to persist in more recent surveys.

Complete survey design details are available elsewhere (see Cantor et al., 2009). Briefly, the 2007 data were collected between January and April of 2008. Respondents were recruited from a sampling frame that was generated using either a Random Digit Dial (RDD) technique or a national listing of U.S. addresses (address). Respondents who were recruited from the RDD sampling frame (N = 4,092) completed a Computer Assisted Telephone Interview (CATI) that was available in either English or Spanish.[1] All adults (N = 3,582) from a household recruited from the address sampling frame were asked to complete a mail-in survey that was only available in English. Eleven respondents from this recruitment wished to complete a Spanish survey and were allowed to complete a CATI. The total sample size of the dataset is 7,674. Sampling weights were used to reflect known demographic and health status characteristics of the U.S. adult population, nonresponse, and survey design.

Analytic Sample

My analysis pertains to just a subset of the total sample. Since the majority of the research documenting racial and ethnic differences in physician trust commonly includes (and at times specifically focuses on) comparisons of black and Latina/o to white respondents (e.g., Boulware et al., 2003; Schnittker & Liang, 2006; Stepanikova et al., 2006), I restricted my sample to just these three groups. The selection criteria I imposed was respondents who reported one of the racial and ethnic groups of interest (i.e., black, Latina/o, white), responded to at least one of the health care user status items, and responded to at least one of the trust items I examined.

After listwise deletion, I had an analytic sample size (*n*) of 4,787. Later in the results section, I report how comparable findings are between complete and incomplete cases. A summary of the weighted analytic sample can be found in Table 1.

Measures

Trust in Health Information Sources

The item asked respondents on a four-point Likert scale, "In general, how much would you trust information about health or medical topics from ..." (1 = "a lot," 4 = "not at all"). Respondents were asked to provide their degree of trust in a total of nine sources of health information. Similar to prior studies that used HINTS to predict trust in sources of health information (e.g., Hesse, Moser, & Rutten, 2010; Richardson, Appleyard, Xiao, & Vallone, 2012), I dichotomized responses (1 = "a lot," 0 = "some" "a little" "none at all"). Thus, the empirical definition of distrust in a source is when a coefficient in a binary logit regression is negative (i.e., lack of agreement with a trust statement, see also Corbie-Smith et al., 2002; Schnittker, 2004). To properly apply binary logit regression, I only included health information sources in the analysis if at least 10% of respondents selected one of the two dichotomous outcomes (Long, 1997). This permitted an analysis of five sources of health information that researchers commonly examine (e.g., Hesse et al., 2010; Nan, Zhao, & Briones, 2013; Richardson et al., 2012): doctor or other physician, family or friends, the Internet, government health agencies, and charitable organizations.

Table 1. Weighted Means (Standard Deviations) and Percentages of Sample Characteristics, by Whether Respondents Trust Physician "a Lot" as Source of Health Information.

	All		Trust Physician Some/a Little/Not at All		Trust Physician a Lot	
% Trust source "a lot" for health information[a]						
Physician	69.3		.0		100.0	
Family/friends	13.3		10.5		14.5	
Government	31.4		16.1		38.2	
Internet	20.7		15.6		22.9	
Charitable organizations	10.1		5.4		12.2	
% Race/ethnicity						
White	74.6		66.2		78.4	
Latina/o	14.3		19.9		11.8	
Black	11.1		13.9		9.8	
% Did not make visit previous 12 months	15.9		24.1		12.3	
% Do not have usual source of care	30.2		41.1		25.4	
% Female	50.2		49.3		50.6	
Mean age (years)	43.65	(16.00)	43.91	(15.00)	43.50	(16.42)
% Education level completed						
< High school	11.0		14.6		9.4	
High school	26.2		26.2		26.2	
≥Some college	62.8		59.2		64.4	
% Household annual income						
<$20,000	32.3		39.2		29.3	
$20,000–$34,999	14.2		14.5		14.1	
$35,000–$49,999	20.1		18.9		20.6	
$50,000–$74,999	12.7		8.2		14.7	
≥$75,000	20.6		19.2		21.3	
% Health insurance	83.1		76.5		86.0	
% Employed	64.4		63.9		64.6	
% Currently married	56.2		53.9		57.2	
Mean self-rated health (1–5)	3.44	(.91)	3.38	(.89)	3.47	(.92)
% Serious psychological distress	7.4		9.3		6.7	
% Current smoker	21.9		24.6		20.7	
Mean confidence in seeking health information (1–5)	3.73	(1.00)	3.44	(1.06)	3.86	(.95)
Mean confidence in self-care (1–5)	3.84	(.84)	3.70	(.88)	3.90	(.81)

$n = 4{,}787$.

[a]Categories are not mutually exclusive from one another.

Race and Ethnicity

I created two dichotomous variables (black, Latina/o) and treated white respondents as the reference group.

Health Care User Status

Two questions assessed different aspects of health care usage. One assessed whether or not a respondent had a usual source of care with the item, "Not including psychiatrists and other mental health professionals, is there a particular doctor, nurse, or other health professional that you see most often?" (Yes/No). I created a dichotomous variable where those with a usual source of care were the reference group. A second asked respondents if they made a non-emergency room visit in the past 12 months (and if so, how many times): "During the past 12 months, not counting times you went to an emergency room, how many times did you go to a doctor, nurse, or other health professional to get care for yourself?" I dichotomized responses, where respondents who reported making at least one of these visits were the reference group. Relying on two indicators separately permits an analysis of whether the presence of generalized distrust is sensitive to the empirical definition of health care user status.

Controls

I prepared two sets of controls to adjust estimates. The first set was designed to control for respondents' socio-demographic background and test H2, whereas the second to control for respondents' health status and test H3. Controls for socio-demographic background included gender (1 = female, 0 = male), age (years) and its squared term, education level completed (less than high school (referent), high school, some college or more), health insurance status (1 = has health insurance, 0 = does not have health insurance), employment status (1 = currently employed, 0 = not currently employed), marital status (1 = currently married; 0 = not currently married), and annual household-level income (less than $20,000 (referent); $20,000–$34,999; $35,000–$49,999; $50,000–$74,999; greater than or equal to $75,000).

The health status controls included indicators of respondents' self-rated health, confidence in self-care, psychological distress, and smoker status.

Self-rated health is a five-point Likert scale (Ware, Kosinski, & Keller, 1996). Confidence in self-care is measured on a five-point Likert scale that asked, "Overall, how confident are you about your ability to take good care of your health?" (1 = "Completely Confident," 5 = "Not Confident at all"), which I reverse-coded so that higher values indicated greater confidence. To measure psychological distress, I used the Kessler-6 non-specific psychological distress scale (Kessler et al., 2002), which asked respondents for the frequency in the past 30 days that they experienced six manifestations of psychological distress (nervous, hopeless, restless, or fidgety, so sad or depressed nothing could cheer respondent up, feeling that everything is an effort, and worthless). For each manifestation, frequency is measured on a 5-point scale (0 = "None of the time," 4 = "All of the time"). The six items are summed to create a score that ranges from 0 to 24 ($\alpha = 0.85$). A score greater than or equal to 13 indicates serious psychological distress, which I captured in a dichotomous variable (1 = serious psychological distress, 0 = no serious psychological distress). To measure smoker status, the survey first asked respondents if they had ever smoked 100 or more cigarettes; of those who responded in the affirmative, the survey asked if they smoke currently (Soulakova, Hartman, Liu, Willis, & Augustine, 2012). I created a dichotomous variable to reflect whether or not the respondent currently smoked (1 = Yes, 0 = No).

Analytic Strategy

The goal is to determine if racial and ethnic minorities have a generalized distrust of physicians, which I outlined exists if (1) racial and ethnic patterns of distrust were equivalent between health care users and non-users; (2) and remained equivalent after the inclusion of relevant controls; and (3) a similar distrust did not manifest in other health information sources. First, I estimated interactions between race and health care user status in binary logit models predicting trusting physicians "a lot." Then I determined if estimates of these interactions changed with the inclusion of the relevant controls. I repeated this step for both empirical definitions of health care user status. Lastly, I compared these interactions across binary logit models predicting trust in other sources of health information, each of which included the relevant controls. I also repeated this step for both definitions of health care user status.

I also conducted two follow-up analyses to assess potential biases in results, which for simplicity are not shown in the tables. First, I examined whether examining only complete cases changed patterns appreciably. Second, I conducted a propensity score analysis to capture some of the bias that a cross-sectional design introduces. Specifically, I considered whether respondents' propensity to use health care (have a regular provider, make a recent visit) changed patterns appreciably.

All models used STATA 13.0 and two-tailed *t*-tests to determine statistical significance. A preliminary analysis (not presented) showed that the sampling frame used (RDD vs. address) was significantly associated with trust in family or friends, government health agencies, and charitable organizations but not physicians or the Internet. All models include the survey weights and survey mode controls appropriate for their respective situations (see Cantor et al., 2009 for additional information).

RESULTS

The first analytic task involved assessing whether racial and ethnic differences in trusting a physician as a source of health information were comparable between health care users and non-users. M1 through M3 in Table 2 build successively toward demonstrating this for the definition of health care user as having made a recent (prior 12 months) non-emergency room visit. M1 shows that Latina/os and blacks were significantly less likely than whites to report trusting physicians "a lot." Differences remained even after controlling for health care user status in M2. As expected, health care non-users were significantly less likely to report trusting physician.

The interactions of interest in this first analytic task – those that adjudicate between H1a and H1b – were introduced in M3. The inclusion of the interactions between racial and ethnic background and health care user status renders the "main effects" of being a Latina/o or black respondent (shown in the first two rows of M3) as representing the racial and ethnic differences in trusting physicians "a lot" only among health care users. Essentially, these main effects reflect the patterns employed commonly in previous research that selects only health care users for analysis. Consistent with this previous research, health care users who identify as Latina/o or black had a significantly lower likelihood of reporting "a lot" of trust in a physician. Missing, however, from the previous research is information on whether these racial and ethnic differences are comparable between health care users and non-users. Rows four and five of M3 show that the

Table 2. Unstandardized Coefficients for Weighted Binary Logit Regression of Trusting Physicians "A Lot" as Source of Health Information on Respondent's Race/Ethnicity, Health Care User Status, and Relevant Controls.

	M1	M2	M3	M4	M5	M6	M7	M8	M9
Latina/o	−.689***	−.557***	−.440*	−.429*	−.373	−.553**	−.675**	−.654**	−.601*
	(.139)	(.140)	(.176)	(.198)	(.212)	(.149)	(.199)	(.214)	(.229)
Black	−.519**	−.456**	−.419**	−.317*	−.373**	−.445**	−.516**	−.447*	−.525**
	(.148)	(.152)	(.137)	(.134)	(.128)	(.153)	(.191)	(.187)	(.183)
No visits		−.720***	−.567**	−.507**	−.516**				
		(.115)	(.159)	(.174)	(.184)				
Latina/o × no visits			−.529	−.444	−.584				
			(.422)	(.421)	(.448)				
Black × no visits			−.210	−.273	−.379				
			(.511)	(.530)	(.580)				
No usual source of care						−.637***	−.714***	−.794***	−.739***
						(.103)	(.131)	(.153)	(.159)
Latina/o × no usual source of care							.273	.321	.246
							(.287)	(.302)	(.327)
Black × no usual source of care							.193	.235	.249
							(.429)	(.432)	(.448)
Socio-demographic controls?	No	No	No	Yes	Yes	No	No	Yes	Yes
Health controls?	No	No	No	No	Yes	No	No	No	Yes
Constant	.985***	1.087***	1.064***	2.071***	.702	1.165***	1.189***	2.493***	1.189**
	(.046)	(.053)	(.053)	(.507)	(.649)	(.054)	(.052)	(.518)	(.681)

Note: Robust standard errors are in parentheses.
$^{*}p < .05$; $^{**}p < .01$; $^{***}p < .001$.

interactions that shed light on this were statistically non-significant, indicating that the racial and ethnic differences in the likelihood of trusting a physician "a lot" were comparable between health care users and non-users. This disconfirms H1a, while tentatively confirming H1b that generalized distrust likely exists among racial and ethnic minorities.

Additional evidence for the existence of generalized distrust and further corroboration for H1b would come in finding support for H2 and H3, which predict that these interactions remain non-significant after accounting for respondents' socio-demographics and health status. As the results summarized in M4 and M5 show, the interactions remained non-significant with the inclusion of the socio-demographic and health status controls, supporting H2 and H3. Although the magnitude of racial and ethnic differences remained comparable between health care users and non-users, the magnitude itself decreased after adjusting for these controls. Specifically, after accounting for socio-demographics in M4, the racial and ethnic main effects decreased slightly, but remained statistically significant. When the health status controls were introduced in M5, the main effect for Latina/os became statistically non-significant, whereas the main effect for blacks actually increased in statistical significance. Not shown in the table is that these changes in the coefficients from M4 to M5 were due largely to the introduction of the confidence in health information seeking measure.

I also examined the similarity of these patterns when using an alternative health care user status definition. M6 through M9 repeated the prior steps for the second definition, which is based on whether respondents report having a usual source of care. M6 shows that the racial and ethnic differences in likelihood of trusting physicians "a lot" remained after controlling for health care user status. Just as in M2, health care non-users were significantly less likely to report trusting physicians. The comparability of these two models shows that this relationship exists, regardless of how health care user is empirically defined. I introduced the interactions of interest in M7, which just as in M3 were non-significant. Racial and ethnic differences in trusting a physician were statistically equivalent among health care users and non-users, offering additional support for H1b. The interactions remain non-significant after adjusting for the socio-demographic and health controls in M8 and M9, respectively, lending additional support for H2 and H3. Just as in M4 and M5, although the interactions remained non-significant, the actual size of the racial and ethnic differences changed. These changes were once again due largely to the inclusion of the confidence in health information seeking measure.

The next analytic step was to determine if patterns were reflecting either a generalized distrust in physicians as sources of health information or a generalized distrust of all sources, which was a test of H4. The first two columns from Table 3 are the same as the full models (M5 and M9) from Table 2, and compares these full models to parallel models predicting trust in the other sources of health information. The comparisons show that the racial and ethnic patterns of distrust only appeared when the source is a physician, regardless of how health care user is defined. Racial and ethnic differences in trusting other sources of health information were either negligible or favored minorities. Notably, racial and ethnic minorities were significantly more likely to trust government health agencies "a lot" as a source of health information than whites, regardless of how health care user was defined. This stands in contrast to prior research documenting distrust in the government among racial and ethnic minorities, which I discuss momentarily. Taken together, the results from Table 3 demonstrated that distrust among racial and ethnic minorities discriminates with respect to source, supporting H4. Combined with the information from Table 2, this attests to the existence of a generalized distrust of physicians as a source of health information among racial and ethnic minorities.

Summarized above are the parsimonious results. I conducted two separate auxiliary analyses (results available upon request) to assess the robustness of the patterns. First, I conducted a propensity score analysis (Rosenbaum & Rubin, 1984; Rubin, 1997) to provide some insight into whether results from Tables 2 and Table 3 were skewed from self-selection into being a health care user or non-user. I conducted separate analyses for each health care user status indicator and incorporated appropriate survey weights in each stage of the analysis. I used all independent variables described earlier to estimate respondents' propensity to be a health care non-user and divided the propensity distribution into quintiles. I generated dichotomous variables to represent respondents' location in the quintile distribution and included these as additional controls in the models described previously. Although not a perfect assessment of selection bias (e.g., self-selection may be associated with variables not included in the propensity estimates), the analyses can direct attention to which results may need to be interpreted cautiously.

First I revisited the models in Table 2 where health care user was defined as having made a recent non-emergency room visit (M2–M5). Across all models, the interactions between health care user status and racial and ethnic background remained non-significant, indicating that racial and ethnic differences in distrust remained equivalent among health care users and

Table 3. Unstandardized Coefficients for Weighted Binary Logit Regressions Comparing Racial/Ethnic Differences in Trusting Health Care Professionals "A Lot" to Differences in Trusting Other Sources of Health Information "A Lot," by Health Care User Status Definition.

	Health Care Professionals		Internet		Family or Friends		Government Health Agencies		Charitable Organizations	
	M1a	M2a	M1b	M2b	M1c	M2c	M1d	M2d	M1e	M2e
Latina/o	−.373	−.601*	.450*	.384	.156	−.006	.466*	.505*	.515*	.377
	(.202)	(.229)	(.213)	(.262)	(.269)	(.256)	(.191)	(.215)	(.246)	(.247)
Black	−.373**	−.525**	.309	.084	−.174	−.370	.392*	.397*	.531*	.455†
	(.128)	(.183)	(.215)	(.211)	(.275)	(.281)	(.162)	(.190)	(.229)	(.235)
No visits	−.516**		.119		.309		.017		.158	
	(.184)		(.188)		(.217)		(.177)		(.252)	
Latina/o × no visits	−.584		−.424		−.424		−.198		−.486	
	(.448)		(.540)		(.540)		(.418)		(.604)	
Black × no visits	−.379		−.089		−.089		.013		.352	
	(.580)		(.871)		(.871)		(.539)		(.592)	
No usual source of care		−.739***		−.263		−.101		−.302*		−.479†
		(.159)		(.204)		(.217)		(.144)		(.254)
Latina/o × no usual source of care		.246		−.058		.076		−.247		.089
		(.327)		(.472)		(.463)		(.354)		(.428)
Black × no usual source of care		.249		.820†		.539		.075		.610
		(.448)		(.422)		(.614)		(.377)		(.477)
Constant	.702	1.189**	−4.852***	−3.610**	−3.554***	−2.799***	−2.154***	−1.125*	−3.588***	−2.497**
	(.649)	(.681)	(1.155)	(1.028)	(.829)	(.757)	(.590)	(.521)	(.797)	(.867)

Notes: Robust standard errors are in parentheses. All models control for respondents' socio-demographic background, health and health care context. Models for family/friends, government agencies, and charitable organizations include adjustments for sampling frame used.
† $p < .10$; * $p < .05$; ** $p < .01$; *** $p < .001$.

non-users. The differences themselves, however, did change in the propensity-adjusted models. The difference in likelihood between Latina/os and whites became only marginal in M3 and M4 (decreased from $p < .05$ to $p < .10$). The result suggests that self-selection into making a recent health care visit overestimated the Latina/o-white difference in these models. The propensity-adjusted M5 (which includes all statistical controls) showed that only blacks have a significantly lower likelihood than whites of reporting trust in physicians, suggesting that the black-white difference remains after accounting for self-selection into making a recent visit.

I also revisited the second set of models in Table 2, where health care user was defined as having a usual source of care (M6–M9), with the propensity score analysis. Once again the interactions of interest remained non-significant, indicating that racial and ethnic differences in the likelihood of trusting a physician "a lot" were equivalent among health care users and non-users. The difference in likelihood among black and white respondents in M9 decreased in significance, but remained within the critical alpha-level ($p < .01$ to $p < .05$), suggesting that self-selection bias overestimated the black-white difference. The patterns for Latina/os remained comparable to the original findings in Table 2.

In a second set of auxiliary analyses, I assessed the extent that patterns of trust differed between complete and non-complete cases. Respondents who were complete cases had a significantly greater likelihood of trusting a physician and the government "a lot." However, the focus of this analysis is on the racial and ethnic differences in these likelihoods. These differences were equivalent among health care users and non-users (both empirical definitions), suggesting that complete case analysis did not bias the relations of conceptual interest (Allison, 2001). Additional support that missingness did not bias results was evidenced when I entered in a dichotomous code to mark which of the respondents were missing values on income, the measure with the greatest missing responses, and found results to be substantively the same. Lastly, there were no significant differences in likelihood of trusting the other three sources (Internet, family/friends, charitable organizations) "a lot."

DISCUSSION

The results imply the existence of a generalized distrust in physicians as a source of health information among racial and ethnic minorities. The findings indicated that racial and ethnic minorities – specifically, blacks and Latina/os – were significantly more likely to distrust physicians than whites, and these differences were comparable between health care users and non-users. The differences were consistent regardless of how I operationalized health care user status (regular vs. recent user), and furthermore were robust to adjustments for respondents' socio-demographic background and health status. These patterns were unique to physicians as a health information source in that they did not manifest when I examined distrust in other information sources. Even accounting for respondents' propensity to be a health care user did not change findings significantly, particularly for black respondents.

The existence of generalized distrust in physicians implies that other processes beyond just differential health care experiences are likely operating to produce racial patterns. One such process may be differential socialization patterns. For example, blacks are generally distrustful of medical research (Chandra & Paul, 2003; Corbie-Smith et al., 2002; Freimuth et al., 2001; Gamble, 1997), perhaps in part because of knowledge of the historical abuse of blacks in this context (Brandon, Isaac, & LaVeist, 2005). The transmission of racially patterned narratives about the medical system can also happen more subtly, such as while observing a parent or guardian interact with a physician as a young child (Cox, Smith, Brown, & Fitzpatrick, 2009; Hammond, 2010; Lareau, 2002). Additional research should unpack these and other processes that contribute to distrust in physicians because such distrust is negatively associated with health and health care outcomes (LaVeist et al., 2009; Piette et al., 2005; Saha et al., 2010; Wileman et al., 2002).

While much research has focused on improving overall health care experience to address disparities, this research offers empirical support for others' contentions that the issue extends beyond the walls of health care (e.g., LaVeist & Nuru-Jeter, 2002; Malat, 2001; Stepanikova et al., 2006). Accordingly, we need to develop more community-based applications to assess and improve racial and ethnic minorities' perceptions of physicians and other health care professionals. For example, one initiative in Chicago works with existing infrastructures to improve community residents' communication with physicians during clinic visits (Peek et al., 2012). A strength of the initiative is that it complements the community-based approach with a traditional approach, physician training, and recognizes the multi-faceted nature of the problem.

It may also be beneficial to leverage the health information sources that racial and ethnic minorities trust. The Internet, for example, showed non-significant racial and ethnic differences. Prior research suggests that minorities tend to use health information from the Internet more often than non-minorities, perhaps to substitute for resources they lack (Mesch, Mano, & Tsamir, 2012). Accessing health information on the Internet is also positively related to future health care use, because individuals find that a physician's expertise is prudent for interpreting and contextualizing the information encountered (Kivits, 2006; Sommerhalder et al., 2009). Government-sponsored campaigns also appear to be a fruitful alternative to emphasize, perhaps also for also improving interactions with physicians. These campaigns may impart skills such as forming and articulating questions for medical visits (such as the "Questions are the Answer" campaign from the Agency for Healthcare Research and Quality, http://www.ahrq.gov/patients-consumers/patient-involvement/ask-your-doctor/index.html).

Relatedly, the finding that racial and ethnic minorities were more likely to trust the government as a health information source "a lot" than whites is unexpected for three reasons. First, one oft-cited reason for distrust in physicians among racial and ethnic minority is the legacy of maltreatment in the health care system, particularly through the Tuskegee syphilis experiment (Brandon et al., 2005; Gamble, 1997). A U.S. government agency (U.S. Public Health Service) conducted the Tuskegee experiment, though medical professionals carried out the actual procedures (Jones, 1993). A second reason for why these results are surprising is because of the prevalence of conspiracy theories among racial and ethnic minorities that the government is intentionally attempting to worsen their health (e.g., Corbie-Smith, Thomas, Williams, & Moody-Ayers, 1999; Ford, Wallace, Newman, Lee, & William Cunningham, 2013; Whetten et al., 2006). The results from this chapter imply that racial and ethnic minorities may be placing blame for maltreatment and conspiracy on the medical profession, while sparing the government. Third, this finding stands in contrast to previous ones showing that racial and ethnic minorities report less trust in the government than whites (e.g., Avery, 2006; Bobo & Gilliam, 1990; Ford et al., 2013). It appears that an exception to this general trend is the case when the government offers health information. Future research should clarify why blacks and Latina/os are more likely than whites to trust in this specific component of government behavior.

Notably, distrust among black respondents exhibited greater signs of generalization than among Latina/os. The Latina/o-white difference in distrust was only significant in models that defined health care user as having a usual source of care. Moreover, propensity-adjusted models erased the

Latina/o-white differences when health care user was defined as having made a recent visit. Most of the research that documents racial patterns of trust in physicians primarily focuses on black-white differences (e.g., Boulware et al., 2003; Cooper et al., 2003; Corbie-Smith et al., 2002; LaVeist et al., 2000), while those few studies that are the exception to this trend and examine Latina/os as well still only include health care users in the analyses (e.g., Doescher et al., 2000; Schnittker, 2004; Stepanikova et al., 2006). Given the heterogeneity within the Latina/o racial category, such as skin tone (Bonilla-Silva, 2004), it is important that future research examine whether a generalized distrust exists for certain subgroups.

The findings should be interpreted in the context of other studies examining trust in physicians. The measure used represents trust in a physician's behavior (providing health information), which is an indirect rating of trust. This is different from direct ratings of trust, such as the following item from the Trust in Physician Scale (Anderson & Dedrick, 1990; Thom, Ribisl, Stewart, Douglas, & The Stanford Trust Study Physicians, 1999): "I trust my doctor to put my medical needs above all other considerations when treating my medical problems." Many agree that there are qualitative differences among trust measures (Anderson & Dedrick, 1990; Hall et al., 2002; Thom et al., 1999), but few have demonstrated that these differences have empirical consequences. One exception is Stepanikova et al. (2006), who found that racial and ethnic differences in trust only manifest when the measure is an indirect, not a direct, rating. They advocate for making this distinction in research examining racial differences in trust to help clarify mixed findings. Accordingly, I caution that the existence of a generalized distrust in physicians among racial and ethnic minorities may only occur when examining indirect measures of trust.

The findings should also be interpreted in light of the study's limitations. Factors that contribute to self-selection into being a health care user are often concurrently related to trust in a physician, resulting in selection bias. I conducted a propensity score analysis that suggested where precisely the selection bias occurs, but outside of longitudinal and experimental research it is difficult to account for selection bias comprehensively. A second limitation is that I am unable to disentangle how provider setting may influence patterns. Racial and ethnic minorities are more likely than whites to cite an emergency department as their usual source of care (Walls, Rhodes, & Kennedy, 2002), and this type of provider setting is least likely to inspire trust (Whetten et al., 2006). This makes information on type of usual source of care relevant for model specification. I would expect that accounting for type of provider setting would further weaken the relationship between having a usual source of care and trust among racial and ethnic minorities.

Future research could not only attempt to address these limitations, but also build on the findings presented here. The cross-sectional nature of the surveys incites the need to understand longitudinal relationships. It is not clear from these data what, if any, would be the racially patterned experiences of health care non-users as they become recent and regular users. Research lines that incorporate comparisons of users and non-users of health care over time are crucial to understanding patient experiences in the contemporary health information setting, and for documenting generalized distrust in physicians.

NOTE

1. In an auxiliary analysis, I determined that the language of the survey did not moderate the relationships of interest among those respondents who completed a CATI.

REFERENCES

Allison, P. (2001). *Missing data*. Thousand Oaks, CA: Sage.

Anderson, L. A., & Dedrick, R. F. (1990). Development of the trust in physician scale: A measure to assess interpersonal trust in patient-physician relationships. *Psychological Reports*, *67*, 1091–1100.

Avery, J. M. (2006). The sources and consequences of political mistrust among African Americans. *American Politics Research*, *34*, 653–682.

Bobo, L., & Gilliam, F. D., Jr. (1990). Race, sociopolitical participation, and black empowerment. *American Political Science Review*, *84*, 377–393.

Bonilla-Silva, E. (2004). From bi-racial to tri-racial: Towards a new system of racial stratification in the USA. *Ethnic and Racial Studies*, *27*, 931–950.

Boulware, L. E., Cooper, L. A., Ratner, L. E., LaVeist, T. A., & Powe, N. R. (2003). Race and trust in the health care system. *Public health reports*, *118*, 358.

Brandon, D. T., Isaac, L. A., & LaVeist, T. A. (2005). The legacy of Tuskegee and trust in medical care: Is Tuskegee responsible for race differences in mistrust of medical care? *Journal of the National Medical Association*, *97*, 951–956.

Cantor, D., Coa, K., Crystal-Mansour, S., Davis, T., Dipko, S., & Sigman, R. (2009). Health Information National Trends Survey (HINTS) 2007 final report. Westat, Rockville, MD.

Chandra, A., & Paul III, D. P. (2003). African American participation in clinical trials: Recruitment difficulties and potential remedies. *Hospital Topics*, *81*, 33–38.

Cooper, L. A., Roter, D. L., Johnson, R. L., Ford, D. E., Steinwachs, D. M., & Powe, N. R. (2003). Patient-centered communication, ratings of care, and concordance of patient and physician race. *Annals of Internal Medicine, 139*, 907–915.

Cooper-Patrick, L., Powe, N. R., Jenckes, M. W., Mhs, Gonzales, J. J., Levine, D. M., & Ford, D. E. (1997). Identification of patient attitudes and preferences regarding treatment of depression. *Journal of General Internal Medicine, 12*, 431–438.

Corbie-Smith, G., Thomas, S. B., & St George, D. M. (2002). Distrust, race, and research. *Archives of Internal Medicine, 162*, 2458–2463.

Corbie-Smith, G., Thomas, S. B., Williams, M. V., & Moody-Ayers, S. (1999). Attitudes and beliefs of African Americans toward participation in medical research. *Journal of General Internal Medicine, 14*, 537–546.

Cox, E. D., Smith, M. A., Brown, R. L., & Fitzpatrick, M. A. (2009). Learning to participate: Effect of child age and parental education on participation in pediatric visits. *Health Communication, 24*, 249–258.

Doescher, M. P., Saver, B. G., Franks, P., & Fiscella, K. (2000). Racial and ethnic disparities in perceptions of physician style and trust. *Archives of Family Medicine, 9*, 1156–1163.

Fiscella, K., Meldrum, S., Peter, F., Cleveland, G. S., Duberstein, P., McDaniel, S. H., & Epstein, R. M. (2004). Patient trust: Is it related to patient-centered behavior of primary care physicians? *Medical Care, 42*, 1049–1055.

Ford, C. L., Wallace, S. P., Newman, P. A., Lee, S.-J., & William Cunningham, E. (2013). Belief in AIDS-related conspiracy theories and mistrust in the government: Relationship With HIV testing among at-risk older adults. *The Gerontologist, 53*, 973–984.

Freimuth, V. S., Quinn, S. C., Thomas, S. B., Cole, G., Zook, E., & Duncan, T. (2001). African Americans' views on research and the Tuskegee syphilis study. *Social Science & Medicine, 52*, 797–808.

Gamble, V. N. (1997). Under the shadow of Tuskegee: African Americans and health care. *American Journal of Public Health, 87*, 1773–1778.

Gordon, H. S., Street, R. L., Sharf, B. F., Kelly, P. A., & Souchek, J. (2006). Racial differences in trust and lung cancer patients' perceptions of physician communication. *Journal of Clinical Oncology, 24*, 904–909.

Halbert, C. H., Armstrong, K., Gandy, O. H., & Shaker, L. (2006). Racial differences in trust in health care providers. *Archives of Internal Medicine, 166*(8), 896–901.

Hall, M. A., Camacho, F., Dugan, E., & Balkrishnan, R. (2002). Trust in the medical profession: Conceptual and measurement issues. *Health Services Research, 37*, 1419–1439.

Hall, M. A., Zheng, B., Dugan, E., Camacho, F., Kidd, K. E., Mishra, A., & Balkrishnan, R. (2002). Measuring patients' trust in their primary care providers. *Medical Care Research and Review, 59*, 293–318.

Hammond, W. P. (2010). Psychosocial correlates of medical mistrust among African American men. *American Journal of Community Psychology, 45*, 87–106.

Hesse, B. W., Moser, R. P., & Rutten, L. J. (2010). Surveys of physicians and electronic health information. *New England Journal of Medicine, 362*, 859–860.

Jacobs, E. A., Rolle, I., Ferrans, C. E., Whitaker, E. E., & Warnecke, R. B. (2006). Understanding African Americans' views of the trustworthiness of physicians. *Journal of General Internal Medicine, 21*, 642–647.

Jones, J. H. (1993). *Bad blood*. New York, NY: Free Press.

Keating, N. L., Gandhi, T. K., Orav, E. J., Bates, D. W., & Ayanian, J. Z. (2004). Patient characteristics and experiences associated with trust in specialist physicians. *Archives of Internal Medicine*, *164*, 1015–1020.

Kessler, R. C., Andrews, G., Colpe, L. J., Hiripi, E., Mroczek, D. K., Normand, S.-L. T., ... Zaslavsky, A. M. (2002). Short screening scales to monitor population prevalences and trends in non-specific psychological distress. *Psychological Medicine*, *32*, 959–976.

Kivits, J. (2006). Informed patients and the internet: A mediated context for consultations with health professionals. *Journal of Health Psychology*, *11*, 269–282.

Kroll, T. L., Richardson, M., Sharf, B. F., & Suarez-Almazor, M. E. (2007). "Keep on truckin" or "It's got you in this little vacuum": Race-based perceptions in decision-making for total knee arthroplasty. *Journal of Rheumatology*, *34*, 1069–1075.

Lareau, A. (2002). Invisible inequality: Social class and childrearing in black families and white families. *American Sociological Review*, *67*, 747–776.

LaVeist, T. A., Isaac, L. A., & Williams, K. P. (2009). Mistrust of health care organizations is associated with underutilization of health services. *Health Services Research*, *44*, 2093–2105.

LaVeist, T. A., Nickerson, K. J., & Bowie, J. V. (2000). Attitudes about racism, medical mistrust, and satisfaction with care among African American and white cardiac patients. *Medical Care Research and Review*, *57*, 146–161.

LaVeist, T. A., & Nuru-Jeter, A. (2002). Is doctor-patient race concordance associated with greater satisfaction with care? *Journal of Health and Social Behavior*, *43*, 296–306.

Long, J. S. (1997). *Regression models for categorical and limited dependent variables*. Thousand Oaks, CA: Sage.

Malat, J. (2001). Social distance and patients' rating of healthcare providers. *Journal of Health and Social Behavior*, *42*(4), 360–372.

McCabe, C. (2004). Nurse–patient communication: an exploration of patients' experiences. *Journal of Clinical Nursing*, *13*, 41–49.

McKnight, D. H., Cummings, L. L., & Chervany, N. L. (1998). Initial trust formation in new organizational relationships. *Academy of Management Review*, *23*, 473–490.

Mechanic, D. (1996). Changing medical organization and the erosion of trust. *The Milbank Quarterly*, *74*, 171–189.

Mesch, G., Mano, R., & Tsamir, J. (2012). Minority status and health information search: A test of the social diversification hypothesis. *Social Science & Medicine*, *75*, 854–858.

Nan, X., Zhao, X., & Briones, R. (2013). Parental cancer beliefs and trust in health information from medical authorities as predictors of HPV vaccine acceptability. *Journal of Health Communication*, *19*(1), 100–114.

O'Malley, A. S., Sheppard, V. B., Schwartz, M., & Mandelblatt, J. (2004). The role of trust in use of preventive services among low-income African-American Women. *Preventive Medicine*, *38*, 777–785.

Parsons, T. (1951). *The social system*. Glencoe, IL: Free Press.

Peek, M. E., Wilkes, A. E., Roberson, T. S., Goddu, A. P., Nocon, R. S., Tang, H., & Chin, M. H. (2012). Early lessons from an initiative On Chicago's south side to reduce disparities in diabetes care and outcomes. *Health Affairs*, *31*, 177–186.

Pescosolido, B. A., Tuch, S. A., & Martin, J. K. (2001). The profession of medicine and the public: Examining Americans' changing confidence in physician authority from the beginning of the 'health care crisis' to the era of health care reform. *Journal of Health and Social Behavior*, *42*, 1–16.

Piette, J. D., Heisler, M., Krein, S., & Kerr, E. A. (2005). The role of patient-physician trust in moderating medication nonadherence due to cost pressures. *Archives of Internal Medicine*, *165*, 1749–1755.

Richardson, A., Appleyard, A. J., Xiao, H., & Vallone, D. (2012). Effects of race/ethnicity and socioeconomic status on health information-seeking, confidence, and trust. *Journal of Health Care for the Poor and Underserved*, *23*, 1477–1493.

Rosenbaum, P. R., & Rubin, D. B. (1984). Reducing bias in observational studies using subclassification on the propensity score. *Journal of the American Statistical Association*, *79*, 516–524.

Rubin, D. B. (1997). Estimating causal effects from large data sets using propensity scores. *Annals of Internal Medicine*, *127*, 757–763.

Saha, S., Jacobs, E. A., Moore, R. D., & Beach, M. C. (2010). Trust in physicians and racial disparities in HIV Care. *AIDS Patient Care & STDs*, *24*, 415–420.

Saha, S., Sanders, D. S., Korthuis, P. T., Cohn, J. A., Sharp, V. L., Haidet, P., ... Beach, M. C. (2011). The role of cultural distance between patient and provider in explaining racial/ethnic disparities in HIV care. *Patient Education and Counseling*, *85*, e278–e284.

Savage, S. V. (2011). Patients, trust, and patient participation: Factors influencing whether patients want to be active health care participants. *Research in the Sociology of Health Care*, *29*, 149–171.

Schnittker, J. (2004). Social distance in the clinical encounter: Interactional and sociodemographic foundations for mistrust in physicians. *Social Psychology Quarterly*, *67*, 217–235.

Schnittker, J., & Liang, K. (2006). The promise and limits of racial/ethnic concordance in physician-patient interaction. *Journal of Health Politics, Policy and Law*, *31*, 811–838.

Schuster, M. A., Collins, R., Cunningham, W. E., Morton, S. C., Zierler, S., Wong, M., & Kanouse, D. E. (2005). Perceived discrimination in clinical care in a nationally representative sample of HIV-infected adults receiving health care. *Journal of General Internal Medicine*, *20*, 807–813.

Sommerhalder, K., Abraham, A., Zufferey, M. C., Barth, J., & Abel, T. (2009). Internet information and medical consultations: Experiences from patients' and physicians' perspectives. *Patient Education and Counseling*, *77*, 266–271.

Soulakova, J. N., Hartman, A. M., Liu, B., Willis, G. B., & Augustine, S. (2012). Reliability of adult self-reported smoking history: Data from the tobacco use supplement to the current population survey 2002–2003 cohort. *Nicotine & Tobacco Research*, *14*, 952–960.

Stepanikova, I., Mollborn, S., Cook, K. S., Thom, D. H., & Kramer, R. M. (2006). Patients' race, ethnicity, language, and trust in a physician. *Journal of Health and Social Behavior*, *47*, 390–405.

Thom, D. H. (2001). Physician behaviors that predict patient trust. *Journal of Family Practice*, *50*, 323–328.

Thom, D. H., Ribisl, K. M., Stewart, A. L., Douglas, A. L., & The Stanford Trust Study Physicians. (1999). Further validation and reliability testing of the trust in physician scale. *Medical Care*, *37*, 510–517.

Van Ryn, M., & Pu, S. S. (2003). Paved With good intentions: Do public health and human service providers contribute to racial/ethnic disparities in health? *American Journal of Public Health*, *93*, 248–255.

Wallace, L. S., Chisolm, D. J., Abdel Rasoul, M., & DeVoe, J. E. (2013). Survey mode matters: Adults' self-reported statistical confidence, ability to obtain health information, and perceptions of patient–health-care provider communication. *Journal of Health Psychology*, *18*, 1036–1045.

Walls, C. A., Rhodes, K. V., & Kennedy, J. J. (2002). The emergency department as usual source of medical care: Estimates from the 1998 national health interview survey. *Academic Emergency Medicine*, *9*, 1140–1145.

Ware, J. E., Jr., Kosinski, M., & Keller, S. D. (1996). A 12-item short-form health survey: Construction of scales and preliminary tests of reliability and validity. *Medical Care*, *34*, 220–233.

Whetten, K., Leserman, J., Whetten, R., Ostermann, J., Thielman, N., Swartz, M., & Stangl, D. (2006). Exploring lack of trust in care providers and the government as a barrier to health service use. *American Journal of Public Health*, *96*, 716–721.

Wileman, L., May, C., & Chew-Graham, C. A. (2002). Medically unexplained symptoms and the problem of power in the primary care consultation: A qualitative study. *Family Practice*, *19*, 178–182.

"IT'S NOT THE DOCTOR – IT'S ME": HOW SELF-BLAME OBSCURES LANGUAGE AND OTHER STRUCTURAL BARRIERS TO DIABETES CARE AMONG LOW-INCOME LATINOS WITH LIMITED ENGLISH PROFICIENCY

Claudia Chaufan, Hegla Fielding, Catherine Chesla and Alicia Fernandez

ABSTRACT

Purpose – *Professional interpreter use improves care in patients with limited English proficiency (LEP) but inequalities in outcomes remain. We explore the experience of US Latinos with LEP and diabetes in language discordant care.*

Education, Social Factors, and Health Beliefs in Health and Health Care Services
Research in the Sociology of Health Care, Volume 33, 187–208

ISSN: 0275-4959/doi:10.1108/S0275-495920150000033013

Methodology/approach – *We conducted in-depth interviews of 20 low-income Latino patients with diabetes and LEP. We interviewed participants in Spanish, digitally recorded and transcribed interviews, and read transcripts to identify themes and interpret meanings using interpretive phenomenology as theoretical framework.*

Findings – *While patients preferred, and experienced greater trust in, language concordant clinical encounters, they did not believe that language discordance affected outcomes because they felt that these depended largely on their compliance with physicians' recommendations. Patients also downplayed structural barriers to care and outcomes. Self-blame was paradoxically encouraged by physicians' praise vis-à-vis favorable outcomes.*

Research limitations/implications – *Limitations include small and convenience sample and limited generalizability. However, findings illustrate communicational dynamics between patients and clinicians with important implications for health care practice and policy. They support the perception that trust develops best within language concordant care, which underscores the importance of recruiting clinicians with diverse language skills. They highlight the importance of sensitizing clinicians to the social determinants of health, which may be overlooked when treating patients with conditions requiring substantial self-management, like diabetes. Language barriers in health care must be understood in the broader context of structural inequalities in health care. The necessary emphasis on self-management may (inadvertently) strengthen the hegemonic view that places responsibility for diabetes outcomes on patients' ability to self-manage their condition to the neglect of social/political determinants of diabetes.*

Originality/value – *Studies have quantitatively examined the effects of language discordant care on diabetes outcomes, yet few have done so qualitatively. To our knowledge, no study has attempted to understand the experience of language discordance from the perspective of LEP patients with diabetes and how this experience may explain observed differences in outcomes.*

Keywords: Hispanic/Latino; diabetes care; diabetes inequalities; language discordant care; interpretive phenomenology; ideology of healthism

INTRODUCTION

Effective communication between physicians and patients is essential to the provision of quality health care. Language barriers encountered in the care of patients with limited English proficiency (LEP), a growing segment of the US population, impair communication and in so doing may adversely affect health care quality and clinical outcomes (Wilson, Chen, Grumbach, Wang, & Fernandez, 2005). LEP patients have decreased access to preventive services (Harlan, Bernstein, & Kessler, 1991; Pearson, Zhao, & Ford, 2011), decreased satisfaction with care (Carrasquillo, Orav, Brennan, & Burstin, 1999; Morales, Cunningham, Brown, Liu, & Hays, 1999), and an increased risk of medical errors and misdiagnoses (Flores, Abreu, Olivar, & Kastner, 1998). A substantial number – 21 out of 52 million – of US Latinos, the fastest growing US minority, report speaking English less than "very well" (Ryan, 2011), thus are particularly vulnerable to the limitations of care across the language divide. Patients with diabetes, a complex disease that requires substantial patient engagement and robust patient-clinician communication, may be particularly vulnerable, and inequalities in diabetes care among Latinos are well documented (Peek, Cargill, & Huang, 2007; Timmins, 2002). Multiple factors produce and perpetuate diabetes inequalities, including class inequalities and varying forms of institutional discrimination (Centers for Disease Control & Prevention, 2011; Institute of Medicine, 2002). Clinicians may inadvertently contribute to these inequalities as they confront the challenge of delivering care to individuals who are not proficient in the language and mores of the dominant culture (Hudelson, Dominice Dao, Junod Perron, & Bischoff, 2013; Schenker, Lo, Ettinger, & Fernandez, 2008; Schouten & Meeuwesen, 2006; Seale, Rivas, & Kelly, 2013).

The use of professional interpreters may improve the quality of care for patients with LEP, by reducing inequalities in utilization rates and increasing patient satisfaction (Karliner, Jacobs, Chen, & Mutha, 2007), characteristically lower among these patients (Carrasquillo et al., 1999; Fernandez et al., 2004). Despite the well-documented utility of professional interpreters, patients who receive language discordant care may nonetheless experience worse clinical outcomes than those who receive language concordant care. Among Latinos patients with diabetes, LEP status is an independent predictor of poor glycemic control only when care is provided by language discordant clinicians yet not when it is provided by language concordant clinicians (Fernandez et al., 2011).

Several studies have quantitatively examined the effects of language discordant care on diabetes care and outcomes, yet far fewer have done so qualitatively. One study using structured observations of doctor-patient interactions found that language discordant care led to significant decreases in the amount of social talk, patient assertiveness, and patient engagement in the consultation, whereas language concordant care involved more discussions of patients feelings, motivations, and lifeworlds (Seale et al., 2013). Nevertheless, and to the best of our knowledge, no study has attempted to probe further into these observations so as to understand the experience of language discordant care from the perspective of patients, and what distinct features of this experience may explain the observed differences in diabetes outcomes. In this qualitative study we explore and interpret patient experience with language discordant care and elaborate on the implications of our findings for health care practice, research and policy, and for the goal of reducing health care inequalities. It is part of a larger project examining patient-clinician communication across the language divide.

METHODS

Sample Description

We interviewed a convenience sample of 20 self-identified Latino patients who receive diabetes care at a major public, urban teaching hospital in the San Francisco Bay Area serving largely minority and low-income populations. Inclusion criteria were self-identified Latino ethnicity, type 2 diabetes as diagnosed by a health professional and limited English proficiency (LEP) as assessed using the following question from the Diabetes Study of Northern California (DISTANCE) survey: "How often do you have difficulty understanding or speaking English?" (Fernandez et al., 2011). If patients replied "usually" or "often" rather than "sometimes" "rarely" or "never" they were considered to have LEP and to be eligible for the study.

Design, Data Collection, and Qualitative Data Analysis

This project was designed using principles of interpretive phenomenology. This qualitative research method assumes that informants, practically engaged and situated within their particular worlds, can ably inform on their experiences using direct concrete narratives of actual events as well as reflections or evaluations of those experiences (Benner, 1994; Chesla, 1995). The interview guide solicited both narratives and reflections (interview guide available upon request).

Participants were recruited from the waiting room of the general medicine clinic at the research site by the first and second authors, who also screened participants for eligibility. In this clinic, patients receive care from a primary care clinician who may or may not speak Spanish. They also have experience of care from a broader clinical team when their primary clinician is not available. Professional health care interpreters who work for the hospital are available via video mediated interpretation during clinic hours; if video interpreters are busy, interpreters are available by phone from a commercial vendor. In rare cases, usually involving complex and sensitive communication such as a new cancer diagnosis, physicians may request that a hospital interpreter participate in person.

Once determined to be eligible, participants were interviewed in a private room on-site at the clinic. Interviews were conducted in Spanish (the first, second, and fourth authors are native Spanish speakers), lasted one hour and a half on average, and were digitally recorded, transcribed, and analyzed. The first and second authors interviewed all participants. After providing written informed consent, participants completed a brief interviewer-administered questionnaire eliciting socioeconomic, demographic, language proficiency, and basic diabetes and health information. This portion of the meeting lasted 20 minutes on average. The remainder of the session was devoted to a semi-structured qualitative interview designed to elicit participants' narratives of direct experience of language discordant care and reflections on this experience, addressing four overarching topics: (a) how language concordant diabetes care differs from language discordant diabetes care; (b) how language concordance/discordance influences their diabetes management and outcomes; (c) informant reflections on what can help improve patient/provider communication; (d) characteristics of providers that patients value in managing their diabetes. Presenting these general topics to patients allowed them to define in their own words their experience of receiving care across the language divide and to share and reflect upon the strategies they used to face the demands of diabetes self management.

Because the sample size was small, we conducted our analysis with the sole aid of a word processor (Microsoft Office Word 2007). The first author read the original Spanish transcripts in their entirety and in the original Spanish version and identified emergent interpretive/analytic themes. Then the second author reviewed the transcripts and identified selected passages that illuminated these themes, while at the same time remaining open to new themes evident in the text. Next, the first and second authors met to discuss emerging themes and texts that illuminated or contradicted those themes, and developed interpretations of the meaning of the selected passages for participants, resolving discrepancies by consensus. The third author, an experienced qualitative researcher and expert in interpretive phenomenology, instructed the first author on the principles of this method, and provided extensive feedback during the initial phase of the analysis. The fourth author, an expert in language discordant care and Latino health, oversaw the investigation, read and interpreted selected transcripts, and made recommendations concerning the implications of the findings for research, policy and practice. The first author translated the selected quotes and wrote the initial and subsequent drafts, which were read by all authors who provided feedback until completion of a manuscript for submission. The Committee for Human Research at the University of California in San Francisco approved the study.

FINDINGS

Out of 20 participants, most (75%, *N*: 15) were women, with ages ranging between 35 and 73 years. All but two had incomes under 200% of the poverty line and half had completed elementary school or less. Most were Salvadorean (50%, *N*: 10) or Mexican (40%, *N*: 8) immigrants, and all lived in urban areas. The majority (65%, *N*: 13) did not receive food assistance, although about a third of these said they had unmet food needs. An important minority (40%, *N*: 8) relied on pantries to satisfy their food needs. Over one third of participants (35%, *N*: 7) either had trouble finding work (25%, *N*: 5) or were too discouraged to look for work (10%, *N*: 2), whereas a similar number (30%, *N*: 6) was not working because holding a job would reduce their benefits (e.g., Social Security).

The duration of participants' diabetes ranged between 1 and 24 years (average duration 11 years), with a Hemoglobin A1C[1] ranging between 5.4% and 11% (average 8%). All participants had been prescribed diet and exercise as a treatment for their diabetes, all but two were on oral medication, a significant minority (45%, *N*: 9) used insulin, and all but two self-monitored their blood glucose.

A majority (60%, *N*: 12) of patients reported that their primary care physicians (and one a nurse practitioner) spoke little (50%, *N*: 10) or no

(10%, *N*: 2) Spanish – this we defined as language discordant care – whereas the remainder reported that their physician's Spanish language skills were acceptable (10%, *N*: 2), good (5%, *N*: 1), very good (10%, *N*: 2), or excellent (15%, *N*: 3), which we defined as language concordant care.

The Dialectic between Trust, Language, and Other Structural Barriers to Care and Self-Blame

Our interpretation of patient interviews yielded two salient findings. First, participants deeply valued having a warm, humane and affectionate doctor-patient relationship and felt that the quality of this relationship was critical to their ability to develop trust with their clinician. Our findings and analysis illustrate some of the specific features of the clinical encounter that support trust from the perspective of patients, confirming what quantitative studies have repeatedly indicated (Ong, Visser, Lammes, & de Haes, 2000; Roter, Hall, & Katz, 1987; Stewart, 1995), yet often failed to articulate for lack of sufficient detail from participants' lives. Second, participants dismissed language and other structural barriers to diabetes care, driven by a conviction that diabetes outcomes depend almost exclusively on their own behaviors. As one participant eloquently put it: "diabetes care [is the responsibility of] the person with diabetes."

Patients' strong preference for language concordant care was due precisely to the fact that they could be more themselves and more able to share their life circumstances ("lifeworlds") when they communicated directly with their physician, which led them to feel greater trust, engage more easily in conversation, and experience a closer, more humane relationship with their clinicians. The ease of communication also encouraged patients to provide detailed information about their lives and circumstances that, even if not medical, appeared relevant to the day-to-day management of their diabetes. In contrast, when care was mediated by an interpreter, communication was reduced in scope and quality, as patients reported being less likely to share information with their physicians, mostly out of discomfort with three-way communication, unease with machine-mediated communication (video or phone), or embarrassment when information related to intimate topics (such as their sexual lives) was shared via a third party that they perceived as nonmedical personnel. Nevertheless, patients tended to trust the medical expertise of their physicians irrespective of their language competence, and seemed to value other features in them, such as humane and respectful treatment, beyond language concordance.

Contrary to our expectations, patients did not believe that language discordance affected diabetes outcomes, largely because they felt that these outcomes depend on their own willingness and ability to adhere to physicians' recommendations, typically involving dietary and exercise regimes. Patients insisted that diabetes outcomes depended on personal responsibility, even as they acknowledged that, for instance, when interacting with doctors who did not speak Spanish they were less likely to seek clarification of medical instructions – a potential barrier to good outcomes (Schouten & Meeuwesen, 2006; Seale et al., 2013). Patients also tended to downplay other structural barriers to treatment, such as family or work obligations, or financial barriers, all of which may be at odds with the demands of the medical and lifestyle treatments of diabetes (Chaufan, Constantino, & Davis, 2011; Piette, Heisler, & Wagner, 2004; Ross, Bradley, & Busch, 2006). Self-blame was paradoxically encouraged by physicians' praise of patients' behaviors when outcomes were favorable. In the following sections, we expand and elaborate on these interpretive/analytic themes.

"I Feel More Open, Calm, Happy": Being One's Authentic Self and Developing Trust

The most salient finding was that patients felt they could be "more themselves" in their own language, thus expressed a strong preference for language concordant care, even if some of them wondered whether it was language concordance rather than other features of their physicians, that we describe later, which explained this difference in their feelings:

> I feel more open when [the physician] speaks my language – I feel calm, happy – and for me it is easier to explain all that I have. [...]. I feel more comfortable ... in peace.

> When you have a doctor who speaks your language, you feel happy coming to the appointment, because if you feel bad about something, you are going to be able to tell them, and they will be able to listen, tell you what to do.

When probing this feeling further, with language discordant care patients reported lesser disposition to share information with their physicians, especially personal, nonmedical information, such as family responsibilities, work demands, or financial constraints that may get in the way of adhering to dietary recommendations, exercise routines, or medication regimes. Language discordant care was seen as particularly problematic when patients had health concerns that they felt embarrassed to share, for example, sensitive information related to their sexual lives. The very presence of the interpreter constituted a third party who, in patients' eyes, lacked the full status of a medical professional and undermined their feelings of ease and comfort.

> It'd feel embarrassed to tell other people to "tell this to the doctor"... let's take an example around, venereal disease, because I would be embarrassed to tell the interpreter.

> Sometimes, one is embarrassed to tell them these things [through an interpreter], or why I am having prostate, or sexual problems.

One patient mentioned the awkwardness of needing to speak to a machine while in an uncomfortable, even painful and intimately vulnerable, position, such as in the course of having a PAP smear, especially when compounded by gender-discordant interpreter services.

> It was one on the phone ... I was having a Pap smear and it is usually not a very good experience, there is always pain, you are complaining [...] and a man is doing the translations ... I felt that ... I did not like it. It was still painful for me, and I was moaning in pain, and while the man ... I think he was ... he cut off the communication and then put a woman.

Furthermore, patients felt a greater closeness with their physician if they were able to speak their own language because they perceived that machine-mediated communication – in the case of phone or video interpreter services – is less human.

> I too feel bad because I'm not paying attention because I'm listening to the machine, and [the doctor] is waiting, then [...] I'm listening to the machine and she is also in a conversation, that is, we are both doing ... I'm asking questions and she is answering, but the machine is the one responding, right?

Patients also felt that during language discordant care they missed aspects of nonverbal communication from physicians, cues that were important to patients, such as their ability to grasp their physician's concern for them, which was critical to their feelings about their physician's professionalism, by which they meant a physician's ability to interact with them "as human beings."

> Because if I had more trust [...] I would feel a lot more open to talk about how I feel [...]. It is not that it is hard, or that I am shy, no. Quite simply, it is because the person I see has an interest, the person is interested, right? Then you feel more open. There is a much higher level of professionalism. So, you open up, you can talk about your life.

> Q: So what does professionalism mean to you?

> Professionalism is when the doctor, when the doctor is aware that they are [...] dealing with human beings, and that each of us [...] is thinking in a different way.

As a result of feeling "more themselves," better understood, and better able to capture the humanity of the physician, and feeling that the physician in turn was able to better capture the patient's humanity and uniqueness, patients also felt greater trust toward physicians with whom they could communicate in their own language. Furthermore, patients also felt that minor interactions with physicians, interactions that patients value, happen in language concordant care that would not happen in language discordant encounters, which reinforced their feelings of trust. Such was the case of one participant who described how a language concordant physician had handed her a business card, inviting the patient to contact her in case of need, an exchange that the patient felt would not have happened had the physician not spoken Spanish.

"We Are in That Triangle": Conversational Dynamics and Inefficiencies

A critical factor accounting for patients' feelings less "themselves," thus less disposed to open up in language discordant encounters, even when quality interpreter services were available, was the awkwardness and inefficiency of three-way conversations. In most circumstances, patients thought that language discordant care required too many steps ("I tell him, he tells her, she tells him, he tells me"), which led to patients refraining from sharing or requesting information and produced feelings of awkwardness in all participants in the encounter.

> For example, the doctor said [...] Talk to the translator, and the translator tells me, I tell the translator what I think, right? And he refers to the doctor. *So we are, well, on that triangle* [...] for me it is a bit difficult [...] sometimes you can't even ask something that you would be interested in.

> Well, sometimes I feel like strange, right? Strange because I would like to explain to my doctor in my own words what I am going through so that he understands, but into a machine, I find that a bit funny, because ... I can't see any face, it's a machine ... It helps because it's telling the doctor what you're feeling, but still, you may get cut off, you need to dial again, so [the doctor] dials, enters my code and my card number, and waits to see if they're available ...

Feelings of awkwardness appeared to be worse for certain types of interpreter mediations (e.g., telephone), but the feeling expressed appeared independent of the modality of interpretation, whether video, in person, or via family members.

"An Interpreter Can Say Anything That Is Not": Barriers to Trust

Not only were patients' openness and disposition to communicate their concerns impaired by the awkward conversational dynamics of interpreted medical encounters, they were also affected by an erosion of trust, especially for patients concerned about the fidelity of the interpretation. Indeed, trust was a constant theme in patients' narratives. Thus, a fair number of patients feared that interpreters would mistranslate, and even if they did not, many of them felt that the nuances of the communication would be lost in translation, as they often believed that interpreters may be less mindful of these nuances than physicians.

> I do not trust an interpreter because they can say anything that is not.
>
> But I've noticed that sometimes [...] one would like to explain something, there's many ways to say something, but interpreters do not capture what we are saying. Sometimes they translate something shorter, or miss details, and one would like the doctor to understand [...]. I often noticed that I mention my symptoms, and hear when the interpreter is translating to the doctor; they say some things but omit others ...

Distrust with inaccurate interpretations was lessened when either patients or doctors had some grasp of each others' language. Indeed, one issue that was salient during our investigation is that language proficiency, whether on the part of providers or patients, was a continuum of skills. Often, patients had a fairly good understanding of English, such that while they could not express themselves in English, their understanding was enough to grasp what a physician was communicating and to develop a feel for the accuracy of the interpretation. For instance, patients would notice whether an interpretation was substantially shorter than the statement the physician made. It was also often the case that the doctor could not speak Spanish but could still partially understand the patient and was able to communicate this understanding to him or her, which contributed to the latter's reassurance and trust in the accuracy of the communication and in the relationship. As one patient put it "Because I can understand a little, I do understand what's going on; what I cannot do is speak English, but [understanding what's going on] reassures me."

"They Assist You Out of Charity": Further Barriers to Trust

In addition to issues around interpreters, feelings of discrimination compounded barriers to trust, especially among patients who had experienced changes in class and insurance status related to the 2008 recession. This point is illustrated by one patient who had been laid off from a well-paid, middle-class job, thus had lost at once her income and her employer-sponsored health care coverage. She was then forced to seek diabetes care in, as she put it, "a medical establishment for low-income people."

> At Kaiser, my doctor was more demanding with me. She would tell me "You need to do this; you need to take your diabetes seriously. Otherwise your kidneys will be in trouble." And she would send me to diabetes classes. I received a lot of support from her. [In these classes] they would talk to me, monitor how I was doing. But here, my doctor does not support me; he only tells me to take my meds.
>
> Q: And how do you feel ...?
>
> Well I don't know, because these are my first times in these hospitals, and I think it is normal, what can I say. I think to myself "maybe it's because ... we have no health insurance, and this is how they treat people." This is how medical establishments for low income people are .... They assist you out of charity.

This patient did not appear to doubt the competence of her physician at the public hospital, yet felt that at the private institution where she used to receive care her physician strove to provide better care. She speculated that her current provider had failed to send her to diabetes classes and to insist that she monitor her blood sugar, and had instead indicated medications because that was the norm when assisting poor patients.

"It's Not the Doctor. It's Me": The Role of Self-Blame

Of note, and despite evidence from quantitative studies, including our own, indicating that language discordant care correlates with worse outcomes, no patient in our sample articulated a clear conviction that language discordance played any role in diabetes management or outcomes. Repeatedly, patients asserted that their physician did their part by instructing them on the medical and lifestyle treatment of diabetes, and that diabetes outcomes depended exclusively on patients themselves and their ability to follow physicians' instructions, or alternatively, put into practice information and advice from educational groups, relatives, or friends. Indeed, patients often downplayed the impact of factors such as family or work obligations, or the financial burden of dietary modifications or medications, even as they acknowledged the existence of such factors in their narratives,

> It is not the doctor – it's me. The doctor tells me a lot, gives good advice. If one does not follow, she is not to blame. It's me.

> Sometimes we only have beans and rice [and] I cannot follow a diet of vegetables, chicken, all that. But when my son is working everything is alright, we have money for chicken ... I exercise, I drink enough water, and I follow my diet. But, I really like chocolate, and I like many things that I cannot eat, and sometimes, I don't follow instructions ("no hago caso").

The idea of patient responsibility was reinforced, however inadvertently, by physicians' praise of patients' engagement in the daily management of their diabetes, and by their positive reaction to patients' achievements concerning dietary, physical activity, or other goals for lifestyle changes. As one patient noted,

> [The doctor] tells me "your tests came down," and I know she feels happy. When I was level [HbA1c] 9, I promised her that I would try to improve, and I reached level 7. She said "yes, with your strong will you can achieve that." And I told them yes, because I have lowered my levels quite a bit [in the past]. And they told me that maybe I could reach level 6, because that was the best. And that motivates me to continue doing what I am doing. It is my goal, as they say; I have to achieve it.

This narrative indicates that the patient's awareness of her physician's feelings about improved test results drives the patient's own feelings of accountability toward both her physician and the achievement of good outcomes. This perceived accountability is reinforced by the physician's feedback as remembered by the patient, strengthening the belief that outcomes depend almost exclusively on what the patient does – or conversely, fails to do. Thus, while patients never reported that physicians blamed them for poor outcomes, attributing good outcomes to patients' intentions and behaviors by implication made patients responsible for the poor ones.

"It Would Be a Dream": The Role of Language Concordance in Doctor-Patient Communication

When we asked patients to imagine that they had a "magic wand" that allowed them to make a wish and request one single change, however implausible, that would improve communication with their physicians, virtually all of them expressed a desire that their physicians speak Spanish, or alternatively, that they themselves be able to speak English.

> It would be a dream, as they say. (...) A dream (...) Yes, because she is an excellent doctor, excellent, and it seems that she is learning Spanish.

And yet, while the idea of learning English felt overwhelming to most patients, even to some who had lived in the United States for decades, many patients also felt that it was both physicians' and patients' duty to learn the language of the other.

> If I had a magic wand, all doctors since early childhood would have to learn Spanish [...] at least the basics. (...) More than anything here in California [...]. I say "children need to learn English and Spanish, because when we are professionals here in California with excellent professionals need to be speaking the two languages."

> Well, study the language. Study the language, English, so that we can understand each other. I should study English and he should study Spanish. Then, we would understand each other better, but to me, it [English] just doesn't stick.

Yet another recurrent wish was that physicians were at least as interested in patients' emotional states as in their physical health.

> If I had found a doctor who [...] looked also at the emotional changes that you have [...] Then, there would have been more communication with the physician [...] on the emotional level.

Patients' wish that physicians be mindful and interested in their emotional states was intertwined with their desire that physicians treat them as persons, a point that we elaborate on in the concluding section.

"Even When They Don't Understand You, They Are Kind": Building Bridges across the Language Divide

Finally, even if all patients expressed a strong and clear preference for language concordant care, it was not the case that they valued their physician's Spanish proficiency over *everything* else. Indeed, many patients felt that some non-Spanish proficient physicians still convey empathy and friendliness through smiles, eye contact, and interest in their personal lives, all of which made a difference to patients' disposition to develop trust toward them.

> There are people who, even when they don't understand you, they are kind, they come in and say "hello, how are you," they tell you their name, they say, "I'll see you right now, I'll send you an interpreter," they try to speak your language, they strive to speak, to make you feel good [...] I think this helps you build trust. Others do not. They simply do their job, as if they were dealing with a piece of furniture.

> Look, I'll tell you one thing, I'm actually not very talkative. I do not feel comfortable [but] with Dr. P. I talk a lot, I have this confidence, I don't know why, but from the first day I saw her I felt this trust, as if I had known her all my life. Like two persons who have never seen each other, and they see each other for the first time, and it's like some chemistry between them. I also have another female doctor who speaks

> Spanish, and yet it is different. She is an American [like Dr. P.], she speaks Spanish very well, and yet it is not the same, not the same connection. A type of person you like at first sight, and then, the interpreter does not matter. It's their personal, human warmth.
>
> Q: So it's not only the language with this doctor …?
>
> No it isn't.

Most patients also mentioned that an important source of trust was to feel that their physician "knew their job," by which they meant that physicians be trained and willing to provide high-quality care that would help patients manage their diabetes.

> When I feel trust I talk more. But let me tell you one thing: it's no good to feel trust, and speak Spanish, if the doctor will not prescribe the right treatment as I have now with a doctor who speaks English, who works hard to see me well, who cares. And even though she speaks English, she explains things to me […]. I have found a good doctor in this respect. But imagine, if I found a Spanish speaking doctor who is very serious, not very friendly, and always too much in a hurry, it would not be useful that he speak Spanish.

This patient, like many others, believed that the language of the clinical encounter, while important, was neither necessary nor sufficient to the delivery of high quality care or to diabetes outcomes. From their perspective, what was critical was that physicians prescribe "the right treatment" and that patients adhere to them.

DISCUSSION

In this study of patient experience of patient physician language concordance and discordance in diabetes care, patients' preference for language concordance – in line with studies showing greater patient satisfaction with language concordant doctor-patient relationships (Carrasquillo et al., 1999; Fernandez et al., 2004; Morales et al., 1999; Schenker et al., 2008) – went beyond mere language comprehension. In fact, patients preferred language concordant care even when interpreter services were available and satisfactory. The reason for their preference was, as patients put it, that they felt "more themselves" in their own language, as a result of which they felt more eager to engage in conversation and share their lifeworlds with their physicians, thus were better able to offer additional information that may help physicians better identify the patient's needs and predicaments.

Feeling more themselves made it easier for patients to engage in conversations that may yield information relevant to the treatment of their condition, even if not clinical information. This becomes especially important with conditions like diabetes, where patients' mastery and implementation of a range of technical, quasi-medical tasks, is inextricably intertwined with everyday life challenges such as job demands, family commitments, socioeconomic constraints, and so forth (Chaufan, 2002, 2008; Dinca Panaitescu et al., 2012). Thus, the ability to gather information that illuminates and helps understand how these challenges may affect diabetes management, and enables the physician to help the patient address these challenges, becomes a critical component of a successful clinical encounter.

As patients felt more themselves, it was easier for them to develop trust with their physicians, a trust that is critical to a strong patient-clinician relationship and concomitantly to clinical outcomes. Among our participants, developing trust went beyond trusting that their message would be accurately conveyed to the recipient by a competent interpreter, not experiencing embarrassment at the presence of a third party, or feeling that the conversational dynamics would not be disrupted by the need to convey their message via an interpreter. For many, trust was grounded on the experience that direct, unmediated communication enhanced the humanity of both participants in the communicative act, even more so when this third party is increasingly not a human presence but a machine.

For patients in this study, developing trust was further complicated by a generalized distrust that members of socially excluded groups may feel toward a health care system in which access to medical services is strongly dependent on employment, income level, and even citizenship status, all of which are critical to having or not having insurance in the United States, and may even determine insurance type. Unlike in other studies, where patients have reported feeling discriminated against by virtue of their race or ethnicity (Hausmann, Kressin, Hanusa, & Ibrahim, 2010), in our study some participants felt discriminated against by virtue of their social class, even as they felt grateful, both toward providers and the medical institution, for the care they received.

Of note, no patient in our sample believed that language discordance negatively influenced diabetes outcomes. This appeared to result from the emphasis placed by patients on their own role in managing diabetes, which made them responsible for their outcomes. Patients reported a great deal of self-blame, specifically when they failed to adhere to their physicians' instructions on lifestyle management. They also tended to overlook other barriers to management and outcomes, such as competing family or work obligations, constrained financial circumstances that limit dietary choices, or the nature of diabetes itself, which may include the progressive deterioration of glycemic homeostasis due to processes such as aging (Fonseca, 2009), regardless of adequate medication adherence.

The feeling of self-blame was often reinforced by well-meaning, positive feedback on the part of physicians who, as patients reported, praised them for "taking charge" of their diabetes and for making successful lifestyle changes. Physicians' positive feedback may inadvertently draw from what in the late 1970s Robert Crawford described as "the emergence of an ideology that blames the individual for his or her illness [...] and sees at-risk behavior as the problem and changing lifestyle as the solution" (Crawford, 1977) (p. 663). This ideology is upheld by national public health messages conveying that to a great extent the evolution of diabetes depends almost solely on lifestyle changes, and that these changes are almost exclusively a matter of individual choice (National Diabetes Education Program, 2013).

Indeed, the self-managed nature of diabetes care requires active patient engagement for the treatment to succeed (Funnell et al., 2008). This salient feature of diabetes presents physicians with the challenge of empowering patients and providing positive feedback without nurturing patient self-blame. Self-blame may also partly explain why LEP patients, in our experience, often remain in medical relationships that may be difficult for them because of language barriers. The belief that success in diabetes care depends almost exclusively on the will and determination of the patient, driven in part by the multipronged nature of the treatment, has resulted in a hegemonic view that puts an inordinate burden of responsibility on persons with diabetes, while downplaying or overlooking multiple, well-documented barriers to good diabetes control, including, yet not limited to, language barriers.

Lastly, over and above the greater difficulty to develop bonds of trust within language discordant care for the reasons described earlier, patients in this study respected their physicians' medical expertise and judgment, and believed that good outcomes depended on being prescribed the right treatment and complying with it. Patients also emphasized how important it was for them to feel treated with respect, empathy, and kindness – in the words of one participant, "like human beings." Patients were also very sensitive to physicians' attitudes and behaviors, noticing eye contact, smiles, and even minor efforts to articulate simple sentences, like "how are you," in the patient's language. Indeed, most patients emphasized that they were satisfied with the clinical encounter when they felt that their physician provided them quality diabetes care and treated them with respect, regardless of physicians' Spanish fluency.

CONCLUSIONS

Our findings suggest that providing language concordant care – by recruiting more Spanish speaking physicians – is central to the success of doctor-patient communication and concomitant success of diabetes care among LEP Latinos. Our findings also suggest that it is important to "professionalize" the profession of medical interpretation and help it gain medical legitimacy vis-à-vis patients (Fernandez & Schenker, 2010). Current norms endorse interpreter's health care role primarily as conduits for communication between clinician and the patient and urge interpreters to refrain from personal involvement in this interaction (Hsieh, 2006; NCIHC, 2005). In combination with the current trend to replace in-person interpreters with video or audio (phone) interpreter services (Azarmina & Wallace, 2005), patients and physicians may find it increasing difficult to develop personal and trusting relationships with individuals they might otherwise experience as part of a medical team. Impersonal interpreter services may be a barrier to quality diabetes care, and health care more generally, at least in some cases, if the patient constructs the interpreter service as lacking professionalism, that is, humanity. This issue may also be culturally and class specific and deserves further investigation.

Significant research supports the contention that providing access to high quality interpretation should significantly improve the quality of health care delivered (Karliner et al., 2007). However, if as our study suggests, interpretation itself impairs the development of an optimal doctor-patient relationship, then it follows that even high-quality interpretation may fail to significantly reduce diabetes inequalities, a finding that underscores the need for language expertise among greater number of clinicians.

We wish to emphasize that patients cared not only about good communication with their physicians but about receiving high quality *technical* care. At least some patients appeared to value this over everything else. This may be particularly important for patients who may feel discriminated against by the health care system by virtue of their class status, that is, who may feel that they receive lower quality care because they are poor. Short of striving for a healthcare system where individuals would not be treated at different establishments or by different doctors depending on their social class or insurance type, or better still striving for a more egalitarian society with lesser class differences, the training of health professionals should include the ability to detect and address these issues.

As to whether language discordance influences outcomes, the views of participants in our study were at odds with what some quantitative studies, including our own work, suggest (Fernandez et al., 2011). In this current study, we found that participants dismissed language barriers and blamed themselves instead for poor outcomes, an attitude that was reinforced by well-meaning, positive feedback from physicians vis-à-vis good outcomes. Physicians should be mindful of this risk and, without refraining from empowering patients or providing positive feedback when outcomes are desirable, they should engage in open conversations with patients about *all* the factors that may influence diabetes outcomes rather than simply stress those dependent on patient agency.

Finally, what emerges from our investigation is that, as numerous scholars before us have shown, it is critical for patients to be treated not as "cases" but as persons, with dignity and respect (Beach et al., 2005; Nápoles, Gregorich, Santoyo-Olsson, O'Brien, & Stewart, 2009), and that even across the language divide, medical education should strengthen practitioners' development of attitudes, dispositions and behaviors that allow patients to know that their physicians are not only willing and able to provide quality care, but also care *for* them in the totality of their human condition.

NOTE

1. A blood test indicating the level of glucose in a patient's blood for the two to three months previous to the test.

ACKNOWLEDGMENTS

The authors thank the patients, medical personnel, and staff who kindly volunteered their time and expertise to our project. Funding was provided by 3R01DK090272-02S1 from the National Institute of Diabetes and Digestive and Kidney Diseases (NIDDK).

REFERENCES

Azarmina, P., & Wallace, P. (2005). Remote interpretation in medical encounters: A systematic review. *Journal of Telemedicine and Telecare, 11*(3), 140–145.

Beach, M. C., Sugarman, J., Johnson, R. L., Arbelaez, J. J., Duggan, P. S., & Cooper, L. A. (2005). Do patients treated with dignity report higher satisfaction, adherence, and receipt of preventive care? *The Annals of Family Medicine, 3*(4), 331–338.

Benner, P. (1994). *Interpretive phenomenology: Embodiment, caring and ethics in health and illness.* Newbury Park, CA: Sage.

Carrasquillo, O., Orav, E. J., Brennan, T., & Burstin, H. (1999). Impact of language barriers on patient satisfaction in an emergency department. *Journal of General Internal Medicine, 14*(2), 82–87.

Centers for Disease Control and Prevention. (2011). *CDC health disparities and inequalities report.* Retrieved from http://www.cdc.gov/mmwr/pdf/other/su6001.pdf. Accessed on December 14, 2013.

Chaufan, C. (2002). Sugar blues: The social (silent) side of diabetes. *Clinical Diabetes, 20*(4), 207–210.

Chaufan, C. (2008). What does justice have to do with it? A bioethical and sociological perspective on the diabetes epidemic. In B. K. Rothman & E. Armstrong (Eds.), *Bioethical issues: Sociological perspectives.* Advances in Medical Sociology. New York, NY: Elsevier.

Chaufan, C., Constantino, S., & Davis, M. (2011). "It's a full-time job to be poor": Understanding barriers to diabetes prevention in immigrant communities in the USA. *Critical Public Health, 22*(2), 147–158. doi:10.1080/09581596.2011.630383

Chesla, C. A. (1995). Hermeneutic phenomenology: An approach to understanding families. *Journal of Family Nursing, 1*(1), 63–78.

Crawford, R. (1977). You are dangerous to your health: The ideology and politics of victim blaming. *International Journal of Health Services, 7*(4), 663–680.

Dinca Panaitescu, M., Dinca Panaitescu, S., Raphael, D., Bryant, T., Pilkington, B., & Daiski, I. (2012). The dynamics of the relationship between type 2 diabetes incidence and poverty: Longitudinal results from Canada's National Population Health Survey. *Maturitas, 72*(3), 229–235.

Fernandez, A., & Schenker, Y. (2010). Time to establish national standards and certification for health care interpreters. *Patient Education and Counseling, 78*(2), 139–140.

Fernandez, A., Schillinger, D., Grumbach, K., Rosenthal, A., Stewart, A., Wang, F., & Pérez-Stable, E. (2004). Physician language ability and cultural competence. *Journal of General Internal Medicine, 19*(2), 167–174.

Fernandez, A., Schillinger, D., Warton, E. M., Adler, N., Moffet, H., Schenker, Y., ... Karter, A. (2011). Language barriers, physician-patient language concordance, and glycemic control among insured Latinos with diabetes: The diabetes study of northern California (DISTANCE). *Journal of General Internal Medicine, 26*(2), 170–176.

Flores, G., Abreu, M., Olivar, M., & Kastner, B. (1998). Access barriers to health care for Latino children. *Archives of Pediatrics & Adolescent Medicine, 152*(11), 1119–1125.

Fonseca, V. A. (2009). Defining and characterizing the progression of type 2 diabetes. *Diabetes Care, 32*(Suppl. 2), S151–S156.

Funnell, M. M., Brown, T. L., Childs, B. P., Haas, L. B., Hosey, G. M., Jensen, B., ... Weiss, M. A. (2008). National standards for diabetes self-management education. *Diabetes Care, 31*(Suppl. 1), S97–S104.

Harlan, L., Bernstein, A., & Kessler, L. (1991). Cervical cancer screening: Who is not screened and why? *American Journal of Public Health, 81*(7), 885–890.

Hausmann, L. R. M., Kressin, N. R., Hanusa, B. H., & Ibrahim, S. A. (2010). Perceived racial discrimination in health care and its association with patients' healthcare experiences: Does measure matter? *Ethnicity & Disease, 20*(Winter), 40–47.

Hsieh, E. (2006). Conflicts in how interpreters manage their roles in provider-patient interactions. *Social Science & Medicine, 62*(3), 721–730.

Hudelson, P., Dominice Dao, M., Junod Perron, N., & Bischoff, A. (2013). Interpreter-mediated diabetes consultations: A qualitative analysis of physician communication practices. *BMC Family Practice, 14*(1), 163.

Institute of Medicine. (2002, March). *An equal treatment: What healthcare providers need to know about racial and ethnic disparities in health care*. Retrieved from http://www.iom.edu/~/media/Files/Report%20Files/2003/Unequal-Treatment-Confronting-Racial-and-Ethnic-Disparities-in-Health-Care/Disparitieshcproviders2008pgFINAL.pdf. Accessed on October 2013, 2013.

Karliner, L. S., Jacobs, E. A., Chen, A. H., & Mutha, S. (2007). Do professional interpreters improve clinical care for patients with limited English proficiency? A systematic review of the literature. *Health Services Research, 42*(2), 727–754.

Morales, L. S., Cunningham, W. E., Brown, J. A., Liu, H., & Hays, R. D. (1999). Are Latinos less satisfied with communication by health care providers? *Journal of General Internal Medicine, 14*(7), 409–417.

Nápoles, A. M., Gregorich, S. E., Santoyo-Olsson, J., O'Brien, H., & Stewart, A. L. (2009). Interpersonal processes of care and patient satisfaction: Do associations differ by race, ethnicity, and language? *Health Services Research, 44*(4), 1326–1344.

National Diabetes Education Program. (2013). *The power to control diabetes is in your hands*. Retrieved from http://ndep.nih.gov/publications/PublicationDetail.aspx?PubId=28. Accessed on December 14, 2013.

NCIHC. (2005). *National standards of practice for interpreters in health care*. Retrieved from http://www.mingweb.org/assets/documents/NCIHC-NationalStandardsofPractice.pdf

Ong, L. M. L., Visser, M. R. M., Lammes, F. B., & de Haes, J. C. J. M. (2000). Doctor–patient communication and cancer patients' quality of life and satisfaction. *Patient Education and Counseling, 41*(2), 145–156.

Pearson, W. S., Zhao, G., & Ford, E. S. (2011). An analysis of language as a barrier to receiving Influenza vaccinations among an elderly Hispanic population in the United States. *Advances in Preventive Medicine*. Article ID 298787. doi:10.4061/2011/298787

Peek, M. E., Cargill, A., & Huang, E. S. (2007). Diabetes health disparities: A systematic review of health care interventions. *Medical Care Research and Review, 64*(Suppl. 5), 101S–156S.

Piette, J. D., Heisler, M., & Wagner, T. H. (2004). Problems paying out-of-pocket medication costs among older adults with diabetes. *Diabetes Care, 27*(2), 384–391.

Ross, J. S., Bradley, E. H., & Busch, S. H. (2006). Use of health care services by lower-income and higher-income uninsured adults. *Journal of the American Medical Association, 295*(17), 2027–2036.

Roter, D. L., Hall, J. A., & Katz, N. R. (1987). Relations between physicians' behaviors and analogue patients' satisfaction, recall, and impressions. *Medical Care, 25*(5), 437–451.

Ryan, C. (2011). *Language use in the United States: 2011*. American Community Surveys Report. Retrieved from http://www.census.gov/prod/2013pubs/acs-2022.pdf

Schenker, Y., Lo, B., Ettinger, K. M., & Fernandez, A. (2008). Navigating language barriers under difficult circumstances. *Annals of Internal Medicine*, *149*(4), 264–269.

Schouten, B. C., & Meeuwesen, L. (2006). Cultural differences in medical communication: A review of the literature. *Patient Education and Counseling*, *64*(1–3), 21–34.

Seale, C., Rivas, C., & Kelly, M. (2013). The challenge of communication in interpreted consultations in diabetes care: A mixed methods study. *British Journal of General Practice*, *63*(607), e125–e133.

Stewart, M. A. (1995). Effective physician-patient communication and health outcomes: A review. *Canadian Medical Association Journal*, *152*(9), 1423–1433.

Timmins, C. L. (2002). The impact of language barriers on the health care of Latinos in the United States: A review of the literature and guidelines for practice. *The Journal of Midwifery & Women's Health*, *47*(2), 80–96.

Wilson, E., Chen, A. H., Grumbach, K., Wang, F., & Fernandez, A. (2005). Effects of limited English proficiency and physician language on health care comprehension. *Journal of General Internal Medicine*, *20*(9), 800–806.

RACE AND SOCIOECONOMIC STATUS: PUBLIC PERCEPTIONS TOWARD QUALITY AND ACCESS TO CARE IN THE AFFORDABLE CARE ACT

Neale R. Chumbler, Samir P. Desai, Justin B. Ingels and Kevin K. Dobbin

ABSTRACT

Purpose – *As the new Patient Protection and Affordable Care Act (ACA) achieves full implementation in 2014–2015, public perceptions regarding improvement in access and quality of care due to the ACA provide a fertile area for sociological research. The aim of this chapter is to determine if race is independently associated with perceptions of quality of care and access to care after ACA implementation. And, secondarily, we examined if such a relationship remained stable after considering SES (education and income) alone and SES with other relevant individual characteristics.*

Education, Social Factors, and Health Beliefs in Health and Health Care Services
Research in the Sociology of Health Care, Volume 33, 209–228

ISSN: 0275-4959/doi:10.1108/S0275-495920150000033009

Methodology/approach – *Data come from a telephone survey of a representative sample of Georgia residents aged 18 years or older. For each domain of the dependent variables (quality of care and access to care), three models were fitted with a nested design. The first model included only race. The second model included only race and SES. Model 3 included race, SES, and the following individual characteristics: (1) self-rated health status; (2) sense of coherence (SOC; a construct used to explain why some people are more disposed than others to illness after stressful situations); (3) travel time to doctor's office; (4) importance of short wait times as doctor's office; (5) political affiliation; and (6) geographic location (rural/non-rural).*

Findings – *Race was significantly associated with both the quality of care and the access to care. Non-White respondents were more likely to perceive improvements to both as a result of the ACA. Likewise, respondents with either higher education or income were also more likely to perceive improvements in quality and access as a result of the ACA. However, these associations were partly explained by respondents' self-reported political affiliations.*

Originality/value – *Results of this study show that public perceptions toward the ACA and its impact on quality and access to care seem to differ based on an individuals' race, income level and political affiliation. This may be a reflection of the media blitzkrieg that surrounds the ACA rather than a direct consequence of the policy itself. A concerted effort to develop communication strategies and outreach efforts by race and SES that can better educate the general population on the ACA may alleviate some of the reservations that are inherent to any major policy implementation, especially in terms of healthcare quality and access.*

Keywords: Race/ethnicity; socioeconomic status; health policy; Affordable Care Act; quality of care; access to care

INTRODUCTION

As we enter the midpoint of the second decade of the twenty-first century, the US healthcare system continues to experience several significant challenges. The number of uninsured individuals continued to increase substantially during the 2000s (Robert Wood Johnson Foundation, 2008). According to the US Census Bureau, 49.9 million individuals were without health insurance in the United States in 2010 (DeNavas-Walt, Proctor, & Smith, 2011). This increased number of US residents without health insurance was one of the major drivers of healthcare reform. To that end, *The Patient Protection and Affordable Care Act* (*ACA*) was signed into law by President Barack Obama on March 23, 2010. Hailed as the most significant overhaul of the US healthcare system since the passage of Medicare and Medicaid in 1965, the ACA aims to decrease the number of uninsured Americans by increasing access to healthcare through guaranteed coverage, reducing healthcare costs, improving healthcare quality and outcomes and streamlining delivery through comprehensive insurance reforms and other measures (Deane, Cho, DiJulio, Brodi, & Kaiser, 2011). In particular, low- and moderate-income uninsured Americans will gain access to coverage either through the expansion of the Medicaid program or through a mixture of government subsidies and increased access to healthcare marketplaces (Deane et al., 2011).

Arguably, one of the most challenging features of our US healthcare system is access to healthcare and this topic of access is largely responsible for initiating the ACA. The United States is the only developed country that does not ensure access to healthcare through universal guaranteed coverage. Among individuals ages 25–64, over 18,000 excess deaths per year can be attributed to the lack of health insurance (Institute of Medicine [IOM], 2002). Analysts have argued that one of the major barriers to controlling healthcare costs is this lack of universal coverage (Andersen, Rice, & Kominski, 2001). Similarly, preserving quality in healthcare is one of the leading issues, especially for healthcare managers and leaders (Andersen et al., 2001). Even though it is a goal to provide access to care for all Americans, it is equally as important that this care is of high quality. To that end, the ACA implemented several processes to improve the quality of care. One action has required that the DHHS establish an Adult Medicaid Quality Measurement Program to fund development, testing, and validation of evidence-based measures to track quality of care for adults enrolled in Medicaid (Horvitz-Lennon et al., 2014). A second measure of the ACA to improve quality of care was to institutionalize the collection of clinical performance data stratified by race, providing encouraging opportunities for organizations to identify health disparities in their patient populations since research has identified racial differences in access to care and quality of care (Clarke et al., 2013).

There is an abundance of sociological literature on the existence of racial differences in health, and these differences are large and persist over time (Williams & Sterntha, 2010). Racial minorities suffer disproportionate morbidity and mortality from chronic diseases (Airhihenbuwa, 1992; Brown, O'Rand, & Adkins, 2012). Indeed, health outcomes can differ markedly across racial groups, with non-White individuals (especially Blacks) experiencing worse health (Lynch & Kaplan, 2000). Sarkin, Groessl, Mulligan, Sklar, Kaplan, & Ganiats (2013) examined the extent to which there were diminishing differences in self-rated health between races from 1972 to 2008. In fact, health ratings for Black individuals were worse between 1995 and 2008 than the late 1980s (Sarkin et al., 2013). US racial health disparities are a consequence of several factors, one of which includes poorer access to care (Shavers et al., 2012). Both the federal government and Private foundations have focused their efforts in recent years to eliminate health disparities. For example, the 2012 National Healthcare Disparities Report indicated that Blacks received worse care than Whites for approximately 40% of quality measures (Agency for Healthcare Research and Quality, 2012). Further, the principal goal outlined in the *Healthy People 2020* publication is to eliminate all health disparities and achieve health equity (i.e., attaining the highest level of health for all people) (Kronenfeld, 2013). Moreover, Private foundations such as the Commonwealth Foundation have programs that center on eliminating health disparities by supporting efforts to improve the quality of care delivered to minorities (Commonwealth Fund, 2013). Efforts to eliminate these racial disparities have been hampered by the lack of a full understanding of all proximal causes including barriers to access of high quality of care, such as SES (Shavers et al., 2012).

As Kronenfeld (2013) cogently pointed out, looking only at data on racial disparities without consideration of SES differences is problematic. That is, if studies focus only on race and ignore SES indicators, one may falsely conclude that differences are linked either specifically to race or are biological and associated with race (Kronenfeld, 2012). It is imperative to consider SES, as higher levels of education and income for non-seniors are generally predictive of better health. In other words, individuals with a lower SES participate in fewer positive health behaviors and more high-risk behaviors (Grzywacz, 2000).

THEORETICAL PERSPECTIVES

Sociological research has long explored the role of social structure and social stratification as a key predictor of health. Social structure is defined as "enduring patterns of social life that shape an individual's attitudes and beliefs, behaviors and actions, and material and psychological resources" (Williams & Sterntha, 2010, pp. S18–19). A principal social structure studied within sociology, socioeconomic status (SES), is especially salient for understanding racial disparities in health (Williams & Sterntha, 2010). The theoretical underpinnings of SES can be traced back to the sociological traditions of both Marx and Weber.

The Marxian tradition views society as separated into "classes" that are determined by exploitative production relations (Lynch & Kaplan, 2000). Indeed, Marx's perspective on social class as one that "reveals the innermost secret, the hidden basis, of the entire social structure" (1894/1991, p. 791). For Marx, "class" was operationalized by the association to the means of production (Lynch & Kaplan, 2000). The Marxian tradition has been further extended and implemented by sociologists such as Wright (1985, 1994). For Wright, this perspective on class distinctions can be underscored by the way in which the middle class is simultaneously exploiting and being exploited. That is, the working class was at a competitive weakness in the marketplace. Wright identified three types of exploitation that is based on ownership of capital assets, control of organizational assets and ownership of skill assets (also see Lynch & Kaplan, 2000).

The Weberian tradition placed more emphasis on the role that the individual played in society. Weber (1922/1958) coined the term "life chances" to describe how classes can be viewed as groups of people who share common sets of beliefs, values and circumstances. Many sociologists have operationalized "life chances" using variables such as occupation, income and education (Lynch & Kaplan, 2000). Our proposed study – similar to most sociological studies – follows more closely this Weberian perspective in that an individual's education and income and wealth are indicators of what resources individuals possess and the "life chances" they have (Kronenfeld, 2013; Lynch & Kaplan, 2000). Therefore, both education and income are important markers of socioeconomic position and we operationalize SES by respondents' education and income.

To our knowledge, there have been no studies that have examined whether differences by race emerge in adults' perceptions of quality of care and access to care after implementation of ACA, especially after controlling for SES and other key variables encompassing measures that assess process of care, health status, coping, and other demographic factors. This void in the literature could lead to biased outcomes and inferences regarding the association of race and SES on perceptions toward important aspects of ACA implementation. The aim of this chapter was to determine if race was independently associated with perceptions of quality of care and access to care after ACA implementation. And, secondarily, we examined if such a relationship remained stable after considering only SES and SES and other relevant non-SES individual characteristics.

DATA AND METHODS

We conducted a random digit dial survey of Georgia residents aged 18 years or older, based on landline telephone exchanges. The sampling frame consisted of random telephone numbers distributed in proportion to their density within all listed telephone households, screened for non-working and business numbers. Participation was voluntary and all participants provided verbal assent.

Interviews were conducted from November 20 to 28, 2012. To participate in the interview, respondents had to be 18 years of age or older and current Georgia residents. A total of 13,988 landline random digit dial numbers were placed using a computer-assisted telephone interviewing system. Among the 1,767 contacts meeting the inclusion criteria, 503 (28.5%) agreed to participate. The median time for survey completion was 12 minutes. The 503 successful interviews provided a margin of error no greater than 4.4% at the 95% confidence level.

Dependent Variables

Respondents were first asked, "As you know, the Affordable Healthcare Act of 2010 (President Obama's healthcare reform or "Obamacare") was approved by the Supreme Court. Do you believe the quality of your healthcare would increase, stay about the same, or decrease as a result of healthcare reform?" We refer to this variable hereafter as "quality of care." We recoded the responses into a binary variable, with 1 representing the perception that quality of care would either increase or stay the same and 0 representing that quality of care would decrease. Respondents were then asked, "Do you believe your access to healthcare would increase, stay the same, or decrease as a result of healthcare reform?" We refer to this variable hereafter as "access to care." Similarly, we recoded the responses into a binary variable, with 1 representing that access for either increase or stay the same and 0 representing that access would decrease.

Independent Variables

Self-perceived race was coded into one of five categories: (1) White; (2) Black (African American); (3) Asian; (4) Hispanic; (5) Multi-racial. Due to the small number of categories, a single dummy variable was created to represent race in both the bivariate and multivariate analyses, with Whites as the reference group (coded "0"), compared to non-Whites (coded "1"). Respondents' educational attainment was operationalized into three categories: no more than a high school diploma some college education and graduate education. In the multivariate models, graduate level education was used as the reference category. Annual household income included 11 different categories (ranging from under $5,000 to $100,000 or more), adjusted based on multiple imputation to account for the 126 missing cases. We created three dummy variables representing income: <$5,000–$24,999; $25,000–$74,999; and $75,000 or more. In the multivariate models, <$5,000–$24,999 was the reference category. These latter two variables represent SES.

Control Variables

Socio-demographic control variables included gender, age, education, political affiliation, and rural-urban residence. Access to healthcare control variables included self-report of travel time to the doctor's office and the importance of convenience and wait times at healthcare facilities. Gender was coded as a dichotomous measure (1 = male). The study respondent's age was treated as a continuous measure. Respondents reported political affiliation as "Democrats," "Republicans," and "Independents." In the multivariate models, "Democrats" was the reference category. Respondent urban/rural residence followed the metropolitan area framework developed in 2003 by the US Office of Management and Budget from 2000 Census data (Hart, Larson, & Lishner, 2005). In previous research, each of these variables has been associated with healthcare quality and access (Haas et al., 2004).

Respondents were also asked, "How long does it take you to get to a particular doctor's office, clinic, health center, or other place that you usually go when you are sick?" Travel time included six different categories, ranging from <15 minutes to more than 120 minutes. These responses were recoded into a binary variable, where 1 represented up to one hour of self-reported travel and 0 represented over 1 hour. To assess the importance of wait times, respondents were asked, "How important is 'convenient travel and short waiting times' to you". This means having short travel times and convenient access to healthcare facilities, and having short waiting times for consultations and hospital admissions. The five response options (ranging from not important to extremely important) were dichotomized into two categories, where 1 represented "very important" ("very important to extremely important") and 0 ("moderately important," "slightly important" and "not important"). Both of these variables have been found to be key correlates in obtaining access to care and achieving quality of care (add refs).

An additional covariate of interest was the respondents' levels of self-rated physical health status (SRHS). The survey posed the following question: "In general, how would you rate your health (including physical and mental health) today?" Respondents answered: 1 "very good" 2 "good" 3 "moderate" 4 "bad" 5 "very bad." In line with existing literature, we recoded the responses into a binary variable, with 1 representing very good or good health and 0 representing moderate, bad, or very bad health. Previous research has found associations between SRHS and community-based individuals' views on their social, environmental, and physical environment and perceptions toward their healthcare (Chumbler & Leech, 2013; Rohrer, Arif, Denison, Young, & Adamson, 2007; Sarkin et al., 2013).

SOC was assessed by an abbreviated three-item version of the SOC scale (Lundberg & Nystrom, 1995). A single question was used to measure each item: (1) "Do you usually feel that the things that happen to you in your daily life are hard to understand?" (*comprehensibility*); (2) "Do you usually see a solution to problems and difficulties that other people find hopeless?" (*management*); and (3) "Do you usually feel that your daily life is a source of personal satisfaction?" (*meaningfulness*). Respondents' answers were "yes, usually" (scored 0); "yes, sometimes" (scored 1); and "no" (scored 2). (Chumbler et al., 2013). Scores were reversed and summed to provide a total SOC scale score in the range of 0–6; a higher score represents a weaker SOC. Following previous research (Surtees, Wainwright, Luben, Khaw, Day, 2003), SOC was recoded as a binary variable, where a score of 0 or 1 represents "strong SOC" and a score of 2–6 "weak SOC" (Chumbler et al., 2013). According to Antonovsky (1987), individuals with a stronger SOC can effectively handle stress and protect their health. Recent research found that a strong SOC protects individuals with impairments including pain (Chumbler et al., 2013). We controlled for SOC because of its strong association with good health and also because SOC has been found to be significantly correlated with individuals' perception of the quality of care they receive (Larsson & Larsson, 1999).

Analytic Strategy

Race and SES were analyzed as the main predictor variables in all analyses. First, univariate associations were evaluated by comparing the dependent variables and the control variables between the Non-White and White respondents. Next, using STATA 12 software, we ran multivariable logistic regression models to test the independent associations of race and SES with the perceptions of ACA as it specifically relates to improving quality of care and access to care. For each domain of these two dependent variables, three models were fitted with a nested design. The first model included only race. The second model included only race and SES. Model 3 included all of the control variables and both race and SES. Separate analyses indicate that there is little reason to be concerned about multicollinearity in the models.

Participants were also given the option of refusing to respond, or to choose "Don't know" as a response for survey items. Survey responses recorded as "refused" or "don't know" were treated as missing values in the final dataset. With the exception of the income variable (see above), the amount of missing data (which included the responses "Refused" and "Don't know," was minimal, ranging from 1% to 3%). The multiple imputation technique was used to account for the missing survey data. This technique allows pooling of the parameter estimates to obtain an improved parameter estimate and also permits incorporation of uncertainty associated with the missing data (Rubin, 1987). Initially, the dataset was explored to determine the pattern of "missingness" and was declared "missing at random" or MAR. The multiple imputation technique was applied because it uses the consistency (or inconsistency) of estimations derived from multiple imputations as additional information, and it can estimate standard errors that are unbiased (Acock, 2005). As a result, all 503 observations were recorded and analyzed for each variable in the survey dataset.

RESULTS

Respondent Characteristics

Of the 503 respondents, 75% were White and of the remaining 121 non-White respondents, nine self-reported to be multi-racial, two as Asian and two as Hispanic and the rest were Black. Nearly two-thirds of respondents were female (62.2%) and had at least a college level education (64%), the mean age was 58.8 years (SD = 17.7; age range, 18–99 years), and 27% resided in rural counties. Respondents self-identified with the following political affiliations: (1) 36% Democrats; (2) 38% Republicans; and (3) 26% Independents. Overall, 60% had a strong SOC (score, 0 or 1), 78% rated their health as good or very good, 81% reported that convenient travel and short waiting times are very important, and 95% reported traveling up to one hour to receive care. Finally, 51% of the respondents reported that the quality of care would increase or stay the same and 56% of the respondents indicated that access to care will increase or stay the same after the implementation of the ACA.

Table 1 summarizes the univariate associations of race with quality of care and access to care. Non-Whites were more likely to be female, have lower incomes, report being Democrat and have a weak SOC than Whites. Moreover, Non-White respondents were more likely to report that both quality of care and access to care would increase/stay the same. No association was observed between race and respondents' level of education, residential location, self-rated health status, travel time, and wait time.

Table 2 summarizes results from the multiple logistic regression of quality of care on race, SES, and the remaining control variables. Model I indicates that race is significantly associated with quality of care. Non-White respondents were more likely to report that the quality of care will increase after ACA implementation. In Model II, education and income each had an independent association with the outcome variable. Respondents with a graduate level degree were more likely to report that the quality of healthcare would increase than those with no more than at least a high school diploma. Both groups of respondents with an income greater than $25,000 were less likely to perceive that the quality of care would increase after ACA implementation compared to lower income respondents. Note that even with the addition of SES the magnitude of the association between race and quality of care changed very little (2%) and remained statistically significant ($p < .001$). Model III includes the rest of the control variables to race and SES. First, there is a 23% reduction in the association between race and quality of care, although the association remains statistically significant ($p < .001$). Second, the significant association between education and quality of care was no longer significant. Third, there were significant reductions in the income coefficients. The $25,000–$74,999 dummy variable was reduced by 32% (log odds −.99, $p < .01$ to −.67, $p > .05$, from models 2 to 3).

Table 1. Descriptive Characteristics of Participants by Race (White vs. Non-White).

Participant Characteristic	White (n = 360)	Non-White (n = 121)	p-value
Age in years, mean (SD)	58.7 (15.4)	51.1 (15)	0.97
Gender, n (%)			
Male	146 (40.5)	32 (26.5)	0.005
Female	214 (59.5)	89 (73.5)	
Education, n (%)			
Graduate level	64 (18)	19 (16)	0.08
College level	172 (48.3)	46 (39)	
High school level	120 (33.7)	53 (45)	
Income, n (%)			
$4,999–$24,999	67 (24.5)	39 (41)	0.001
$25,000–$74,999	97 (35.5)	37 (39)	
$75,000 and above	110 (40)	19 (20)	
Rural/urban, n (%)			
Rural	101 (28)	30 (25)	0.48
Urban	259 (72)	91 (75)	
Political affiliation, n (%)			
Democrat	72 (22.5)	85 (81)	0.00
Republican	158 (49)	4 (4)	
Independent	91 (28.5)	16 (15)	
Sense of coherence			
Weak	134 (37.3)	57 (47.1)	0.055
Strong	226 (62.7)	64 (52.9)	
Self-rated health status			
Poor	81 (22.5)	24 (20)	0.56
Good	279 (77.5)	96 (80)	
Travel time			
Up to 1 hour	344 (95.8)	113 (93.3)	0.27
More than 1 hour	15 (4.2)	8 (6.7)	
Wait time			
Extremely to very important	281 (79.2)	101 (85.6)	0.12
Moderately to not important	74 (20.8)	17 (14.4)	
Quality of healthcare			
Decrease	211 (63.4)	5 (4.8)	0.00
Increase/stay the same	122 (36.6)	101 (95.2)	
Access to healthcare			
Decrease	190 (56.2)	6 (5.4)	0.00
Stay the same	148 (43.8)	105 (94.6)	

Fourth, two additional control variables were statistically significant – political affiliation and travel time. Respondents who traveled one hour or less to receive care from their provider believed that the quality of healthcare would increase after ACA implementation. As compared to

Table 2. Results of Multiple Logistic Regression Models for Quality of Healthcare.

Quality of Care (Dependent Variable)	Model 1 Coefficient (S.E)	Model 2 Coefficient (S.E)	Model 3 Coefficient (S.E)
Race	3.54*** (0.47)	3.48*** (0.48)	2.7*** (0.51)
Education			
Graduate level		Reference category	Reference category
College level		−0.42 (0.31)	−0.23 (0.34)
High school level		−0.90* (0.37)	−0.80 (0.41)
Income			
\$4,999–\$24,999		Reference category	Reference category
\$25,000–\$74,999		−0.99** (0.35)	−0.67 (0.408)
\$75,000 and above		−1.28*** (0.35)	−1.0* (0.43)
Age			−0.02 (0.27)
Gender			0.37 (0.26)
Political affiliation			
Democrat			Reference category
Republican			−2.36*** (0.34)
Independent			−1.53*** (0.36)
Rural/urban			0.31 (0.29)
Sense of coherence			0.16 (0.25)
Self-rated health status			−0.11 (0.32)
Travel time			1.29* (0.63)
Wait time			−0.06 (0.31)
Constant			0.49 (0.86)

Note: Reference category for the following variables are as follows: (1) race – White; (2) gender – female; (3) rural/urban – rural; (4) SOC = poor SOC; (5) SRHS –poor SRHS; (6) travel time – >1 hour; (7) wait time – moderately to not important.

$^{*}p < 0.05$; $^{**}p < 0.01$; $^{***}p < 0.001$.

Democrats, respondents who identified themselves as Republican and Independent were each independently associated with a perception that the quality of healthcare would decrease after ACA implementation.

Table 3 summarizes results from the multiple logistic regression analysis of access to care on race, SES, and the remaining control variables. Model I indicates that non-White respondents were more likely to perceive that access to care will increase after ACA implementation. Model II includes SES and the magnitude of race was minimally affected. Moreover, education and income each had an independent association with access to care. Respondents with a graduate level degree were more likely to report that

Table 3. Results of Multiple Logistic Regression Models for Access to Healthcare.

Access to Care (Dependent Variable)	Model 1 Coefficient (S.E)	Model 2 Coefficient (S.E)	Model 3 Coefficient (S.E)
Race	3.12*** (0.43)	3.00*** (0.43)	2.09*** (0.47)
Education			
Graduate level		Reference category	Reference category
College level		−0.66* (0.31)	−0.506 (0.34)
High school level		−0.92* (0.36)	−0.81* (0.405)
Income			
$4,999–$24,999		Reference category	Reference category
$25,000–$74,999		−0.66* (0.33)	−0.27 (0.403)
$75,000 and above		−1.19** (0.35)	−0.88* (0.44)
Age			−0.15 (0.26)
Gender			0.38 (0.25)
Political affiliation			
Democrat			Reference category
Republican			−2.52*** (0.37)
Independent			−1.45*** (0.36)

Table 3. *(Continued)*

Access to Care (Dependent Variable)	Model 1 Coefficient (S.E)	Model 2 Coefficient (S.E)	Model 3 Coefficient (S.E)
Rural/urban			0.34 (0.28)
Sense of coherence			0.29 (0.24)
Self-rated health status			−0.17 (0.31)
Travel time			1.07 (0.62)
Wait time			0.004 (0.31)
Constant			0.97 (0.85)

Note: Reference category for the following variables are as follows: (1) race – White; (2) gender – female; (3) rural/urban – rural; (4) SOC – poor SOC; (5) SRHS – poor SRHS; (6) travel time – >1 hour; (7) wait time – moderately to not important.
$^*p < 0.05$; $^{**}p < 0.01$; $^{***}p < 0.001$.

access to healthcare would increase than those with no more than a high school diploma. As compared to respondents who reported an annual income of <$25,000, those with an income of ≥$75,000 were less likely to perceive that access to healthcare would increase after ACA implementation. In Model III, which includes the control variables, only one of the two education variables remained statistically significant (high school education). Similarly one of the two income categories (≥$75,000) remained statistically significant, but was reduced in magnitude. Respondents who identified themselves as Republican or Independent were more likely to report a perception that access to care would decrease after ACA implementation.

DISCUSSION AND CONCLUSION

The primary purpose of this chapter was to determine if race was independently associated with perceptions of quality of care and access to care after ACA implementation. And, secondarily, we examined if such a relationship remained stable after considering SES alone and SES with other relevant individual characteristics. Hypotheses were grounded in theories with original underpinnings of the classic work of Marx and Weber, and in turn, culminated in more contemporary review of the scientific literature. This chapter capitalized on recent secondary data from a representative sample of community-dwelling adult Georgians that queried specific perceptions regarding the quality of care and access to care after ACA implementation. A key goal of ACA is to reduce the number of uninsured through Medicaid expansion and the creation of health insurance exchange marketplaces (organizations established to expedite the purchase of health insurance in each state) with premium tax credits. Even after the enrollment surge of over eight million people by March 31, 2014, which has used health insurance exchanges to enroll in the ACA, there remain misperceptions of the actual realities of the ACA (Healthcare.gov, 2014). The latest Kaiser Health Tracking Poll reported that 46% of the public had an unfavorable impression of ACA, while 38% had a favorable one (Kaiser Health Tracking Poll, 2014). It is imperative to understand if race is correlated with perceptions toward quality of care and access to care for at least two reasons. One, people of color are at disproportionate risk of being uninsured and having low incomes (Kawachi, Daniels, & Robinson, 2005). Therefore, the ACA coverage expansions could benefit non-White individuals and advance efforts to eliminate disparities (Kaiser Family Foundation, 2013). Two, programs and interventions can be tailored by race to improve communication and enrollment into the ACA. This tailoring is particularly important because the ACA has dramatically increased the number of low-income nonelderly adults eligible for Medicaid. Beginning in 2014, states now can elect to offer Medicaid coverage to adults whose incomes do not exceed an effective threshold of 138 percent of the federal poverty level (Hill, Abdus, Hudson, & Selden, 2014).

Results supported our primary aim. We found that race was independently associated with perceptions of quality of care and access to care after ACA implementation. A secondary aim of this chapter was to determine if such a relationship remained stable after considering only SES (as operationalized by respondent income and education) and SES along with other relevant non-SES individual characteristics. Specifically, we found that non-White respondents were more likely to report that both the quality of care and access to care will increase after ACA implementation. This significant association was not attenuated and was of similar magnitude after adjusting for the participants' SES (as operationalized by respondent income and education) and after adjusting for a variety of other control variables including process of care, health status, coping, political affiliation, and other socio-demographic factors. In other words, the racial differences in the perceptions of quality of care and access to care were not mediated by SES, self-report health status, coping mechanisms, self-report processes of care, political affiliation, and other socio-demographic factors. These findings are consistent with a growing body of literature showing racial differences in access to care, quality of care received and health status, independent of SES and other factors (Brown et al., 2012; Haas et al., 2004; LeCook, McGuire, & Zaslavsky, 2012; Michael, Schaffer, Egan, Little, & Pritchard, 2013; Prentice, Fincke, Miller, & Pizer, 2011). Racial-ethnic minorities are more likely than their White counterparts to experience interpersonal discrimination (Brown et al., 2012). Individuals who reside in predominantly minority neighborhoods have lower quality medical care and have more challenges accessing care (Williams & Collins, 2001). Indeed, some recent research found that health disparities between Blacks and Whites persist after controlling for SES, but were eliminated after adjusting for perceived discrimination (Bratter & Gorman, 2011; Brown et al., 2012). Future research should add a perceived measure of discrimination when examining perceptions toward quality of care and access to care.

We did perform some additional analyses by running interaction effects of race by some of the significant variables in Models 2 and 3 (results not shown). With reference to quality of care, it appears that part of the effect of race reflects an individual's political affiliation and experience with travel time to their health provider. As compared to White Republicans, White Democrats were associated with perceptions toward quality of care would increase. As compared to White respondents with poor SRHS, non-White individuals with poor SRHS had stronger perceptions that quality of care would increase. As compared to White respondents with a graduate school education, non-Whites with a graduate school education were associated with quality of care increasing, a finding congruent with the work of Bratter and Gorman (2011). In this work, Bratter and Gorman (2011) found that SRHS is more sensitive to socioeconomic standing among Whites. More specifically, poorer health is more likely to occur among Whites when they reflect at least daily on their own racial status – but only when it happens in tandem with med-range educational achievement (Bratter & Gorman, 2011). These findings with reference to political affiliation are supported by Henderson and Hillygus (2011) who investigated individual level dynamics in healthcare attitudes toward ACA between 2008 and 2010. These authors found that self-interest strongly predict change in healthcare attitudes, with Republicans growing more opposed to universal health insurance coverage between 2008 and 2010. Henderson and Hillygus (2011) also found that preferences around universal coverage were associated with race.

Further analyses (not shown) revealed important differences in the relationships between race and perceptions of access of care by political affiliation and by rural versus urban location, as indicated by significant coefficients for interaction effects. As compared to White Republicans, White Democrats were associated with perceptions toward access to care would increase. This suggests that differences in perception regarding access to care between *some* Whites and non-Whites can be explained by political affiliation. As compared to Whites living in rural areas, non-White respondents living in rural areas perceived that access to care would increase. These findings are consistent with a body of literature that argues that the racial composition of the place where an individual lives could determine access to care, particularly Blacks and Latinos (Haas et al., 2004). For non-White individuals (e.g., Black; Latino), residing in an area with others who share similar language and culture can facilitation the dissemination of information and communication about healthcare and perhaps offer some refuge against discrimination, especially if more minority healthcare providers practice in these areas. These factors have been reported to facilitate access to care (Haas et al., 2004). On the other hand, more segregated areas have fewer economic opportunities, worse physical environments and fewer public resources, all of which impede access to care (Haas et al., 2004).

We acknowledge the following caveats specific to the present study. First, our data consists exclusively on self-report information regarding the healthcare system and health status at the individual level. For instance, administrative data is available to calculate actual travel times and wait times that patients experience in the healthcare system. Second, one of the control variables that we employed in the study is SRHS. SRHS is a fundamental measure of health status employed in the sociological and public health literature. It has been found to have high predictive and concurrent validity with several key outcome variables including (morbidity, mortality, and utilization of health services) (Idler & Benyamini, 1997). However, there are no other health related data in this analysis. Future research should use other self-rating measures of health status in addition to SRHS. Indeed future research should use measures of well-being, presence of chronic conditions and measures of mental health. Third, with the self-report nature of the study, some of the variables may be subject to recall or response bias and may limit the ability to assess the perceptions of quality of care and access to care. Fourth, our sample was a representative sample of Georgians. Due to this sole geographical location and the fact that this is a sample of Georgia residents where non-Whites are far more likely to be Democrat and Whites Republican or Independent is important. Due to this fact, it is unclear how generalizable our findings are to a broader population of older adults. However, the strength of our sample is that it contained a heterogeneous group of older adults in terms of race and SES.

Despite these limitations, this chapter makes contributions in sociology and has relevant policy implications. The fact that our study identified racial disparities in perceptions toward access to care and quality of care will contribute to the policy debate regarding racial disparities in health by emphasizing these differences in health have substantial economic costs to society (Williams & Sterntha, 2010). LaVeist, Gaskin, and Richard (2009) estimated that the medical care and lost productivity costs for racial disparities in health amount to $309 billion annual loss to the economy. These economic costs are a convincing additional policy justification for eliminating health disparities (Williams & Sterntha, 2010).

REFERENCES

Acock, A. (2005). Working with missing values. *Journal of Marriage and Family*, *67*, 1012–1028.

Agency for Healthcare Research and Quality. (2012). *National healthcare disparities report*. Rockville MD: AHRQ. Publication No. 13-0002. Retrieved from http://www.ahrq.gov/research/findings/nhqrdr/index.htm. Accessed on May 2, 2014.

Airhihenbuwa, C. O. (1992). Health promotion and disease prevention strategies for African Americans: A conceptual model. In R. L. Braithwaite & S. E. Taylor (Eds.), *Health issues in the Black community* (pp. 267–280). San Francisco, CA: Jossey-Bass.

Andersen, R. M., Rice, T. H., & Kominski, G. F. (2001). Introduction and overview. In R. M. Andersen, T. H. Rice, & G. F. Kominski (Eds.), *Changing the US health care system: Key issues in health services policy and management* (pp. xxxi–xliii). San Francisco, CA: Jossey-Bass.

Antonovsky, A. (1987). *Unraveling the mystery of health*. San Francisco, CA: Jossey-Bass.

Bratter, J., & Gorman, B. (2011). Is discrimination an equal opportunity risk? Racial experiences, socioeconomic status and health status among black and white adults. *Journal of Health and Social Behavior*, *52*, 365–382.

Brown, T. H., O'Rand, A. M., & Adkins, D. E. (2012). Race-ethnicity and health trajectories: Tests of three hypotheses across multiple groups and health outcomes. *Journal of Health and Social Behavior*, *53*, 359–377.

Chumbler, N. R., Kroenke, K., Outcalt, S., Bair, M. J., Krebs, E., Wu, J., & Yu, Z. (2013). Association between sense of coherence and health-related quality of life among primary care patients with chronic musculoskeletal pain. *Health and Quality of Life Outcomes*, *11*, 216.

Chumbler, N. R., & Leech, T. (2013). The impact of neighborhood cohesion on older individuals' self-rated health status. In J. J. Kronenfeld (Ed.), *Social determinants, health disparities and linkages to health and health care* (Vol. 31, pp. 41–55). Research in the Sociology of Health Care. Bingley, UK: Emerald Group Publishing Limited.

Clarke, A. R., Goddu, A. P., Nocon, R. S., Stock, N. W., Chyr, L. C., Akuoko, J. A. S., & Chin, M. H. (2013). Thirty years of disparities intervention research: What are we doing to close racial and ethnic gaps in health care? *Medical Care*, *51*, 1020–1026.

Commonwealth Fund. (2013, March). Retrieved from http://www.commonwealthfund.org/Program-Areas/Archived-Programs/Health-Care-Disparities.aspx

Deane, C., Cho, S., DiJulio, B., Brodi, M., & Kaiser, H. J. (2011). Public opinion on the affordable care act at one year: Continuities and contradictions. *The California Journal of Politics & Policy*, *3*, 1–15.

DeNavas-Walt, C., Proctor, B. D., & Smith, J. C. (2011). US census bureau, current population reports, P60-239. *Income, poverty, and health insurance coverage in the United States: 2010*. Washington, DC: U.S. Government Printing Office.

Grzywacz, J. G. (2000). Socioeconomic status and health behaviors among Californians. In J. J. Kronenfeld (Ed.), *Health, illness, and use of care: The impact of social factors* (Vol. 18, pp. 121–149). Research in the Sociology of Health Care. New York, NY: Elsevier.

Haas, J. S., Phillips, K. A., Sonneborn, D., McCulloch, C. E., Baker, L. C., Kaplan, C. P., ... Liang, S. (2004). Variation in access to healthcare for different racial/ethnic groups by the racial/ethnic composition of an individual's county of residence. *Medical Care*, *42*, 707–714.

Hart, L. G., Larson, E. H., & Lishner, D. M. (2005). Rural definitions for health policy and research. *American Journal of Public Health*, *95*, 1149–1155.

Healthcare.gov. (2014). *Get covered: A one-page guide to the health insurance marketplace*. Retrieved from healthcare.gov/get-covered-a-1-page-guide-to-the-health-insurance-marketplace. Accessed on May 15.

Henderson, M., & Hillygus, D. S. (2011). The dynamics of health care opinion, 2008–2010: Partisanship, self-interest, and racial resentment. *Journal of Health Politics, Policy and Law*, *36*, 946–960.

Hill, S. C., Abdus, S., Hudson, J. L., & Selden, T. M. (2014). Adults in the income range for the affordable care act's medicaid expansion are healthier than pre-ACA enrollees. *Health Affairs*, *33*, 691–699.

Horvitz-Lennon, M., Volya, R., Donohue, J. M., Lave, J. R., Stein, B. D., & Normand, S. T. (2014). Disparities in quality of care among publicly insured adults with schizophrenia in four large U.S. States, 2002–2008. Health Services Research *[Epub ahead of print]*, *49*, 1121–1144. doi:10.1111/1475-6773.12162

Idler, E. L., & Benyamini, Y. (1997). Self-rated health and mortality: A review of twenty-seven Community Studies. *Journal of Health and Social Behavior*, *38*, 21–37.

Institute of Medicine. (2002). *Care without coverage: Too little, too late*. Washington, DC: National Academies of Press.

Kaiser Family Foundation. (2013). *Health coverage by race and ethnicity: The potential impact of the affordable care act*. Washington, DC: KFF.

Kaiser Health Tracking Poll. (2014). The Henry J. Kaiser Family Foundation, May 30, 2014.

Kawachi, I., Daniels, N., & Robinson, D. E. (2005). Health disparities by race and class: Why both matter. *Health Affairs*, *24*, 343–352.

Kronenfeld, J. J. (2012). Health care system issues and race/ethnicity, immigration, SES and gender as sociological issues linking to health and health care. In J. J. Kronenfeld (Ed.), *Issues in health and health care related to race/ethnicity, immigration, SES and gender* (Vol. 30). Research in the Sociology of Health Care. Bingley, UK: Emerald Group Publishing Limited.

Kronenfeld, J. J. (2013). Social determinants and health disparities. In J. J. Kronenfeld (Ed.), *Social determinants, health disparities and linkages to health and health care* (Vol. 31, pp. 3–19). Research in the Sociology of Health Care. Bingley, UK: Emerald Group Publishing Limited.

Larsson, W., & Larsson, G. (1999). Patients' views on quality of care: Do they merely reflect their sense of coherence? *Journal of Advanced Nursing*, *30*, 33–39.

LaVeist, T. A., Gaskin, D. J., & Richard, P. (2009). *The economic burden of health inequalities in the United States*. Washington, DC: Joint Center for Political and Economic Studies.

LeCook, B., McGuire, T. G., & Zaslavsky, A. M. (2012). Measuring racial/ethnic disparities in health care: Methods and practical issues. *Health Services Research*, *47*, 1232–1254.

Lundberg, O., & Nystrom, M. (1995). A simplified way of measuring sense of coherence experiences from a population survey in Sweden. *European Journal of Public Health*, *5*, 56–69.

Lynch, J., & Kaplan, G. (2000). Socioeconomic position. In L. Berkman & I. Kawahi (Eds.), *Social epidemiology* (pp. 13–35). New York, NY: Oxford University Press.

Marx, K. (1894/1991). Chapter 47. Genesis of Capitalist Ground-Rent. In F. Engels, (Ed.). *Capital: A critique of political economy* (D. Fernbach, Trans., 1981, Vol. 3, pp. 917–951). London: Penguin Classics.

Michael, M., Schaffer, S. D., Egan, P. L., Little, B. B., & Pritchard, P. S. (2013). Improving wait times and patient satisfaction in primary care. *Journal for Healthcare Quality*, *35*(2), 50–60.

Prentice, J. C., Fincke, B. G., Miller, D. R., & Pizer, S. D. (2011). Outpatient wait time and diabetes care quality improvement. *American Journal of Managed Care*, *17*(2), e43–e54.

Robert Wood Johnson Foundation. (2008). *Percentage of nonelderly Americans without health insurance coverage, 1987–2006*. Retrieved from http://covertheuninsured.org/factsheets/display.php?FactSheetID=101

Rohrer, J. E., Arif, A., Denison, A., Young, R., & Adamson, S. (2007). Overall self-rated health as an outcome indicator in primary care. *Journal of Evaluation in Clinical Practice*, *13*, 882–888.

Rubin, D. B. (1987). *Multiple imputation for nonresponse in surveys*. New York, NY: Wiley.

Sarkin, A. J., Groessl, E. J., Mulligan, B., Sklar, M., Kaplan, R. M., & Ganiats, T. G. (2013). Racial differences in self-rated health diminishing from 1972 to 2008. *Journal of Behavioral Medicine*, *36*, 44–50.

Shavers, V. L., Fagan, P., Jones, D., Klein, W. M. P., Boyington, J., Moten, C., & Rorie, E. (2012). The state of research on racial/ethnic discrimination in the receipt of health care. *American Journal of Public Health*, *102*, 953–966.

Surtees, P., Wainwright, N., Luben, R., Khaw, K. T., & Day, N. (2003). Sense of coherence and mortality in men and women in the EPIC-Norfolk United Kingdom prospective cohort study. *American Journal of Epidemiology*, *158*, 1202–1209.

Weber, M. (1922/1958). Class status, party. In H. H. Gerth & C. W. Mills (Eds.), *Max Weber: Essays in sociology* (pp. 180–195). New York, NY: Routledge and Kegan Paul.

Williams, D. R., & Collins, C. (2001). Racial residential segregation: A fundamental cause of racial disparities in health. *Public Health Reports*, *116*, 404–415.

Williams, D. R., & Sterntha, M. (2010). Understanding racial-ethnic disparities in health: Sociological contributions. *Journal of Health and Social Behavior*, *51*(Suppl.), S15–S27.

Wright, E. O. (1985). *Classes*. London: Verso.

Wright, E. O. (1994). *Interrogating inequality*. London: Verso.

A PLACE TO TRUST: BLACK PROTESTANT AFFILIATION AND TRUST IN PERSONAL PHYSICIANS

Abigail A. Sewell and Rashawn Ray

ABSTRACT

Purpose – *Past research indicates that blacks are less trusting of physicians than are whites; yet, researchers have not examined within group differences in physician trust by religious denomination – an effort that is complicated by the high correlated nature of race and religion. To better understand black-white differences in physician trust, this chapter examines heterogeneity in trust levels among blacks associated with religious designations that distinguish Black Protestants from other ethnoreligious groups.*

Methodology/approach – *Using data from the 2002 and 2006 General Social Surveys, this study adopts an intersectional (i.e., race x religion) typology of religious denomination to understand the black-white gap in physician trust. Weighted multivariate linear regression is employed.*

Findings – *Black-white differences in physician trust are identified only when religious affiliation is considered but not when religious affiliation is omitted. Blacks who are affiliated with Black Protestant churches are*

Education, Social Factors, and Health Beliefs in Health and Health Care Services
Research in the Sociology of Health Care, Volume 33, 229–249

ISSN: 0275-4959/doi:10.1108/S0275-495920150000033010

more trusting than other religious groups, including Evangelical Protestants, Mainline Protestants, and blacks who are affiliated with other faiths.

Originality/value – *This chapter indicates that there is more heterogeneity in trust levels among blacks than between blacks and whites. Moreover, the findings suggest that religion can play an important role in bridging the trust gap between blacks and the medical sciences.*

Keywords: Race; religion; Black Protestant; trust; physicians

Social science research indicates that blacks are less likely than whites to trust "most people," racial outgroup members, and institutional actors (Alesina & La Ferrara, 2002; Glaeser, Laibson, Scheinkman, & Soutter, 2000; Hibbing & Theiss-Morse, 2001; Hughes & Thomas, 1998; LaVeist, Nickerson, & Bowie, 2000; Simpson, McGrimmon, & Irwin, 2007). One key institutional bond that has implications for health outcomes is the patient-physician relationship. Yet, researchers have not examined how social factors, such as religion, serve as important moderators of black-white differences in trusting personal physicians. This chapter draws from the prior research that shows that religion may buffer the effect of discrimination on psychological distress (Ellison, Musick, & Henderson, 2008) and, subsequently, trust attitudes toward physicians. The study attends to one dimension of religion that has been found to be associated with how an individual views and responds to racial discrimination (Lincoln & Mamiya, 1990) – religious affiliation.

Discrimination in the medical encounter and, specifically, the patient-physician relationship may be a culprit for a lack of trust among blacks (LaVeist et al., 2000; Smedley, Stith, & Nelson, 2003). For instance, although only 14 percent of blacks indicate that they personally have been treated unfairly in medical encounters due to their race or ethnicity, 35 percent indicate that either a family member or someone they know has been treated unfairly (Lillie-Blanton, Brodie, Rowland, Altman, & McIntosh, 2000). Comparable figures of 1 and 14 percent among whites, respectively, are of a decidedly smaller magnitude. Furthermore, blacks are over three times more likely than whites to be concerned about future discrimination toward themselves, friends, and/or their family members during medical encounters (Lillie-Blanton et al., 2000). Prior research has found that religious affiliation and orientations predict both adherence to discriminatory attitudes toward minority groups (Kirkpatrick, 1993) as well as reactions to discriminatory views by others (Byrnes & Kiger, 1992). Fundamentalist affiliates are more likely to hold discriminatory attitudes toward minority groups but less likely to react against discriminatory views. No research, however, has examined how social factors, such as religious affiliation, are implicated in the link between discriminatory experiences in the medical encounter and trust in personal physicians.

This study situates affiliations with faith-based communities as a key moderator in the relationship between racial group membership and attitudes toward personal physician. Faith-based affiliations may be a moderating mechanism because it transforms the relationship between trusting attitudes and perceived discrimination against the individual or the group due to race. Specifically, this study works from the premise the affiliates of Black Protestant communities may harbor more trust in personal physicians because the conditions of community within these faith-based communities foster more positive views of physicians. These conditions include higher levels of religious participation, more contact with the medical system via faith-based community partnerships with physicians and public health professionals, and more contact with high-status professionals within the faith-based organization. Using data from the 2002 and 2006 General Social Survey, this study examines whether black-white differences in trust are contingent upon the type of faith-based affiliation one has. The next section reviews extant research regarding heterogeneity in blacks' views of personal physician by way of religious affiliation.

BACKGROUND RESEARCH

Researchers posit that historical instances of discriminatory practices toward blacks within social institutions, such as health care, serve as sources of collective memories regarding racial inequities transmitted across institutions and through social networks of friends, family members, and blood and non-blood relatives (Gamble, 1997; Lipset & Schneider, 1987; Washington, 2006). Furthermore, aspects of systemic racism throughout American history may contribute to distrust among blacks, including lynchings, unsolved killings in sundown towns, and the rise of the "prison industrial complex" (Alexander, 2012, Blalock, 1967; Bobo & Thompson, 2006; Marable, 1983; Roediger, 1999). Simply put, the history of racial discrimination is as long as, and embedded within, the history of America

(Feagin, 2006). Incidents such as the Tuskegee Syphilis Study and other medical abuses of blacks speak directly to the patient–physician relationship and give credence to blacks' present-day distrust in medicine and inequities perceived in other institutions and interactional spaces (Gamble, 1997; Washington, 2006). Accordingly, blacks may be less trusting of physicians not only because of present-day inequities in the quality of treatment in the health care system, but also because of collective memories stemming from a legacy of medical abuse and experimentation on black people.

Faith-based communities in the Black community serve as a key social location wherein collective memories of inequitable treatment are given space (Cone, 1984; Lincoln & Mamiya, 1990; Taylor, Thornton, & Chatters, 1987). While such collective memories can serve to buttress feelings of group discrimination, they can also serve to build community through shared experiences of constrained opportunity structures within and across institutions. By fostering social contact and identity construction, collective memories catalogue and interweave a group's historical timeline and contemporary lived experiences (Halbwachs, 1992; Zerubavel, 2003). Institutions where the networks of blacks are more dense and racially homogenous, such as faith-based organizations, may facilitate the cultural transmission of collective memories that also foster trust. Religion has always been a source of support and strength for the black community (Du Bois, 1903; Frazier, 1964; Lincoln, 1974; Taylor, Chatters, & Levin, 2004). The Black Protestant church, specifically, is a space that is often owned and operated by other blacks who are invested in the progression of the black community (Lincoln & Mamiya, 1990; Taylor, Thornton, & Chatters, 1987; Thomas, Quinn, Billingsley, & Caldwell, 1994). In fact, black churches and their leaders (e.g., Southern Christian Leadership Conference (SCLC), Martin Luther King, Jr.) were influential in shaping the discourse of the Civil Rights Movement (Morris, 1986, 1996; Williams, 1987).

Accordingly, faith-based affiliations offer an opportunity to examine whether blacks may be more likely to trust physicians in certain sociopolitical contexts, such as Black Protestant churches. There are several reasons to expect higher levels of trust among blacks who are affiliated with Black Protestant churches than among blacks who are not affiliated with Black Protestant churches. First, while integrated churches often do not incorporate the customs, leadership potentials, and/or theological preferences of blacks (Edwards, 2008), Black Protestant churches are more likely to have black clergy and leadership (Lincoln & Mamiya, 1990). Since blacks are more likely to trust ingroup members (Simpson et al., 2007), blacks affiliated with Black Protestant churches may be more likely than blacks affiliated with other types of churches to extend trust to other institutional gatekeepers (e.g., physicians) as well. From this perspective, blacks affiliated with Black Protestant churches extend trust toward physicians because the Black Protestant arena creates a safe space that elicits trustworthy behaviors, attitudes, and norms toward institutional gatekeepers. Attachment to one institution (religion) may foster attachment to another institution (medicine) – an argument that has been made in regards to the effects of religious affiliation among working class whites (Wilcox, Cherlin, Uecker, & Messel, 2012). Second, Black Protestant churches may have historically rooted patterns of coping with discrimination from society in general (Bierman, 2006) that may lead them to, in the end, exhibit a higher level of trust than African Americans not involved in Black Protestant churches, including trust in physicians.

Third, Blacks who are affiliated with Black Protestant churches may be more trusting of physicians because recommendations to healthcare providers who treat black patients equitably may pass through the social networks of church members whom they are more likely to trust. Fourth, Black Protestant churches may be hubs for faith-based public health initiatives (Levin, 1984). In this case, black pastors may vouch for physicians and public health scholars who are conducting interventions in black communities (Levin, 1986). Fifth, black Protestants may trust physicians more because they are of lower socioeconomic status than blacks of other religious traditions (Sherkat, 2001, 2002), and persons of lower socioeconomic status have been found in some studies to exhibit more trust toward physicians than persons of higher socioeconomic status (Chu-Weininger & Balkrishnan, 2006).

Yet, prior research that has examined racial differences in physician trust and religious affiliation has not found evidence of black-white differences in physician trust (Hall, Camacho, Dugan, & Balkrishnan, 2002), even holding constant faith-based affiliations (Benjamins, 2006). We argue this is because prior research has not used a measure of religious affiliation that distinctly identifies the levels of trust among Black Protestants as distinguishable from the levels of trust among blacks who are affiliated with other faith-based organizations. Were Black Protestants to be distinguished from blacks who are affiliated with other faith-based organization, racial differences in physician trust may be identified. Specifically, heterogeneities in levels of trust among blacks might be revealed.

This chapter provides new insight over and beyond existing studies by interrogating the link between religious denomination and racial inequalities in trusting physicians. We examine whether Black Protestant affiliation influences the race gap in physician trust between blacks and whites in the United States. This interrogation is done in a way that highlights a serious methodological challenge in studying the intersections of two correlated social conditions – ethnoracial status and religious denomination. Methodologically speaking, we reconsider the black-white physician trust gap by distinguishing religious groups by racial status using an intersectional model of ethnoreligiousity. Generally, we ask: Are blacks who attend Black Protestant churches more likely to trust physicians than other ethnoreligious groups? Accordingly, we propose three hypotheses for this study.

Hypothesis 1. Blacks are less likely to trust physicians than whites.

Hypothesis 2. Blacks who attend Black Protestant churches, compared to blacks who do not, are more likely to trust physicians.

Hypothesis 3. Blacks who attend Black Protestant churches, compared to whites, are more likely to trust physicians.

The first hypothesis extends from the long line of research that predicts lower levels of trust among blacks when compared to whites. The second hypothesis specifically focuses on heterogeneities in trust among blacks. The third hypothesis, meanwhile, entails that Black Protestants will be so different from blacks that their views on physicians are also distinct from whites. Together, these hypotheses indicate that the black-white physician trust gap is contingent upon faith-based affiliations and that faith-based affiliations, in general, are a moderator of race differences in physician trust.

DATA

Data for this study come from the 2002 and 2006 General Social Surveys (GSS) conducted by the National Opinion Research Center (Davis, Smith, & Marsden, 2007). The 2002 and 2006 GSS used a full probability sample of persons of 18 years of age or older living in non-institutional arrangements within the 48 contiguous states of the United States. Face-to-face interviews of approximately 1.5 hours were conducted between March and May of 2002 and 2006. Assessments of primary care physicians are derived from a random sub-sample of 2,728 respondents given questions that were assessed during the Mental Health Module. Black and white respondents with invalid data on the dependent and independent variables are excluded from the analysis. Latinos, Asians, other races, and persons who do not report their race are also omitted from the analysis. The final sample size is 2,209.

Dependent Variable

This study examines racial differences in trust toward physicians using a shortened Trust in Physician Scale (Anderson & Dedrick, 1990). Trust in physicians is measured by asking a series of statements about the medical care they are receiving now (or would expect if they sought care). Anderson and Dedrick's Trust in Physician scale focuses primarily on physicians treating general health conditions (Anderson & Dedrick, 1990). The scale includes five indicators of trust: Honesty; Fiduciary Ethic; Technical Judgment; Cultural Authority; and Interpersonal Competence.

The *Honesty* dimension is assessed by agreement with the statement, "I trust my doctor to tell me if a mistake was made about my treatment." The *Fiduciary Ethic* dimension is assessed by agreement with the statement, "I trust my doctor to put my medical needs above all other considerations when treating my medical problem." The *Technical Judgment* dimension is assessed by agreement with the statement, "I trust my doctor's judgment about my medical care." The *Cultural Authority* dimension is assessed by agreement with the statement, "My doctor is a real expert in taking care of medical problems like mine." The *Interpersonal Competence* dimension is assessed by disagreement with the statement, "I doubt my doctor really cares about me as a person."

Each of the aforementioned statements was coded originally on a five-point scale (1 = strongly agree, 2 = agree, 3 = neither agree nor disagree, 4 = disagree, and 5 = strongly disagree). Respondents' answers were coded "don't know" only if they volunteered this response; these respondents are dropped from subsequent analyses. Respondents who refused to provide a response to the statements are also dropped from the analyses. Items are coded so that more positive responses reflect greater trust in physicians. Factor analysis of the five items indicates a single underlying dimension with little variation in the factor loadings (Cronbach's alpha (α) = .75). A summary scale was constructed by dividing the sum of responses by five. Table 1 presents descriptive statistics for the dependent variable and the independent and control variables detailed below.

Racial Group Membership

Racial group membership is measured by a dummy indicator variable – 1 = black non-Latino ("black"); 0 = white non-Latino ("white"). Racial group membership is classified by the respondent using procedures followed in the decennial U.S. Census. Seventeen percent of the sample is classified as black.

Religious Affiliation

Religious affiliation is measured in three ways. The first way that religious affiliation is measured is with RELTRAD designations (Steensland et al., 2000), which identifies six religious denominations – Evangelical Protestant, Mainline Protestant, Black Protestant, Catholic, Jew, Other Faith, and Non-Affiliated. The second way that religious affiliation is measured is with a simplified RELTRAD designation, which identifies four religious affiliations – Black Protestant, Protestant-Affiliated, Other-Affiliated, and Non-Affiliated. RELTRAD designations are simplified in this way due to unbalanced cell sizes by race. The simplified RELTRAD designation collapses the distinctions between Evangelical Protestants and Mainline Protestants (as Protestant-Affiliated) and the distinctions between Catholics, Jews, and members of other faiths (as Other-Affiliated). The third way that religious affiliation is measured is with an intersectional religious affiliation designation – ethnoreligious groups. This typology allows for the effect of four simplified RELTRAD religious affiliations (Black Protestant, Protestant-Affiliated, Other-Affiliated, and Non-Affiliated) to be distinct by racial group. Whites who are classified as Black Protestant using RELTRAD designations are removed from the analysis due to small sample size ($n = 31$). This leaves seven ethnoreligious groups to be evaluated.

Control Variables

To account for sources of measurement error associated with differences in the coding of the middle trust response category between the two surveys, a dummy indicator for the 2002 survey year is included as a control variable (reference category = 2006 survey year). Supplemental analyses indicate that the survey year indicator captures the effects of survey measurement error. Though the effect of year was significant ($F = 20.04$, $p < 0.001$), the effects of correlates of trust were consistent across years of the GSS (F = 0.67, p = 0.733). Thus, the 2002 and 2006 GSS samples are pooled for the following analyses.

To assess the role of racial differences in sociodemographic correlates of trust, covariates for marital, work, and parental status, household size, gender, age, education, subjective class identification, region, parental nativity, religious service attendance, voting behavior, and political party affiliation are included (Table 1). Measures that tap sociodemographic differences between blacks and whites include marital status (1 = married, 0 = other); work status (1 = full-time worker, 0 = other); parental status (1 = have children, 0 = no children); household size (family sizes more than 10 collapsed into highest category); gender (1 = females, 0 = males); age (1st and 2nd order polynomial term for years of life lived); education (years of school completed); a categorical measure of lower or working class identification (reference category = middle or upper class); region (1 = Southerner, 0 = non-Southerner); and parental nativity (1 = has two native parents, 0 = has one or two non-native parents). Racial differences in religious attendance are measured using a nine-category ordinal variable assessing frequency of religious service attendance (0 = never, 1 = less than one time a year, 2 = about 1–2 times a year, 3 = several times a year, 4 = about once a month, 5 = 2–3 times a month, 6 = nearly every week, 7 = every week, 8 = several times a week). Racial differences in political factors are measured by voting behavior (1 = ever voted, 0 = never voted) and a categorical measure of Democratic or Republican political party affiliation (reference category = Independent or Other party).

METHODS OF ANALYSIS

Weighted multivariate regression is employed to adjust for differential sampling probabilities among individuals across survey year (WTSSALL). Robust standard errors are also employed. First, this study examines unadjusted and adjusted racial differences in trusting physicians using a dummy indicator for black respondents (white respondents are the reference category). Racial differences are then adjusted by holding constant sociodemographic characteristics. Second, religious denomination differences in trusting physicians are examined using RELTRAD designations (Steensland et al., 2000), holding constant racial differences and then sociodemographic characteristics. Third, unadjusted and adjusted religious denomination differences in trusting physicians are examined using simplified RELTRAD

Table 1. Descriptive Statistics by Race and for the Combined Sample, $N = 2,209$.

	Black (N = 369)				White (N = 1,840)				Combined (N = 2,209)			
	Mean	SD	Min	Max	Mean	SD	Min	Max	Mean	SD	Min	Max
Outcomes												
Trust in physician scale	3.93	0.75	1.00	5.00	3.98	0.76	1.00	5.00	3.97	0.76	1.00	5.00
Religious affiliation												
RELTRAD designations												
Black Protestant	0.58		0.00	1.00	–		–	–	0.10		0.00	1.00
Evangelical Protestant	0.15		0.00	1.00	0.29		0.00	1.00	0.27		0.00	1.00
Mainline Protestant	0.05		0.00	1.00	0.23		0.00	1.00	0.20		0.00	1.00
Catholic	0.07		0.00	1.00	0.24		0.00	1.00	0.21		0.00	1.00
Jewish	0.00		0.00	1.00	0.03		0.00	1.00	0.02		0.00	1.00
Other faith	0.05		0.00	1.00	0.05		0.00	1.00	0.05		0.00	1.00
Non-affiliated	0.11		0.00	1.00	0.16		0.00	1.00	0.15		0.00	1.00
Affiliation designations												
Black Protestant	0.58		0.00	1.00	–		–	–	0.10		0.00	1.00
Protestant-affiliated	0.19		0.00	1.00	0.53		0.00	1.00	0.47		0.00	1.00
Other-affiliated	0.12		0.00	1.00	0.31		0.00	1.00	0.28		0.00	1.00
Non-affiliated	0.11		0.00	1.00	0.16		0.00	1.00	0.15		0.00	1.00
Control variables												
Married (0 = unmarried)	0.30		0.00	1.00	0.51		0.00	1.00	0.48		0.00	1.00
Full-time worker (0 = not full-time worker)	0.53		0.00	1.00	0.50		0.00	1.00	0.50		0.00	1.00
No. of people in household	2.40	1.49	1.00	10.00	2.33	1.33	1.00	11.00	2.34	1.36	1.00	11.00
Parent (0 = no children)	0.80		0.00	1.00	0.71		0.00	1.00	0.72		0.00	1.00
Female (0 = male)	0.63		0.00	1.00	0.56		0.00	1.00	0.57		0.00	1.00
Age of respondent	44.22	15.82	18.00	89.00	48.14	17.38	18.00	89.00	47.48	17.19	18.00	89.00
South (0 = non-south)	0.62		0.00	1.00	0.33		0.00	1.00	0.38		0.00	1.00
Two parents born in the United States (0 = other)	0.90		0.00	1.00	0.87		0.00	1.00	0.88		0.00	1.00
Years of education	12.80	2.66	2.00	20.00	13.77	2.76	2.00	20.00	13.61	2.77	2.00	20.00

Subjective class identification												
Lower class (0 = other)	0.13		0.00	1.00	0.05		0.00	1.00	0.06		0.00	1.00
Working class (0 = other)	0.50		0.00	1.00	0.40		0.00	1.00	0.42		0.00	1.00
Middle/upper class (reference category)	0.37		0.00	1.00	0.55		0.00	1.00	0.52		0.00	1.00
Has ever voted (0 = never voted)	0.68		0.00	1.00	0.78		0.00	1.00	0.77		0.00	1.00
Political party affiliation												
Republican (0 = other)	0.06		0.00	1.00	0.35		0.00	1.00	0.30		0.00	1.00
Independent/other (0 = other)	0.31		0.00	1.00	0.38		0.00	1.00	0.36		0.00	1.00
Democrat (reference category)	0.63		0.00	1.00	0.27		0.00	1.00	0.33		0.00	1.00
Religious service attendance	4.58	2.65	0.00	8.00	3.57	2.77	0.00	8.00	3.74	2.77	0.00	8.00

Source: 2002 and 2006 General Social Survey.
Note: SD = Standard deviation.

designations. Last, unadjusted and adjusted ethnoreligious differences in trusting physicians are examined using an intersectional conceptualization of religious affiliation designations that distinguishes Black Protestants who are black from other race-specific religious affiliation designations codified with simplified RELTRAD designations.

RESULTS

Table 2 shows regression models for the effect of racial group membership on physician trust. The first model in Table 2 implies that blacks are not less trusting than whites of physicians ($b = -0.073$; $p = 0.196$). This finding counters Hypothesis 1 that blacks are less likely to trust physicians than

Table 2. Weighted Linear Regression for the Effect of Race and Religious Denomination on Physician Trust, $N = 2{,}209$.

	Model 1	Model 2	Model 3	Model 4
Racial group membership (ref. White)				
Black	−0.07	−0.10	−0.25**	−0.25**
	(0.06)	(0.06)	(0.09)	(0.09)
Religious affiliation: RELTRAD (ref. evangelical protestant)				
Black Protestant			0.28*	0.26*
			(0.11)	(0.11)
Mainline Protestant			0.01	0.02
			(0.05)	(0.06)
Catholic			0.03	0.05
			(0.05)	(0.05)
Jewish			−0.24*	−0.22*
			(0.10)	(0.10)
Other faith			−0.06	−0.02
			(0.10)	(0.10)
Non-affiliated			−0.11	0.02
			(0.06)	(0.07)
Controls		Included		Included
Constant	3.97***	4.07***	3.99***	4.06***
	(0.02)	(0.15)	(0.04)	(0.16)
Observations	2,209	2,209	2,209	2,209

Source: 2002 and 2006 General Social Survey.
Notes: Unstandardized beta coefficients shown; standard errors in parentheses. Reference category for RELTRAD is Evangelical Protestant. Models with controls include adjustments for subjective class identification, worker status, household size, parental status, female gender, age of respondent, Southern regional location, parental nativity, years of education, civic participation, political party identification, and religious service attendance.
*$p < 0.05$; **$p < 0.01$; ***$p < 0.001$ (two-tailed test).

whites. Model 2 indicates that this non-significant relationship holds even when considering black-white differences in sociodemographic characteristics. These findings suggest that blacks are actually more heterogeneous than the literature has implied.

Model 3 in Table 2 includes variables for church affiliation using RELTRAD designations. RELTRAD designations allow a specification for members of Black Protestant churches that are not otherwise possible using other church affiliation typologies. As mentioned in the methods section, whites who could be designated as Black Protestant are not included in the sample due to small sample sizes. As such, the Black Protestant coefficient refers only to blacks who are affiliated with Black Protestant churches. When RELTRAD designations are considered, the coefficient for black group membership becomes significant and negative ($b = -0.248$; $p = 0.005$), which indicates that blacks are significantly less likely to trust physicians than whites when religious affiliation is taken into consideration. Meanwhile, the coefficient for Black Protestant church affiliation is significant and positive ($b = 0.283$; $p = 0.012$). This finding implies that blacks who attend Black Protestant churches are more likely to trust physicians than Evangelical Protestants. Collectively, these findings support Hypothesis 2 that blacks who attend Black Protestant churches, compared to blacks who do not, are more likely to trust physicians. It also suggests that Black Protestants may actually be more likely to trust physicians than whites. These findings also provide qualified support for Hypothesis 1: holding constant religious affiliation, blacks are less trusting of physicians than whites.

Fig. 1 shows unadjusted levels of physician trust by race and religious affiliation using an intersectional typology of church affiliation, as shown in Model 3 of Table 3. In this typology of religious affiliation, the differences between evangelical Protestants and mainline Protestants are collapsed, as well as the differences among Catholics, Jews, and members of other faiths. Accordingly, racial distinctions are considered for three religious groups in comparison to blacks who are Black Protestant – Protestant-affiliated, other-affiliated, and non-affiliated. Fig. 1 reveals that Black Protestants are actually more likely to trust physicians than all other groups including all other types of blacks and all other types of whites.

To further highlight this pattern, Table 3 shows regression models for the effect of religious affiliation on physician trust using a simplified RELTRAD classification scheme that collapses distinctions between Evangelical Protestants and Mainline Protestants (Protestant-Affiliated) and between Jews, Catholics, and other faiths (Other-Affiliated). White respondents who are classified as Black Protestants were removed from the sample for this study, as such by default the reference category for all

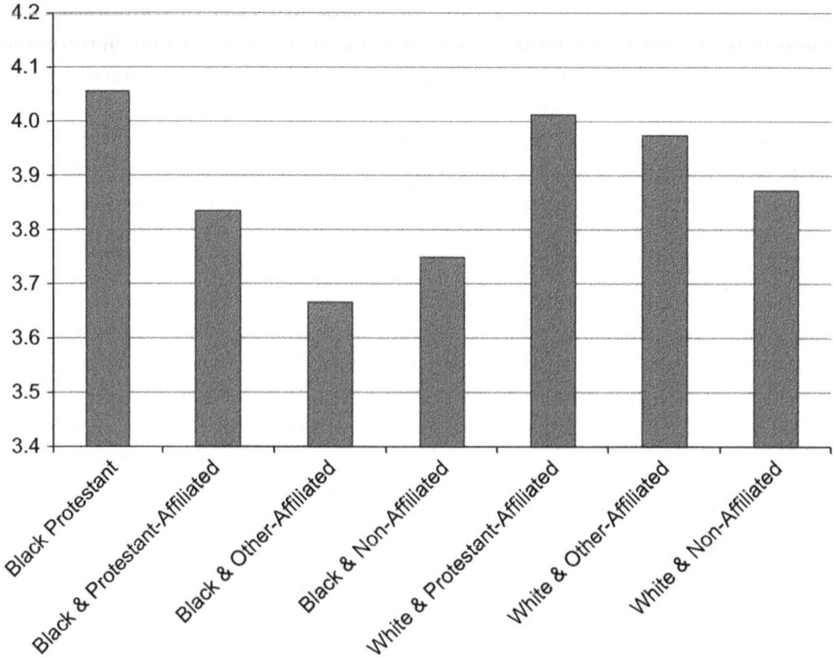

Fig. 1. Physician Trust by Race and Religious Affiliation, $N = 2{,}209$.

models in Table 3 is black respondents who are classified as Black Protestants. The black coefficient in Model 1 of Table 3 indicates that blacks who are not Black Protestant exhibit less trust than blacks who are Black Protestant ($b = -0.250$; $p = 0.004$). As such, Hypothesis 2 is confirmed.

Moreover, the simplified RELTRAD religious affiliation coefficients in Model 1 of Table 3 indicate that Black Protestants exhibit more trust than respondents of any race or of any other religious affiliations ($F[3,2204] = 4.49$; $p = 0.004$). Specifically, Black Protestants are more trusting than persons who are affiliated with other Protestant groups ($b = -0.280$; $p = 0.011$), persons who are affiliated with other faiths ($b = -0.291$; $p = 0.010$), and persons who are non-affiliated ($b = -0.397$; $p = 0.001$). These findings hold when controlling for religious differences in sociodemographic characteristics (Table 3, Model 2). Black Protestants are more trusting of physicians than other religious groups even when individual characteristics are considered.

Models 3 and 4 of Table 3 employ an intersectional typology of ethnoreligious affiliations to more explicitly examine Black Protestant's levels of

Table 3. Weighted Linear Regression for the Effect of Ethnoreligious Affiliation on Physician Trust, $N = 2{,}209$.

	Model 1	Model 2	Model 3	Model 4
Racial group membership (ref. White)				
Black	−0.25**	−0.25**		
	(0.09)	(0.09)		
Religious affiliation: simplified RELTRAD (ref. Black Protestant)				
Protestant-affiliated	−0.28*	−0.26*		
	(0.11)	(0.11)		
Other-affiliated	−0.29**	−0.26*		
	(0.11)	(0.11)		
Non-affiliated	−0.40***	−0.26*		
	(0.11)	(0.11)		
Ethnoreligious affiliation (ref. Black Protestant)				
Black and Protestant-affiliated			−0.22	−0.20
			(0.14)	(0.14)
Black and other-affiliated			−0.46**	−0.38*
			(0.17)	(0.16)
Black and non-affiliated			−0.32	−0.22
			(0.18)	(0.17)
White and Protestant-affiliated			−0.04	−0.02
			(0.07)	(0.07)
White and other-affiliated			−0.03	0.01
			(0.08)	(0.08)
White and non-affiliated			−0.16	−0.01
			(0.08)	(0.09)
Controls		Included		Included
Constant	4.27***	4.31***	4.02***	4.07***
	(0.11)	(0.19)	(0.07)	(0.16)
Observations	2,209	2,209	2,209	2,209

Source: 2002 and 2006 General Social Survey.
Notes: Unstandardized beta coefficients shown; standard errors in parentheses. Reference category for religious affiliation and ethnoreligious affiliation is Black Protestant. Models with controls include adjustments for subjective class identification, worker status, household size, parental status, female gender, age of respondent, Southern regional location, parental nativity, years of education, civic participation, political party identification, and religious service attendance.
$^*p < 0.05$; $^{**}p < 0.01$; $^{***}p < 0.001$ (two-tailed test).

physician trust in relation to race-specific religious (i.e., ethnoreligious) groups. The main coefficient for black racial group status is interacted with the four-category simplified RELTRAD designation variable. Model 3 reveals that blacks who are affiliated with non-Protestant places of worship are significantly less trusting of physicians than blacks who attend Black Protestant churches ($b = -0.462$; $p = 0.007$). Moreover, supplemental tests for the joint significance of ethnoreligious groups (available upon request) indicates that Black Protestants hold distinct views of personal physicians than other ethnoreligious groups ($F[6,2202] = 2.86$; $p = 0.009$), other black ethnoreligious groups ($F[3,2202] = 3.35$; $p = 0.018$), and other-affiliated persons ($F[2,2209] = 3.85$; $p = 0.0213$). The negative value of the beta coefficients in Model 3 suggests that Black Protestants are more trusting of personal physicians than white ethnoreligious groups. Still, while Black Protestants have higher levels of trust in personal physicians than whites on average, the difference between Black Protestants and whites is not statistically significant ($F[3,2202] = 2.06$; $p = 0.1039$). Hypothesis 3 is not confirmed: Black Protestants hold similar views towards physicians as do whites.

Model 4 of Table 3, which includes covariates for pertinent sociodemographic factors, show similar patterns. Differences in levels of physician trust between Black Protestants and other black respondents are partly attenuated once sociodemographic factors are considered ($F[3, 2186] = 2.46$; $p = 0.061$). Supplemental analysis (available upon request) indicates that the sociodemographic factors responsible for the attenuation of the distinction between Black Protestants and other black ethnoreligious groups are a combination of political factors and religious service attendance. Holding all else constant, differences in physician trust between Black Protestants and other-affiliated black respondents remain statistically significant, ($b = -0.384$; $p = 0.016$). Hypothesis 2 is partly supported.

Meanwhile, Hypothesis 3 is not supported. Although Model 3 of Table 3 indicates that blacks who attend Black Protestant churches are slightly more likely to trust physicians than whites who are not affiliated ($b = -0.155$; $p = 0.059$), Black Protestants are not more likely to trust physicians than whites who are affiliated with Protestant or non-Protestant organizations. These findings indicate that there are more similarities between Black Protestants and whites in regards to physician trust (though they may be referencing different physicians) than between Black Protestants and non-Protestant blacks. Altogether, the results show that blacks who attend Black Protestant churches trust differently than blacks who do not attend black Protestant churches.

DISCUSSION

This chapter examined the role of religious affiliation in attenuating racial differences in physician trust. We found that Black Protestants are more trusting of physicians than other ethnoreligious groups. Our findings have implications for highlighting how the public health intervention model can be more successful – that is, by working through the safe spaces of Black Protestant churches. We argue that public health and health services researchers will be more effective at breaking down black distrust by working through churches and other faith-based organizations.

Black distrust in physicians must be recognized as rooted in a distinct racialized history characterized by institutional and individual acts of discrimination that can be traced back to American slavery and Jim Crow and linked to the current sociohistorical ramifications of being racially marginalized in America. Gamble's conceptualization of collective memories (Gamble, 1997) identifies how the very fabric of institutionalized social relationships are shaped by American race relations that systemically produce racialized spaces of disadvantage and opportunity (Feagin, 2006). As a social condition, race shapes the formation and maintenance of relationships (Link & Phelan, 1995; Williams & Collins, 1995), thereby serving as a key axis by which affective bonds develop that facilitate the extension of trust in the behaviors of institutional actors.

Black Protestant churches are effective at reducing racial differences in trust because these sites already have trust embedded in the makings of the social institution. Since the 1700s, churches have been one of the few places where blacks can find refuge (Frazier, 1964). Black pastors are community trustees (Levin, 1986) who in many ways have "a symbolic key to the Black community" (Ray, 2014). The literature on health and religion shows that Black Protestant churches serve not only as intervention sites but also as hubs that increase healthcare utilization by connecting church members with trustworthy practitioners who will show a high level of care and concern for their health and the health of their loved ones (Blank, Mahmood, Fox, & Guterbock, 2002; DeHaven, Hunter, Wilder, Walton, & Berry, 2004; Levin, 1984, Ray, 2014; Young & Stewart, 2006). Black Protestant churches can be found in all areas throughout the country regardless of racial composition, whether this is rural Indiana or the plains of Kansas. As some of the first owned and fully operated black establishments, Black Protestant churches are not only places of faith, but also places of safety, leadership, and trust for a host of black communities (Lincoln, 1974; Lincoln & Mamiya, 1990; Ray, 2014; Taylor et al., 2004).

Methodologically, we go beyond simply identifying the unique contributions race and religion to variations in physician trust. Instead, we describe physician trust levels by ethnoreligiosity – a two dimensional social condition that reflects an individual's concurrent positionality within a racialized society divided by religious groupings. From this perspective, we do not seek to decompose the "race gap" per se. Rather, we sort the population by levels of physician trust in ways that capture the unique intersections of race and religion. Similar approaches have been taken by Idler and Kasl (1997) in their decision to bifurcate Protestants by race. Yet, the formulization of a Black Protestant category by Steensland et al. (2000) allows us to take a further step by dividing other religious groupings by ethnoraciality. Moreover, our racialization of religious groupings occurs within the context of the analytical model rather than in the context of the research design. In these ways, our interactional approach to race and religion represents a fundamental reconsideration of traditional categorization methods in studies of race and religion.

Admittedly, our analysis does not reflect the multi-ethnic environment of the United States. Past research employing the GSS has found it difficult to untangle the effect of race from that of ethnicity because of small sample sizes. Still, Latinos have been found to have lower levels of trust than whites (Stepanikova, Mollborn, Cook, Thom, & Kramer, 2006) and qualitatively different perspectives on social attitudes (Hunt, 2007). Also, our analysis relies on a shortened version of the Trust in Physician scale (Anderson & Dedrick, 1990). Black Protestant effects are unable to be evaluated with the longer version of the Trust in Physician scale, which was only asked in the 1998 GSS, due to small sample sizes. As such, this study provides preliminary evidence that blacks affiliated with Black Protestant churches exhibit higher levels of physician trust than other ethnoreligious groups.

Future research would benefit from understanding the similarities and points of departure in ethnoreligious determinants of trusting attitudes among and between Latinos and Asians as compared to blacks and whites. Future research would also benefit from examining ethnoreligious differences in physician trust using a broader range of items to determine trust in physicians. Further, exploring intraracial diversity in the correlates of trust will provide a more nuanced understanding of how historic and contemporary forces interweave to produce unique collective memories across and within racial and ethnic groups.

ACKNOWLEDGMENTS

The authors would like to thank Ellen Idler for helpful feedback on this manuscript. This manuscript was written while the first author was a Vice

Provost's Postdoctoral Fellow in the Population Studies Center at the University of Pennsylvania.

REFERENCES

Alesina, A., & La Ferrara, E. (2002). Who trusts others? *Journal of Public Economics, 85*, 207–234. doi:10.1016/S0047-2727(01)00084-6

Alexander, M. (2012). *The New Jim Crow: Mass incarceration in the age of colorblindness*. New York, NY: The New Press.

Anderson, L. A., & Dedrick, R. F. (1990). Development of the trust in physician scale: A measure to assess interpersonal trust inpatient-physician relationships. *Psychological Reports, 67*, 1091–1100.

Benjamins, M. R. (2006). Religious influences on trust in physicians and the health care system. *The International Journal of Psychiatry in Medicine, 36*, 69–83.

Bierman, A. (2006). Does religion buffer the effects of discrimination on mental health? Differing effects by race. *Journal for the Scientific Study of Religion, 45*(4), 551–565.

Blalock, H. M., Jr. (1967). *Toward a theory of minority-group relations*. New York, NY: Wiley.

Blank, M. B., Mahmood, M., Fox, J. C., & Guterbock, T. (2002). Alternative mental health services: The role of the black church in the south. *American Journal of Public Health, 92*, 1668–1672. doi:10.2105/AJPH.92.10.1668

Bobo, L. D., & Thompson, V. (2006). Unfair by design: The war on drugs, race, and the legitimacy of the criminal justice system. *Social Research: An International Quarterly, 73*, 445–472.

Byrnes, D. A., & Kiger, G. (1992). Social factors and responses to racial discrimination. *The Journal of Psychology, 126*(6), 631–638.

Chu-Weininger, M. Y., & Balkrishnan, R. (2006). Consumer satisfaction with primary care provider choice and associated trust. *BMC Health Services Research, 6*(1), 139.

Cone, J. H. (1984). *For my people: Black theology and the black church*. Maryknoll, NY: Orbis Books.

Davis, J. A., Smith, T. W., & Marsden, P. V. (2007). *General social surveys, 1975–2006: Cumulative codebook*. Chicago, IL: National Opinion Research Center.

DeHaven, M. J., Hunter, I. B., Wilder, L., Walton, J. W., & Berry, J. (2004). Health programs in faith-based organizations: Are they effective? *American Journal of Public Health, 94*, 1030–1036.

Du Bois, W. E. B. (1903). *The souls of black folk*. New York, NY: Oxford University Press.

Edwards, K. L. (2008). Bring race to the center: The importance of race in racially diverse religious organizations. *Journal for the Scientific Study of Religion, 47*, 5–9. doi:10.1111/j.1468-5906.2008.00387.x

Ellison, C. G., Musick, M. A., & Henderson, A. K. (2008). Balm in gilead: Racism, religious involvement, and psychological distress among African-American adults. *Journal for the Scientific Study of Religion, 47*(2), 291–309.

Feagin, J. R. (2006). *Systemic racism: A theory of oppression*. New York, NY: Routledge.

Frazier, E. F. (1964). *The Negro church in America*. New York, NY: Schocken Books.

Gamble, V. N. (1997). Under the shadow of tuskegee: African Americans and health care. *American Journal of Public Health, 87*, 1773–1778. doi:10.2105/AJPH.87.11.1773

Glaeser, E. L., Laibson, D. I., Scheinkman, J. A., & Soutter, C. L. (2000). Measuring trust. *The Quarterly Journal of Economics, 115*, 811–846. doi:10.1162/003355300554926

Halbwachs, M. (1992). *On collective memory*. Chicago, IL: University of Chicago Press.

Hall, M. A., Camacho, F., Dugan, E., & Balkrishnan, R. (2002). Trust in the medical profession: Conceptual and measurement issues. *Health Services Research, 37*(5), 1419–1439. doi:10.1111/1475-6773.01070

Hibbing, J. R., & Theiss-Morse, E. (2001). *What is it about government that Americans dislike?* Cambridge: Cambridge University Press.

Hughes, M., & Thomas, M. E. (1998). The continuing significance of race revisited: A study of race, class, and quality of life in America, 1972 to 1996. *American Sociological Review, 63*, 785–795. doi:10.2307/2657501

Hunt, M. O. (2007). African American, Hispanic, and white beliefs about black/white inequality, 1977–2004. *American Sociological Review, 72*, 390–415. doi:10.1177/000312240707200304

Idler, E. L., & Kasl, S. V. (1997). Religion among disabled and nondisabled persons I: Cross-sectional patterns in health practices, social activities, and well-being Ellen. *The Journals of Gerontology Series B: Psychological Sciences and Social Sciences, 52B*(6), S294–S305. doi:10.1093/geronb/52B.6.S294

Kirkpatrick, L. A. (1993). Fundamentalism, Christian orthodoxy, and intrinsic religious orientation as predictors of discriminatory attitudes. *Journal for the Scientific Study of Religion*, 256–268.

LaVeist, T. A., Nickerson, K. J., & Bowie, J. V. (2000). Attitudes about racism, medical mistrust, and satisfaction with care among African American and white cardiac patients. *Medical Care Research and Review, 57*, 146–161. doi:10.1177/1077558700574007

Levin, J. S. (1984). The role of the black church in community medicine. *Journal of the National Medical Association, 76*, 477.

Levin, J. S. (1986). Roles for the black pastor in preventive medicine. *Pastoral Psychology, 35*, 94–103. doi:10.1007/BF01768709

Lillie-Blanton, M., Brodie, M., Rowland, D., Altman, D., & McIntosh, M. (2000). Race, ethnicity, and the health care system: Public perceptions and experiences. *Medical Care Research and Review, 57*, 218–235. doi:10.1177/1077558700574010.

Lincoln, C. E. (1974). *The black church since Frazier*. New York, NY: Schocken Books.

Lincoln, C. E., & Mamiya, L. H. (1990). *The black church in the African American experience*. Duke University Press.

Link, B. G., & Phelan, J. (1995). Social conditions as fundamental causes of disease. *Journal of Health and Social Behavior, 35*, 80–94.

Lipset, S. M., & Schneider, W. (1987). The confidence gap during the reagan years, 1981–1987. *Political Science Quarterly, 102*, 1–23. doi:10.2307/2151482

Marable, M. (1983). *How capitalism underdeveloped black America: Problems in race, political economy, and society*. Cambridge, MA: South End Press.

Morris, A. D. (1986). *Origins of the civil rights movements*. New York, NY: Simon and Schuster.

Morris, A. D. (1996). The black church in the civil rights movement: The SCLC as the decentralized, radical arm of the black church. In C. Smith (Ed.), *Disruptive religion: The force of faith in social movement activism* (pp. 29–46). New York, NY: Routledge.

Ray, R. (2014). An intersectional analysis to explaining a lack of physical activity among middle class black women. *Sociology Compass, 8*(6), 780–791.

Roediger, D. R. (1999). *The wages of whiteness: Race and the making of the American working Class*. New York, NY: Verso.

Sherkat, D. E. (2001). Investigating the sect-church-sect cycle: Cohort-specific attendance differences across African-American denominations. *Journal for the Scientific Study of Religion, 40*(2), 221–234. doi:10.1111/0021-8294.00052

Sherkat, D. E. (2002). African–American religious affiliation in the late 20th century: Cohort variations and patterns of switching, 1973–1998. *Journal for the Scientific Study of Religion, 41*(3), 485–493. doi:10.1111/1468-5906.00132

Simpson, B., McGrimmon, T., & Irwin, K. (2007). Are blacks really less trusting than whites? Revisiting the race and trust question. *Social Forces, 86*, 525–552. doi:10.1093/sf/86.2.525

Smedley, B. D., Stith, A. Y., & Nelson, A. R. (Eds.). (2003). *Unequal treatment: Confronting racial and ethnic disparities in health care*. Washington, DC: National Academies Press.

Steensland, B., Robinson, L. D., Wilcox, W. B., Park, J. Z., Regnerus, M. D., & Woodberry, R. D. (2000). The measure of American religion: Toward improving the state of the art. *Social Forces, 79*, 291–318. doi:10.1093/sf/79.1.291

Stepanikova, I., Mollborn, S., Cook, K. S., Thom, D. H., & Kramer, R. M. (2006). Patients' race, ethnicity, language, and trust in a physician. *Journal of Health and Social Behavior, 47*, 390–405. doi:10.1177/002214650604700406

Taylor, R. J., Chatters, L. M., & Levin, J. (2004). *Religion in the lives of African Americans: Social, psychological, and health perspectives*. Thousand Oaks, CA: Sage.

Taylor, R. J., Thornton, M. C., & Chatters, L. M. (1987). Black Americans' perceptions of the sociohistorical role of the church. *Journal of Black Studies, 18*, 123–138. doi:10.2307/2784547

Thomas, S. B., Quinn, S. C., Billingsley, A., & Caldwell, C. (1994). The characteristics of northern black churches with community health outreach programs. *American Journal of Public Health, 84*, 575–579. doi:10.2105/AJPH.84.4.575

Washington, H. A. (2006). *Medical apartheid: The dark history of medical experimentation on black Americans from colonial times to the present*. New York, NY: Doubleday.

Wilcox, W. B., Cherlin, A. J., Uecker, J. E., & Messel, M. (2012). No money, no honey, no church: The deinstitutionalization of religious life among the white working class. In L. A. Keister, J. Mccarthy, & R. Finke (Eds.), *Religion, work and inequality* (Vol. 23, pp. 227–250). Research in the Sociology of Work. Bingley, UK: Emerald Group Publishing Limited.

Williams, D. R., & Collins, C. (1995). U.S. socioeconomic and racial differences in health: Patterns and explanations. *Annual Review of Sociology, 21*, 349–386. doi:10.2307/2083415

Williams, J. (1987). *Eyes on the prize: America's civil rights years, 1954–1965*. New York, NY: Viking.

Young, D. R., & Stewart, K. J. (2006). A church-based physical activity intervention for African American women. *Family & Community Health, 29*, 103–117.

Zerubavel, E. (2003). *Time maps: Collective memory and the social shape of the past*. Chicago, IL: University of Chicago Press.

PART VI
SPECIAL TYPES OF CARE SETTINGS

SUPPORT FOR HIV TESTING AND HIV CRIMINALIZATION AMONG OFFENDERS UNDER COMMUNITY SUPERVISION[☆]

Brad Barber and Bronwen Lichtenstein

ABSTRACT

Purpose – *U.S. health policy promotes HIV testing and linkage to care (test-and-treat) with an emphasis on high risk groups such as convicted offenders. We sought to identify whether or not laws for mandatory HIV disclosure to sexual partners are a barrier to HIV testing among offenders under community supervision.*

Methodology/approach – *A total of 197 probationers and parolees were surveyed in a closed/item-open-ended item methodology on two reporting days in Alabama. Three main questions were asked: (1) What do offenders know about HIV? (2) What do they know about the law? (3) Do they support mandatory disclosure and HIV testing? Data for*

[☆] We are indebted to the Alabama Department of Pardons and Paroles for facilitating the study, the Birmingham Field Office for physical space and material assistance, and to the interviewees for their willing participation.

Education, Social Factors, and Health Beliefs in Health and Health Care Services
Research in the Sociology of Health Care, Volume 33, 253–273

ISSN: 0275-4959/doi:10.1108/S0275-495920150000033011

the quantitative items were analyzed with SPSS and matched with open-ended responses for explanatory purposes.

Findings – *Testing and criminalization of non-disclosure were fully supported as key elements of HIV prevention. This support was framed by conceptions of HIV as a killer disease, of people with HIV as potential murderers, and by low self-awareness of HIV risk.*

Social implications – *While the study involved only a single group of convicted offenders in a southern state, the results suggest that disclosure laws legitimize HIV stigma and undermine test-and-treat strategies among communities at risk.*

Originality/value – *The research is the first of its kind to investigate possible links between HIV criminalization and barriers to HIV prevention and care among convicted offenders.*

Keywords: Convicted offenders; support of HIV testing; HIV criminalization

In 2010, the U.S. National Office of AIDS Policy (ONAP) developed the National HIV/AIDS strategy with three major related goals: (1) to reduce HIV incidence through routine testing, (2) to decrease HIV-related disparities and stigma, and (3) to provide access to HIV care (ONAP, 2010a). For the first and third goals, the strategy focuses on outreach to vulnerable communities for HIV testing and linkage to care, an approach that is referred to as test-and-treat. Convicted offenders are included in the goal for targeted HIV outreach. The strategy acknowledges a variety of potential barriers to this goal, including state laws for mandatory HIV disclosure to sexual partners. As stated in the document, people living with HIV/AIDS (PLWHA) have little incentive to be frank with sexual partners if they face increased HIV stigma and fear of arrest after being legally framed as medically dangerous (ONAP, 2010a). HIV criminalization laws therefore appear to be at odds with scaled-up efforts for HIV testing in communities at risk (Center for HIV Law and Policy, 2010).

The origins of HIV-specific laws, such as mandatory disclosure to sexual partners are seated in legislative responses to the rapid spread of HIV in the 1980s (Jürgens et al., 2009). Although the laws are controversial (Jürgens et al., 2009; Kaplan, 2012), they are also increasingly common throughout the United States. Following one HIV-related prosecution in

1986 (Center for HIV Law and Policy, 2010), at least eight states enacted HIV disclosure laws shortly afterward (Turkewitz, 2011). By 2008, 24 states had enacted HIV-specific codes for mandatory disclosure (Galletly & Pinkerton, 2008), with 13 more states creating statutes for this purpose in 2010 (Movement Advancement Project, 2014). Despite this law enforcement approach to HIV prevention, new HIV cases have remained steady at around 50,000 per year since 2010 and infection rates among Young Black Men who have Sex with Men (YBMSM) have risen sharply in recent years (Centers for Disease Control and Prevention [CDC], 2013a).

HIV prevention strategies for former inmates involve a variety of ancillary services such as discharge planning, transitional case management, housing, mental health services, and drug treatment (Robillard, Gallito-Zaparaniuk, Braithwaite, Arriola, & Kennedy, 2009). In the current test-and-treat era, employees in AIDS service agencies and health departments provide HIV-specific services such as counseling for mandatory disclosure, testing, and referrals or treatment for HIV/AIDS. However, access to HIV care is often affected by a variety of factors that involve convicted offenders, such as stigma, mental illness, substance abuse, and distrust of authorities (Ulett et al., 2009). Since sociological perspectives can help policymakers to understand sociocultural barriers to HIV prevention, it is useful to identify whether or not offenders under community supervision, as a target population, are receptive to HIV testing, and if laws for mandatory disclosure affect their willingness to participate in test-and-treat strategies for HIV control.

This chapter presents the results of a study that assessed knowledge and attitudes toward mandatory HIV disclosure and HIV testing among 197 offenders under community supervision in Alabama, the United States. The demographic characteristics of this population reflect racial disparities in the U.S. criminal justice system and regional disparities of HIV risk. For example, while African Americans comprise 26 percent of the total population of Alabama (U.S. Census Bureau, 2012), almost twice as many state-supervised probationers and parolees are Black (49 percent) (Alabama Board of Pardons and Paroles, 2013). On a broader scale, African Americans represent 13 percent of the total U.S. population (U.S. Census Bureau, 2013) and 30 percent of community supervised populations nationally (U.S. Bureau of Justice Statistics, 2011). Because HIV risk and criminal justice involvement are closely related (Epperson, El-Bassel, Gilbert, Orellana, & Chang, 2008), laws for HIV control and targeted policies for HIV testing should be examined in terms of how communities at risk perceive or respond to them. Toward this end, four main questions were asked of our sample: (1) What did the participants know about HIV/AIDS? (2) What did they know about Alabama's disclosure law? (3) Did they consider mandatory disclosure to be a barrier to HIV testing? (4) Should offenders be tested for HIV/AIDS? Few studies have addressed these questions empirically; even fewer have been conducted among convicted offenders who are stakeholders in scaled-up efforts for HIV prevention in the United States. This study offers new information on the intersection between HIV laws and HIV testing among offenders under community supervision in a region with the highest rates of HIV/AIDS in the United States (CDC, 2013b).

HEALTH DISPARITIES, SOCIAL JUSTICE, AND HIV CONTROL

HIV disparities are the product of social difference according to intersections of gender, race/ethnicity, poverty, sexual identity, and other markers of social status. In sociological terms, HIV disparities exemplify the social-constructivist paradigm in which patterns of disease and death are shaped by history, social structure, and the lived environment (Weitz, 2012). Parker and Aggleton (2003) argued that power and domination are at the crux of the matter, with stigma being the means by which social inequality is strengthened and reinforced through moral judgments about who becomes infected or ill. This argument is in line with sociological understandings of health disparities more broadly. For example, Wilkinson and Pickett (2009) found that, despite stigmatizing tropes about poor people's bad health habits, national and cross-national variance in morbidity and mortality are closely related to income disparities, even when controlling for smoking, lack of physical exercise, and poor diet. Just as the unequal distribution of wealth is directly responsible for shorter life spans among low-income people, the unequal distribution of social power, including wealth, also produces disproportionately greater HIV rates among society's most vulnerable or least valued actors (Link and Phelan, 2002). Thus, while blame for illness is commonly attributed to lifestyle, societies create their own patterns of disease for transmissible infections such as HIV/AIDS, as well as chronic health conditions that disproportionately affect low-income groups and people of color. HIV disparities were shaped most notably by the U.S. war on drugs which created "[a] penal system so large that it is now an important part of a uniquely American system of social stratification" (Western, 2006, p. 11). Large-scale incarceration has hollowed out communities of color, creating gender ratio disparities that promote sexual concurrency as a risk factor for HIV (Lichtenstein, Desmond, & Schwebke, 2008) and women's disempowerment in initiating condom use with male partners (Ferguson, Quinn, Eng, & Sandelowski, 2006).

Health disparities also involve barriers to health care. Sociology has identified the interplay of socioeconomic and cultural factors in these barriers, which include mistrust of medical professionals who are often socially different from the patients they treat (ONAP, 2010b). The reference to social difference is particularly relevant to this study. In writing about illness and identity, Karp (1999, p. 83) referred to chronic illness as a career in which "the person holds a position, engages in routine activities, and takes on certain perspectives." In extending this concept to AIDS-affected communities, such perspectives include historical distrust of a health system that recruited unsuspecting African American men for experimentation in the Tuskegee Syphilis Study of 1932–1972 (Jones, 1993). Because African Americans are disproportionately affected both by HIV/AIDS and criminal justice involvement, and distrust for the health system is seated in the *habitus* (collective dispositions) of black Americans (Gamble, 1997), it is important to identify how HIV testing is perceived in an era of HIV criminalization. If Karp's career trajectory holds for AIDS-affected communities that have been targeted for test-and-treat strategies, then the perspectives and positions of participants in this study could include resistance to scaled-up HIV testing on the basis of community-based distrust for U.S. public health policy.

Two related issues in terms of HIV disparities involve prosecutions for non-disclosure and a widening gap between law and medicine over prosecuting exposure to sexual partners. First, people who are poor or homeless, immigrant, or engaged in sex work have been prosecuted disproportionately on a global scale (Jürgens et al., 2009). In the United States, minority groups are more likely than Whites to be convicted under HIV laws for exposure, as well for posing a threat to public safety. To illustrate, after analyzing data on 56 criminal convictions under Michigan's HIV disclosure law, Hoppe (2012) found that African American men were more likely to be convicted than Whites or Hispanics, especially if they had not disclosed to women partners. Galletly and Lazzarini's (2013) analysis of 25 arrests for HIV exposure in Tennessee revealed a similar overrepresentation of African American men who received longer sentences than whites for the same crime.

Second, scientific knowledge about HIV/AIDS has advanced so that HIV laws appear to be outdated and punishment under such laws to be unnecessarily punitive, especially if HIV transmission does not occur.

Nevertheless, prosecutions for HIV-related crimes have escalated in recent years (Center for HIV Law and Policy, 2010). Criminal sanctions in such cases can be particularly harsh. In Texas, one PLWHA who spat on a police officer was charged with assault and sentenced to 35 years in prison (Center for HIV Law and Policy, 2010), even though saliva is not a mode of HIV transmission. In Iowa, a man with an undetectable viral load, who used a condom during intercourse, was sentenced to 25 years for non-disclosure (National Alliance of State and Territorial Directors [NASTAD], 2011). The lengthy sentence in this and other cases does not recognize that PLWHA with undetectable viral loads are unlikely to infect sexual partners (Donnell et al., 2010). Such legal approaches typically affect underserved populations who are often the locus of surveillance for sexual disease as well as for crime control in the United States.

METHODS

Recruitment and Sampling

Recruitment of probationers and parolees took place after IRB approvals were obtained from The University of Alabama and the Alabama Board of Pardons and Paroles. A total of 77 probationers and 120 parolees ($N = 197$) were recruited over two mandatory reporting days at the Probation and Parole Office in Birmingham, the largest site for offenders under community supervision in Alabama. All supervisees were eligible to participate in the research if they were 19 years or older, and all were given an opportunity to participate on a voluntary basis. The decision to recruit supervisees at one site centered on the practicality of collecting data from a central location and the need to obtain a sizeable sample so that both groups could be compared on study variables of interest. The site was a substantial distance from the authors' home institutions, which afforded the participants a measure of anonymity in addition to other protections, such as omitting names, addresses, and other identifying information from completed questionnaires.

For the purpose of comparison, offenders who had ever served time in prison were categorized as parolees, and offenders who never served time in prison were categorized as probationers. The only supervisory difference between these two groups was that the parolees were under the jurisdiction of the state Board of Pardons and Paroles and probationers were under the jurisdiction of Alabama's Circuit Courts. Unless a special condition is ordered by the Parole Board (for the parolees) or the presiding judge (for the probationers), the terms of supervision are the same.

Instrument

The participants completed a self-administered questionnaire at the 5th grade reading level. The instrument had five sections, for a total of 34 items. Section 1 consisted of 11 true/false items about how HIV could be prevented (e.g., condom use) or transmitted (e.g., mosquitoes; shared needles for drug use). Section 2 consisted of five Likert-scaled items to assess participants' perceptions of HIV risk and who should be tested for HIV. An additional item asked if participants knew anyone with HIV/AIDS but, as stipulated by the Alabama Board of Pardons and Paroles, we could not ask about participants' own HIV status. Section 3 consisted of three yes/no items about the HIV law and one scaled item about how much participants knew about the law (a lot, some details, or nothing). Four open-ended items then assessed knowledge of the law. For example, by asking "What do you know about the Alabama HIV law?" we wanted to find out if participants knew that HIV non-disclosure to sexual partners is a misdemeanor crime punishable by a fine of $500.00 and up to three months in jail. Other items in this section asked about the source of this knowledge, what they said about the law, and opinions about whether or not the law was fair. This closed-item/open-ended item technique is often used to elicit the meaning of responses to closed items in public opinion research (Zaller & Feldman, 1992). Section 4 consisted of two yes/no items about whether or not participants had ever attended a HIV prevention class and if they were offered these classes while being supervised. Section 5 consisted of eight demographic items for gender, age, race/ethnicity, marital status, education, income levels, arrest charge, and offender status (probation or parole).

Procedures

Recruitment and data collection occurred simultaneously on the two mandatory reporting days. Procedures involved setting up a table in a corner of the central waiting area of the Probation and Parole Office with a signboard and university insignia in order to avoid any appearance of being affiliated with the office or supervisees' conditions for probation or parole. Recruitment consisted of asking each individual who attended the office if he or she wished to participate in the study. About 85 percent of attendees agreed to participate, with refusals citing lack of interest or being pressed for time. After participants were formally consented and allotted a questionnaire to complete, we helped to interpret items if asked (some participants had minimal literacy), checked each protocol for any missing responses, and stored the protocols in a lock-box. Each participant received a $5.00 Wal-Mart gift card and a copy of the consent form to take home. On both days, the target sample of 100 surveys was administered and collected before the office closed at 5:00 p.m. Three surveys were discarded because they lacked an identification number for coding purposes for a total sample of 197 participants.

Characteristics

The participants were similar demographically to the overall population of offenders in Alabama. Most participants were African Americans (73 percent), male (65 percent), aged between 26 and 50 years old (65 percent) and unmarried (58 percent). More than two-thirds had a 12th grade education or lower (67 percent), and 80 percent of the sample had earned $20,000 or less in the past year. However, probationers and parolees differed significantly by gender, age, income, and the offense for which they were being supervised. Parolees were more likely than probationers to be male (73 percent vs. 56 percent), older than 35 years (64 percent vs. 37 percent), and to have earned less than $10,000 in the past year (69 percent vs. 46 percent). They were also more likely to have been convicted of violent or sex-related crimes (35 percent vs. 13 percent). Table 1 compares the sociodemographic characteristics of the two groups.

Analysis

The quantitative data were coded for SPSS analysis. First, we scored responses in the knowledge section of the survey instrument by dividing the number of correct responses by the 11 items for percentages of the total. Then, we organized these percentages into low, medium, and high scores. Next, chi-square tests were performed to identify relationships between sociodemographic characteristics, ordinal scores for HIV knowledge, and responses for Likert-scaled items relating to knowledge of the HIV law and attitudes toward HIV testing and mandatory disclosure. We also used

Table 1. Demographic Characteristics by Offender Status ($N = 197$).[a]

Variable	Probationers ($N = 77$)	Parolees ($N = 120$)	p
Gender			*.016*
% Male	56	73	
% Female	44	28	
Race/ethnicity			NS[a]
% African American	66	79	
% White	34	20	
% Hispanic	0	1	
Age			*.001*
% 19–25	29	10	
% 26–35	33	27	
% 36–50	20	46	
% Over 50	17	18	
Marital status			NS
% Unmarried	58	59	
% Married	27	18	
% Divorced/widowed	14	22	
Education			NS
% HS or less	58	75	
% Some college	29	20	
% College degree	13	6	
Income			*.015*
% Below $10,000	46	69	
% $10,001–$20,000	27	16	
% $20,001–$30,000	19	11	
% Over $30,000	8	4	
Arrest charge			*.007*
% Drugs	48	33	
% Theft	23	23	
% Violent	10	30	
% Sex	3	5	
% Other	16	10	

NS = not significant at $p < .05$.
[a]Totals may not sum to 100% due to rounding.

chi-square tests in order to compare responses on HIV knowledge and attitudes towards mandatory disclosure and HIV testing by offender status (probation or parole). Finally, we compared responses to yes/no or scaled items on HIV law and HIV testing to open-ended items on these topics for explanatory purposes. For example, scaled responses to "How much do you know about Alabama's HIV law?" were linked to narrative details about knowledge of the law prior to taking the survey, and yes/no responses to the item "Do you think the law is fair?" were linked to details about why the law was fair or unfair. These responses were organized according to themes that emerged from perspectives on HIV testing and the law. As reported by Reja, Manfreda, Hlebec, and Vehovar (2003, p. 169), the "richness of responses" in linking closed- and open-ended items for designated topics helps to explain the participants' rationale or frame of reference according to sociodemographic characteristics or circumstances. This mixed analytical technique was used to inform the results that are discussed next.

RESULTS

Knowledge about HIV/AIDS and Mandatory Disclosure HIV Law

Most participants answered the 11 true/false items on the HIV knowledge section correctly, with an average test score of 80 percent. Nevertheless, more than one-third of the sample (38 percent) believed incorrectly that mosquitoes transmitted HIV and more than half (59 percent) did not know that bleach could be used to sterilize needles for injection drug use. When converted to high/medium/low scores, two-thirds (65 percent) of participants earned a high score (9–11 knowledge items answered correctly). Most participants (69 percent) had also heard about Alabama's HIV law for mandatory disclosure, but only 19 percent overall knew any details beyond the threat of being arrested or jailed for non-disclosure. Little variation existed in terms of offender status or demographic characteristics such as gender, race/ethnicity, level of education, and HIV knowledge. However, parolees were more likely than probationers to know someone with HIV (45 percent vs. 22 percent), perhaps because they were older, more socially disadvantaged, and had served time in prison. Although the relationship between knowing someone with HIV and offender status was significant at the $p < .01$ level, personal acquaintance did not influence test scores for knowledge about HIV/AIDS ($p = .116$), or Alabama's HIV law ($p = .639$). Table 2 compares the results on knowledge about HIV, mandatory disclosure, and knowing someone with HIV/AIDS by offender status.

Narrative comments about Alabama's HIV law indicated that participants' knowledge related mostly to hearsay about people in the community being arrested for non-disclosure. The source of this information involved church, friends, or the workplace for probationers (83 percent) and jail,

Table 2. Knowledge of HIV/AIDS, Mandatory Disclosure, and PLWHA by Offender Status.

Item	Score	Probationers ($n = 77$) %	Parolees ($n = 120$) %	Total ($n = 197$) %	*p*
a. Knowledge of HIV/AIDS[a]	High	61	68	65	NS
	Medium	35	27	30	
	Low	4	5	5	
b. Knowledge of disclosure law[b]	High	17	20	19	NS
	Medium	53	49	50	
	Low	30	31	31	
c. Knows someone with HIV/AIDS	Yes	22	45	37	*.001*
	No	78	55	63	

NS = not significant at $p < .05$.
[a]HIV/AIDS scores: Out of a maximum of 11 items, high scorers were correct on 9–11 items, medium scorers were correct on 6–8 items, and low scorers were correct on 1–5 items.
[b]HIV law scale: "a lot" = high; "some details" = medium, "none" = low.

prison or family and friends for parolees (78 percent). Several misconceptions about the law were apparent after taking the narrative responses into account. Of the 53 participants who described what they knew about Alabama's HIV law (e.g., "You can go to jail" "You can be arrested"), nine were under the impression that the law falls under a murder charge and 17 thought that having HIV was a crime. Only one participant provided detailed information about the law (e.g., it is a misdemeanor crime; it is rarely prosecuted in Alabama), stating that he had learned these details from a case worker at a county health department. In sum, participants' knowledge about mandatory disclosure was perfunctory and obtained primarily from anecdotal sources.

Mandatory Disclosure as a Barrier to HIV Testing

Two-thirds of participants (66 percent) stated that mandatory disclosure was a barrier to HIV testing. The level of belief did not vary significantly by offender status or sociodemographic characteristics. In terms of why the law was a barrier to testing, a few participants again cited "fear of arrest" and "fear of arrest/going to jail" or, tangentially, "they don't want to be told they have HIV/AIDS, so they don't get tested." One participant believed that "The law does not reduce the spread of HIV/AIDS because so many people conceal their HIV status from their partners." Twelve percent of the sample was acquainted with someone who had been arrested for non-disclosure. While this percentage is relatively low, it helps to explain participants' beliefs about the consequences of HIV testing for someone who receives a positive diagnosis.

Participants were also asked if they thought the law was fair or unfair. Paradoxically, despite believing that criminalization was a barrier to HIV testing, 85 percent of the 109 participants who responded to this item believed that the law was fair, and that prosecuting violators was warranted. Once again, this agreement did not vary significantly by offender status or sociodemographic characteristics, with the law receiving broad support from all quarters. Explanations for this result centered on a collectivist perspective and moral certitude about the necessity of protecting sexual partners from infection. Five themes were identified in narrative responses to this item:

(1) People have a right to know their partners' HIV status ($n = 39$)
(2) Not disclosing harms/kills others ($n = 25$)
(3) The law protects the public/reduces the spread of HIV ($n = 17$)
(4) It is morally wrong not to disclose ($n = 7$)
(5) The law provides justice ($n = 5$).

As evident from summary comments in Table 3, beliefs about fairness were sometimes expressed in moral outrage for non-disclosure as an act of murder. The intensity of these expressions helps to explain why such laws have gained traction in the United States, including among people with a criminal record themselves. Only nine participants, all African Americans, questioned the fairness of the law in terms of the burden of responsibility for PLWHA and communities at risk.

Who Should Be Tested?

The question of whether or not offenders should be tested for HIV (testing is mandatory in Alabama prisons) met with similar approval. Almost all participants (98 percent) agreed that inmates in jail and prison should be tested for HIV. Although less likely to agree that probationers or parolees should be tested for HIV, most participants supported testing as a public health measure for offenders under community supervision (68 percent). This result did not vary significantly by race, gender, or offender status. However, despite a history of drug use and other risk factors, only

Table 3. Support for Alabama's HIV Law for Mandatory Disclosure ($N = 109$).[a]

a. The Law is Fair ($n = 93$, 85%)	b. The Law is Unfair ($n = 9$, 8%)
"Your ass needs to go to jail for that."	"The law protects those who are not infected but violates the privacy of those who are."
"They should be required to put their HIV status on drivers' licenses."	"Some laws don't make sense."
"The law helps them to stop and think."	"People shouldn't have to go to jail for having sex with HIV."
"Yes, because people want to spread AIDS."	"It's unfair because everyone don't know about the law."
"I don't want them around, so it's fair."	"Only poor people are being prosecuted for it."
"It's fair because it's the law."	"It should be a personal choice to disclose your status to a partner."
"The law is fair because it stops the killing."	"We are living in times when [partners] don't listen to you."
"HIV is deadly and to conceal is criminal."	
"If you have AIDS and don't tell your partner, that's murder."	
"The law will help to save the next generation."	

[a]Seven participants (6%) who answered this question were undecided about whether or not they supported the law; they are not included here.

17 percent of participants realized or admitted that probationers and parolees were at greater risk of HIV than members of the general public. Further, only 16 percent agreed that parolees, who generally are older and have served time in prison, were at greater risk than probationers whose criminal justice involvement is often minimal. These results are summarized in Table 4.

One result was more encouraging in terms of realistic appraisals of individual HIV risk. Risk awareness was highest among participants who had attended HIV classes (46 percent of parolees vs. 15 percent of probationers). These participants were significantly more likely than non-attendees to agree that offenders under community supervision are at greater risk than the general public ($p = .03$), suggesting that HIV programs in correctional settings, drug treatment programs and other points of contact are useful for HIV risk awareness and prevention. Further, more than one-third of participants (38 percent) who were offered HIV prevention classes had taken them compared to only 14 percent of people who were never offered classes ($p = .001$). Providing HIV education classes to offenders could be the key to participation rather than expecting offenders to

Table 4. HIV Testing, Risk, and Education ($N=197$).[a]

Item	Agree %	Disagree %	Undecided %
a. Who should be tested for HIV?			
Probationers/parolees	68	15	18
Inmates in jail	98	1	1
Inmates in prison	98	1	1
b. Who is at greater risk of HIV?			
Probationers over general public[a]	17	68	17
Parolees over general public	20	68	14
Parolees over probationers	16	69	17

[a]Totals may not total 100% because of rounding.

volunteer on their own accord. Most attendees had taken HIV classes in prison rather than in community settings, which suggests greater availability to such programs when incarcerated, but also fewer opportunities for offenders under community supervision. Only 21 percent of the entire sample had been offered HIV classes while on probation or parole.

DISCUSSION

The study revealed strong support for HIV testing and mandatory HIV disclosure among a sample of offenders under community supervision in Alabama. By focusing on these two elements of HIV control, we were able to identify if target groups, which include convicted offenders, were receptive to HIV testing in an era of criminalization for non-disclosure. As noted in the introduction, policymakers, health providers, and community activists are increasingly concerned about HIV laws for mandatory disclosure because, as reported by Turkewitz (2011): "Who wants to know their status if they can be arrested?" We will discuss the findings of our study within this dialectical framework, with a particular focus on results that could inform test-and-treat strategies for HIV control among convicted offenders.

Participants were asked what they knew about HIV/AIDS in segue to our primary focus on attitudes and beliefs toward HIV testing and mandatory disclosure. We found that awareness of how HIV is acquired and prevented was reasonably good. The average score of 80 percent was similar to 82 percent correct answers on HIV risk behavior knowledge among

1,050 students at historically Black colleges and universities (Sutton et al., 2011), and 84 percent correct responses among 800 felony probationers in rural states (Oser, Leukefeld, Cosentino-Boehm & Havens, 2006). By contrast, knowledge of Alabama's HIV disclosure law was only fair, although most participants knew that non-disclosure was a crime. Other statements about the law, including that people who do not disclose could be charged with murder under Alabama's HIV code, were more vengeful than true. Some participants believed that HIV itself was crime, which raises the question of whether or not HIV criminalization helps to promote such beliefs at a time when policymakers seek to end stigma and discrimination toward PLWHA and to build stronger rapport with health providers, including by revisiting laws for HIV exposure that are not supported by medical evidence (ONAP, 2010b).

The results were mixed on fairness of the law versus the law as a barrier to testing. Although most participants cited fear of arrest and going to jail as barriers to testing, an even larger majority believed that the law was fair, referring to non-disclosure as an act of murder or death sentence. These responses are likely to reflect ideas about HIV transmissibility that are rooted in the panics of the 1980s, before the advent of antiretroviral medicines made HIV treatable and reduced the likelihood of transmission to sexual partners (Donnell et al. 2010). Such views might be common in constituencies that are being targeted for HIV testing, as suggested by Horvath, Weinmeyer, and Rosser's (2010) finding that 65 percent of 1,725 MSM supported the criminalization of non-disclosure. The idea that PLWHA carry a death sentence exists among other publics as well. For example, Djokic et al. (2009, p. 27) reported that 75 percent of 500 U.S. housing authority residents believed that PLWHA die within a year of being diagnosed, a result that the authors attributed to "serious adverse stigmata." Educational efforts are clearly needed in order to counter the perception that HIV is a certain death sentence for anyone who receives a positive diagnosis.

HIV testing was supported as a public health measure for HIV control. Participants' beliefs that inmates, in particular, should be tested might reflect Alabama's policy of mandatory testing prisoners as required by state law, or the idea that prisoners are more likely to have HIV/AIDS. While approval of HIV testing was unequivocal, participants were more likely to believe that inmates should be tested rather than community-based offenders like themselves. This high level of support for testing could be interpreted as receptiveness to test-and-treat programs among offenders under community supervision; however, additional findings of this study suggest otherwise. For example, most participants did not believe that probationers and parolees were at greater HIV risk than the U.S. general population, a misconception that could reduce voluntary HIV testing (see "Implications"). Participants also held stigmatizing ideas about PLWHA and supported HIV criminalization by a wide margin, both of which could deter voluntary testing in order to avoid being stigmatized. On this point, Levy et al. (2014) found that stigma was a barrier to HIV prevention self-efficacy among BMSM and that HIV testing itself was stigmatized in their social networks.

An unexpected finding of the study relates to the importance of HIV classes in achieving goals for HIV prevention. One-third of participants had taken HIV classes in prison or drug treatment programs, a higher proportion than in other correctional settings in the United States (see Belenko, Langley, Crimmins, & Chaple, 2004; Collica, 2007; Oser et al., 2006). Participants in the current study were significantly more aware that offenders under community supervision were at greater risk of HIV/AIDS than the general public, although they were also older than the 15–29 years at which people are typically diagnosed with HIV/AIDS (CDC, 2013c). This age discrepancy affirms the urgency of implementing HIV prevention programs for young people at risk, particularly offenders under community supervision who were never incarcerated or enrolled in drug treatment programs.

As a final point, participants' beliefs that structural interventions (HIV laws, HIV testing) were beneficial for HIV control raises the question of support for laws that are deemed to be a barrier to testing. Other researchers have identified stigma as a bridging factor between the two domains. For example, Mahajan et al. (2008), NASTAD (2011), Block (2014), and Jürgens et al. (2009), to name a few, identified stigma as an obstacle in testing for HIV, and as noted earlier, policymakers have framed HIV criminalization in terms of prejudice toward PLWHA (ONAP, 2010a). In the present case, stigma was expressed in views about HIV/AIDS as a deadly disease and non-disclosure as an act of murder. This response helps to solve a riddle: the law was supported because of a basic premise ("non-disclosure is murder"), and was a barrier to testing for the same reason – PLWHA are "murderers in the making." This logic is likely to reflect attitudes toward PLWHA in the community at large.

Limitations

The results should be interpreted with caution. Although the self-administered questionnaires were worded at a fifth grade reading level, about 20 percent of participants needed help in order to interpret or complete some items. While every attempt was made to be as neutral and non-directive as possible, such hands-on help might have produced socially desirable answers. Future research with offenders could use "talk" methods such as focus groups or personal interviews that do not require participants to answer survey items. However, qualitative methods might not be as practical as brief surveys that can be completed at short notice on reporting days when large numbers of offenders are in attendance. While our research is novel in exploring the knowledge and attitudes of U.S. probationers and parolees on HIV control measures, the study also did not fully explore why HIV laws were a barrier to HIV testing. Further research could identify the effects of incarceration, probation, or parole on willingness to be tested, investigate the dynamics of race and gender in relation to testing and the law, and examine relations between mandatory disclosure, penalties for HIV exposure, and uptake of testing and HIV care.

IMPLICATIONS FOR THE SOCIOLOGY OF HEALTH CARE

The sociological implications of the results center on health beliefs and dispositions in relation to U.S. policy for scaled-up HIV testing among communities at risk. The participants' beliefs that convicted offenders are *not* at greater HIV risk than members of the general public suggest low rates of voluntary HIV testing in such groups, despite high levels of support for this measure. In public opinion surveys, people who believe that they are not at risk of HIV/AIDS are unlikely to be tested on a voluntary basis (Henry J. Kaiser Family Foundation, 2014). In relation to the Southeastern states, Gay, Napravnik, and Eron (2006) and Krawczyk et al. (2006) found that an alarming number of non-diagnosed PLWHA do not get tested prior to becoming symptomatic or being hospitalized with an AIDS-defining illness. Such delays in care-seeking, which are among the worst in the nation, are likely to contribute to the region's disproportionately high HIV rates as a cause of excess morbidity and mortality among African Americans. The testing-related *habitus* of the South, as shaped by low self-awareness of HIV risk, low health literacy among communities at risk (Parikh, Parker, Nurss, Baker, & Williams, 1996), and the moral geography of a socially conservative region, casts doubt on the efficacy of national strategies to reduce HIV rates through early testing and linkage to care.

A question that was raised earlier in this chapter involves barriers to scaled-up HIV testing on the basis of historical distrust for U.S. health policy among African Americans. The issue is relevant to HIV control because most participants – as well as 78 percent of Alabama's incarcerated offenders – involve people of color (Mauer & King, 2007). If distrust for public health policy is a salient factor among African Americans, then high levels of support for HIV testing and criminalization must be explained in terms of the context in which participants supported punitive sanctions for HIV non-disclosure and distanced themselves from PLWHA in them-and-us polarities. We contend that such responses reflect the power of HIV stigma to create social distance from the "other," even among convicted offenders who have a discredited identity of their own. The attitudes and beliefs that were expressed here place convicted lawbreakers in the role of defenders of the status quo and of hegemonic power in the workings of social inequality through HIV stigma (Parker & Aggleton, 2003). The harshness of these responses indicates that HIV holds a special place in the hierarchy of social stigma, and that convicted offenders represent the generalized other in terms of beliefs and attitudes toward HIV/AIDS in communities at risk. The implications of these findings are that HIV stigma may, in fact, be particularly harsh in HIV-affected communities, thereby helping to explain the discrepancy between support for HIV testing and criminalization of non-disclosure among participants, as well as delays in testing and care-seeking for HIV in southeastern states.

A conundrum for public health is how to reconcile the growing rift between law and medicine in approaches to HIV control. If HIV laws serve to legitimize prejudice and discrimination against PLWHA, then efforts should be made to synchronize HIV codes or policies with statutes for notifiable sexually transmitted infections such as syphilis or gonorrhea, and to review health care practices that appear too legalistic or alienating for people with a history of involvement with coercive authority. Since the sociology of health care looks critically at institutional goals and actions that contribute to health inequalities, the results of this study could be used to help destigmatize HIV/AIDS, advocate for reform, and make HIV testing more socially acceptable according to public health strategies that explicitly seek the voluntary participation of high risk populations. It is important to acknowledge that HIV laws for mandatory disclosure were generated by widespread fear and moral outrage after so-called "monstrous sexualities" were blamed for the HIV epidemic in the 1980s (Persson & Newman, 2008). Medical advances have since transformed HIV from a fatal disease to a manageable one, thereby creating a discursive space for reconceptualizing HIV/AIDS in less stigmatizing terms, and also making it possible to contest outdated laws that appear to be more about punishment than prevention among communities at risk.

REFERENCES

Alabama Board of Pardons and Paroles. (2013). *Demographic statistics by race/ethnicity for probationers and parolees in Alabama.* Unpublished data. May 24, 2014.

Belenko, S., Langley, S., Crimmins, S., & Chaple, M. (2004). HIV risk behaviors, knowledge, and prevention education among offenders under community supervision: A hidden risk group. *AIDS Education and Prevention, 16*(4), 367–385.

Block, R. G. (2014). Is it just me? Experiences of HIV-related stigma. *Journal of HIV/AIDS and Social Services, 8*(1), 1–9.

Center for HIV Law, & Policy. (2010). *Ending and defending against HIV criminalization: A manual for advocates.* Retrieved from http://www.hivlawandpolicy.org/resources/view/563. Accessed on November 13, 2013.

Centers for Disease Control and Prevention (CDC). (2013a). *HIV in the United States: At a glance.* Retrieved from http://www.cdc.gov/hiv/statistics/basics/ataglance.html. Accessed on January 10, 2014.

Centers for Disease Control and Prevention (CDC). (2013b). *HIV and AIDS in the United States by geographic distribution.* Retrieved from http://www.cdc.gov/hiv/statistics/basics/geographicdistribution.html. Accessed on February 12, 2014.

Centers for Disease Control and Prevention (CDC). (2013c). *HIV among youth.* Retrieved from http://www/cdc/gov/hiv/risk/age/youth/. Accessed on June 5, 2014.

Collica, K. (2007). The prevalence of HIV peer programming in American prisons: An opportunity wasted. *Journal of Correctional Health Care, 143*(4), 278–288.

Djokic, D., Englund, J., Daum, R., Martin, R., Dozier, T., Potts, S., ... Marcinak, J. (2009). HIV knowledge and attitudes toward HIV testing of South side Chicago housing authority residents. *AIDS Patient Care and STDs, 23*(1), 23–28.

Donnell, D., Baeten, J. M., Kiarie, J., Thomas, K. K., Stevens, W., Cohen, C. R., ... Celum, C. (2010). Heterosexual HIV-1 transmission after initiation of antiretroviral therapy: A prospective cohort analysis. *The Lancet, 375*, 2092–2098.

Epperson, M. W., El-Bassel, N., Gilbert, L., Orellana, E. R., & Chang, M. (2008). Increased HIV risk associated with criminal justice involvement among men on methadone. *AIDS and Behavior, 12*(1), 51–57.

Ferguson, Y., Quinn, S. C., Eng, E., & Sandelowski, M. J. (2006). The gender ratio imbalance and its relationship to risk of HIV/AIDS among African American women at historically black colleges and universities. *AIDS Care, 18*(4), 323–331.

Galletly, C. L., & Lazzarini, Z. (2013). Charges for criminal exposure to HIV and aggravated prostitution filed in the Nashville, Tennessee prosecutorial region 2000–2010. *AIDS and Behavior.* doi:10.1007/s10461-013-0408-1

Galletly, C. L., & Pinkerton, S. D. (2008). Preventing HIV transmission via HIV exposure laws: Applying logic and mathematical modeling to compare statutory approaches to penalizing undisclosed exposure to HIV. *Journal of Law, Medicine, & Ethics, 36*(3), 579–584.

Gamble, V. N. (1997). Under the shadow of Tuskegee: African Americans and health care. *American Journal of Public Health*, *87*(11), 1773–1778.

Gay, C. L., Napravnik, S., & Eron, J. J. (2006). Advanced immunosuppression at entry to HIV care in the Southeastern United States and associated risk factors. *AIDS*, *20*(5), 773–782.

Henry J. Kaiser Family Foundation. (2014). *HIV testing in the United States*. Retrieved from http://kff.org/hivaids/fact-sheet/hiv-testing-in-the-united-states/. Accessed on July 30, 2014.

Hoppe, T. (2012). Punishing HIV: How Michigan trial courts frame criminal HIV disclosure cases. Paper presented at the 19th International AIDS Conference, Washington, DC, July 22.

Horvath, K. J., Weinmeyer, R., & Rosser, S. (2010). Should it be illegal for HIV-positive persons to have unprotected sex without disclosure? An examination of attitudes among US men who have sex with men and the impact of state law. *AIDS Care*, *22*(10), 1221–1228.

Jones, J. H. (1993). *Bad blood: The Tuskegee syphilis experiment*. New York, NY: The Free Press.

Jürgens, R., Cohen, J., Cameron, E., Burris, S., Clayton, M., Elliott, R., ... Cupido, D. (2009). Ten reasons to oppose the criminalization of HIV exposure or transmission. *Reproductive Health Matters*, *17*(34), 163–172.

Kaplan, M. (2012). Rethinking HIV exposure crimes. *Indiana Law Journal*, *87*(4), 1517–1570.

Karp, D. A. (1999). Illness and identity. In K. Charmaz & D. A. Paterniti (Eds.), *Health, illness, and healing: Society, social context, and self* (pp. 83–94). Los Angeles, CA: Roxbury.

Krawczyk, C. S., Funkhouser, E., Kilby, J. M., Kaslow, R., Bey, A. K., & Vermund, S. H. (2006). Factors associated with delayed initiation of HIV medical care among infected persons attending a southern HIV/AIDS clinic. *Southern Medical Journal*, *99*(5), 472–481.

Levy, M. E., Wilton, L., Phillips II, G., Glick, S. N., Kuo, I., Brewer, R. A., ... Magnus, M. (2014). Understanding structural barriers to accessing HIV testing and prevention services among Black Men who have Sex with Men (BMSM) in the United States. *AIDS Behavior*, *18*(5), 972–996.

Lichtenstein, B., Desmond, R. A., & Schwebke, J. R. (2008). Partnership concurrency status and condom use among women diagnosed with T. Vaginalis. *Women's Health Issues*, *18*(5), 369–384.

Link, B. G., & Phelan, J. (2002). Conceptualizing stigma. *Annual Review of Sociology*, *27*, 365–385.

Mahajan, A. P., Sayles, J. N., Patel, V. A., Remien, R. H., Ortiz, D., Szekeres, G., & Coates, T. J. (2008). Stigma in the HIV/AIDS epidemic: A review of the literature and recommendations for the way forward. *AIDS*, *22*, S67–S79.

Mauer, M., & King, R. S. (2007). *Uneven justice: State rates of incarceration by race and ethnicity*. The Sentencing Project. Retrieved from http://www.sentencingproject.org/doc/publications/rd_stateratesofincbyraceandethnicity.pdf. Accessed on July 29, 2014.

Movement Advancement Project. (2014). *HIV criminalization laws*. Retrieved from http://www.lgbtmap.org/equality-maps/hiv_criminalization_laws. Accessed on May 25, 2014.

National Alliance of State and Territorial Directors [NASTAD]. (2011). *National HIV/AIDS strategy imperative: Fighting stigma and discrimination by repealing HIV-specific criminal statutes*. Retrieved from http://www.nastad.org/Docs/020213_NASTAD%20Decriminalization%20Master%20Document.pdf. Accessed on January 26, 2014.

Office of National AIDS Policy [ONAP]. (2010a). *National HIV/AIDS policy for the United States*. Retrieved from http://www.whitehouse.gov/sites/default/files/uploads/NHAS.pdf. Accessed on December 13, 2013.

Office of National AIDS Policy [ONAP]. (2010b). *National HIV/AIDS strategy for the United States: Federal implication plan*. Retrieved from http://www.whitehouse.gov/files/documents/nhas-implementation.pdf. Accessed on December 13, 2013.

Oser, C. B., Leukefeld, C. G., Cosentino-Boehm, A., & Havens, J. R. (2006). Rural HIV: Brief interventions for felony probationers. *American Journal of Criminal Justice*, *31*(1), 125–143.

Parikh, N. S., Parker, R. M., Nurss, J. R., Baker, D. W., & Williams, M. V. (1996). Shame and health literacy: The unspoken connection. *Patient Education and Counseling*, *27*(1), 33–39.

Parker, R., & Aggleton, P. (2003). HIV and AIDS-related stigma and discrimination: A conceptual framework and implications for action. *Social Science and Medicine*, *57*(1), 13–24.

Persson, A., & Newman, C. (2008). Making monsters: Heterosexuality, crime and race in recent western media coverage of HIV. *Sociology of Health & Illness*, *30*(4), 632–646.

Reja, U., Manfreda, K. L., Hlebec, V., & Vehovar, V. (2003). Open-ended vs. close-ended questions in web questionnaires. *Developments in Applied Statistics*, *19*, 159–177.

Robillard, A. G., Gallito-Zaparaniuk, P., Braithwaite, R., Arriola, K. J., & Kennedy, S. (2009). Providing HIV services for incarcerated and ex-offender populations: Perspectives of frontline staff. *Journal of HIV/AIDS & Social Services*, *8*(1), 95–113.

Sutton, M. Y., Hardnett, F. P., Wright, P., Wahi, S., Pathak, S., Warren-Jeanpiere, L., & Jones, S. (2011). HIV/AIDS knowledge scores and perceptions of risk among African American students attending historically black colleges and universities. *Public Health Reports*, *126*(5), 653–663.

Turkewitz, J. (2011). U.S. money spurs spread of HIV criminalization laws. *The Indypendent*. Retrieved from http://www.indypendent.org/2011/08/11/us-money-spurs-spread-hiv-criminalization-laws. Accessed on March 9, 2014.

Ulett, K. B., Willig, J. H., Lin, H.-Y., Routman, J. S., Abroms, S., Allison, J., … Mugavero, M. J. (2009). The therapeutic implications of timely linkage and early retention in HIV care. *AIDS Patient Care and STDs*, *23*(1), 41–49.

U.S. Bureau of Justice Statistics. (2011). *Probation and parole in the United States, 2010*. Retrieved from http://bjs.ojp.usdoj.gov/index.cfm?ty=pbdetail&iid=2239. Accessed on January 20, 2014.

U.S. Census Bureau. (2012). *State & county quick facts: Alabama*. Retrieved from http://quickfacts.census.gov/qfd/states/01000.html. Accessed on February 19, 2014.

U.S. Census Bureau. (2013). *State & county quick facts*. Retrieved from http://quickfacts.census.gov/qfd/states/00000.html. Accessed on February 5, 2014.

Weitz, R. (2012). *The sociology of health, illness, and health care* (6th ed.). Boston, MA: Wadsworth.

Western, B. (2006). *Punishment and inequality in America*. New York, NY: Sage.

Wilkinson, R., & Pickett, K. (2009). *The spirit level: Why greater equality makes societies stronger*. New York, NY: Bloomsbury Press.

Zaller, J., & Feldman, S. (1992). A simple theory of the survey response: Answering questions versus revealing preferences. *American Journal of Political Science*, *36*(3), 579–616.

BECOMING AN EXPERT AUTISM CAREGIVER: HEALTH LITERACY AND COMMUNITY CATALYSTS

Cara A. Chiaraluce

ABSTRACT

Purpose – *The purpose of this study is to investigate the informal micro-level mechanisms through which caregivers maximize their health literacy and caregiving skill-set, particularly in cases of emergent, pervasive health disorders. Specifically, I investigate how important micro-level social factors, such as lay self-education and local community networks, mitigate extensive experiences of medical uncertainty that are associated with caring for a child with autism. This study theorizes a series of processes of becoming lay health care professionals (HCP), which serve as effective health care interventions and ways to secure vital resources for patients and their families.*

Methodology/approach – *This study uses qualitative research methods in the form of 50 individual intensive interviews with primary caregivers of at least one child under the age of 18 with an official autism diagnosis, as well as two years of participant-observation at two primary sites that are autism parent and caregiver resource meetings, both located in Northern California.*

Education, Social Factors, and Health Beliefs in Health and Health Care Services
Research in the Sociology of Health Care, Volume 33, 275–296

ISSN: 0275-4959/doi:10.1108/S0275-495920150000033012

Findings – *This study first demonstrates the major institutional limits and gaps involved in health-related caregiving for children with autism. Next, I define the processes through which caregivers challenge these institutional constraints and fight for life altering resources for their families, which include becoming a lay diagnostician and expert caregiver. Here, I demonstrate a sophisticated set of health literacy skills and key local community-based ties that caregivers develop and rely on, which affords families the tools to overcome diverse institutional obstacles in health-seeking and health care access.*

Research limitations/implications – *The families in this study are predominantly white, middle-class, and reside in California. For future research, the scope of the study could be expanded by increasing the sample size and including greater geographic and demographic diversity.*

Originality/value – *This study contributes vital, yet missing, pieces to the autism puzzle, which currently focuses on prevention, the fight for a so-called "cure," and the role of vaccines in disorder prevalence. In the meantime, families are living with autism each day and are struggling for understanding and knowledge, and to secure adequate support services. In doing so, this study sheds light on current institutional gaps and limits in health care and delivery for children with autism, and suggests specific effective health care interventions applicable to other cases of emergent illnesses and disorders.*

Keywords: Autism; caregiving; health literacy; family; lay expert; patient networks

INTRODUCTION

Autism is a bio-neurological developmental disorder that varies in severity, though is characterized by persistent deficits in social communication and social interaction, and repetitive patterns of behavior, interests, or activities (*Diagnostic and Statistical Manual of Mental Disorders* (*DSM-5*)). Currently, there exists no definitive etiology, "cure," or uniform treatment schedule proven to recover, rehabilitate, or minimize autism symptoms. It is precisely because of the emergent and pervasive nature of autism that makes it more difficult to diagnosis and to treat children, as well as involves a very different social and cultural caring experience for caregivers and their families.

The demonstrated inability of medical professionals and formal health care infrastructure to address the wide-ranging uncertainties involved in the autism caring experience is paramount to understanding why parents go to the extreme lengths that they do to educate themselves in order to help their children; why they turn to a diverse set of non-medical allies to do so, and how. In this study, I investigate the key role of caregiver health literacy and informal lay networks in accessing health services and catalyzing each family's diagnostic and caring journey with autism.

In order to gain the skills, knowledge, and resources necessary to mitigate extensive experiences of uncertainty, to receive an appropriate diagnosis for their child, and to secure the resources necessary to support their child's well-being, caregivers embark on a series of embodied educational processes, or processes of becoming lay health care professionals (HCP). Throughout the distinct processes of becoming lay-experts, caregivers gather different contacts and resources and learn entirely new skills, bodies of knowledge, and ways of interacting and communicating, which allow them to overcome obstacles in the caring experience.

First, the story begins rooted firmly on the micro-level – within each patient family's isolated home and private doctor-patient interactions. Here, many parents observe "red-flag" behaviors in their children, which are dismissed or minimized by their pediatricians during well-baby visits. Then, to follow-up on their concerns, parents turn outwardly – away from the medical institution – to their local lay community for any information or answers that their physicians are unable to provide. Through the process of becoming various health care lay-experts, a sophisticated set of health literacy skills are developed, and with the help of particular community individuals, families begin to overcome diverse institutional obstacles in health-seeking and access to care.

THE EXPERT PATIENT MODEL

This chapter is situated in the contemporary trend in health care of the "expert patient" or "reflexive patient." The expert patient is one who can manage his/her own illness through an emphasis on self-esteem building, maximizing one's health literacy and skills, and user-led health services (Department of Health, 2001; Fox, Ward, & O'Rourke, 2005; Shaw & Baker, 2004). The expert patient paradigm parallels the "patient-centeredness" approach in medicine (Balint, 1969; Mead & Bower, 2000; Stewart, 1984), which emphasize doctor mindfulness and cultural competence in an attempt to reform traditional paternalistic doctor patient relationship. Both approaches emphasize the importance of health literacy as a way to challenge the traditional model of patients as passive, uncritical recipients of medical knowledge and practice.

However, many scholars provide strong critiques of this model in health care, citing it as simply the medical gaze repackaged or as a tool to increase patient compliance (Dixon-Woods, 2001; Fox et al., 2005), that it lacks cultural competency, and assumes that patients are rational actors who want to be empowered and have access to the resources and cultural capital to do so (Henwood, Wyatt, Hart, & Smith, 2003). As Lupton (1997) adds, "late modernist notions of reflexivity ... fail to recognize the complexity and changeable nature of the desires, emotions, and needs that characterize the patient-doctor relationship" (p. 373). Others, critique the negotiation model presented by Kleinman (1988), as overly idealistic since in many cases of illness, medical deference and opinion is required to achieve diagnosis or to receive treatment and access to healing resources (Massé, Legare, Cote, & Dodin, 2001).

To contribute to this conversation, I demonstrate how the most effective means through which caregivers are able to meet their child's health care needs are education-based, as well as localized and grounded in micro-level social dynamics (i.e., intimate social ties, the workplace, peer networks, and local playgrounds). Accordingly, I show why studies of health-seeking behaviors and the expert patient need to take seriously the different informal mechanisms through which caregivers maximize their education and skills as lay-experts, outside of formal institutions and professional ties.

DATA AND METHODS

This study is based on observation and in-depth interviews with mothers and is centered physically and theoretically within the home and family. In total, I conducted fifty in-depth semi-structured interviews with the primary caregiver of a dependent child, under 18 years old, diagnosed with autism, Autism Spectrum Disorder, and/or Asperger's Syndrome and living within Northern California in order to meet face-to-face for an interview. It is important to note that my entire sample includes children whose primary diagnosis would now fit under the Autism Spectrum Disorder diagnosis, according to the latest DSM-V (May 2013). All children ranged in age from 5 to 17 years, though the median age was 10 years old. An overwhelming majority of the children in this sample were under 12 years old and male. Of the total 50 interviews, only 20% of mothers had daughters diagnosed with autism; the remaining 80% had sons with autism, which is representative of the disproportionate diagnosis for boys. Nationally, autism is five times more common in boys than girls (Centers for Disease Control and Prevention, 2014). Additionally, 10% of the total families had more than one child diagnosed with autism, and four of the children in this study were adopted.

All interviewee participants ranged in age from 27 to 52 years, with a median age of 36 years. The overwhelming majority of interviewees self-identify as middle-class. A disproportionate number of mothers had a higher-education and all but two mothers were married. Of the 48 married women, their husbands all worked full-time outside of the home. Of the women I interviewed, 31 were stay-at-home mothers, 11 worked part-time outside of the home, 2 worked part-time within the home, and 6 worked full-time outside of the home. The racial composition of my sample is as follows: 75% Caucasian, 13% Latina, and 12% Bi-Racial (6% Latina-White, 4% Asian-White, 2% Latina-African American). However, autism does affect children from all races and classes; therefore, this shows a limitation of this study to discuss issues of diversity, particularly in terms of race and social class.

All interviews lasted from one to three hours, averaging two hours in length, and were audio recorded and later transcribed verbatim. The majority of interviews were conducted in mother's homes throughout Northern California; the minority were conducted in local public places, such as a coffee shop, public library, or mother's office space. In all interviews, I roughly followed a standard schedule of questions, though I allowed participants to guide our conversations and to focus our discussion on areas that were of most importance to them personally.

Two years of ethnographic fieldwork supplements these interviews and includes observation of monthly autism caregiver resource meetings, which lasted for two hours and were located in Northern California. Meetings are attended by on average 30 caregivers, most of whom are women between the ages of 30 and 55, and most of whom who are mothers. I also observed a variety of autism-related informational meetings, fundraisers, public talks and educational community events, all open to the public and located in Northern California.

MAKING SENSE OF RED FLAGS: BECOMING A LAY DIAGNOSTICIAN

The road to the autism diagnosis is winding and paved by each family. Only 8 out of 50 children (16%) in my sample were diagnosed with autism before the age of three, although they presented symptoms since infancy. The remaining 42 families embarked on a journey to the autism diagnosis, which lasted anywhere from six months to five years. These cases provide valuable insight into what sparks their health literacy-seeking behaviors, and how and where lay families gain greater institutional access and control.

Dana, a mother of a now five-year-old boy, describes her son's complicated road to the diagnosis and her personal coping mechanisms:

> I would describe this process, mainly at the beginning, as a battle. I felt like I was constantly fighting for something – an appointment, to get off a wait-list, for a referral to someone, to get into a research study, for my family to understand, for my boss to let me cut back to part-time and keep my job. A battle, I tell ya! But we found our way, and we got there and it's a lot less rocky now, we have a system .... Throughout this whole process, educating myself was my priority. I threw myself into reading everything, listening to every podcast I could find, spending days on Google searching and searching and emailing every contact I could get my hands on. My family always knew where to find me – sitting at the computer!

Like Dana, most mothers coped with frustrating interactions in the clinic by becoming a lay diagnostician, or a non-medical expert or scientific professionals who actively observes, tracks, diagnoses, and treats a group of symptoms as a medical condition. Shaw et al.'s (2008) analysis of how individuals decide to seek health care, they find that "In order to make decisions about health care, patients take on the role of lay-diagnostician and information-seeking is their first activity" (p. 1517). Similarly, Davison, Smith and Frankel (1991) use "lay epidemiology" to describe lay theorizing about health and illness by drawing on local observations, daily experience, scientific evidence, and health education messages.

Caregivers take on the role of lay diagnostician by carefully and closely observing, noting, and analyzing their child's behavior – in what contexts do their behaviors change (i.e., when and where do the tantrums most often occur)? When and where do his repetitive behaviors seem to intensify? What exactly does he do or not do when around other children that makes him stand-out? At what age did he start losing vocabulary and no longer retains word? Then, the data compiled from these questions and the careful analysis of the child's symptoms (i.e. their patient case) is then presented to the appropriate medical professional.

For example, Rachel described the response by her pediatrician to her concern that her son was acting "differently from her older daughter" and not talking at the age of two:

> It was just kind of like, "Oh, well, he's not talking yet but that's, you know, within the range of normal." We just kind of went through the regular checkup and shots and nothing came-up. So that's when we sought out a speech therapist on our own for the nonverbal and communication issues.

Rachel interprets her son's atypical behaviors as a medical problem – as a verbal and communication issue – which she then treated in its matching medical form, through speech therapy. Similarly, Brynn, a mother of a two-year-old child with autism, describes similar experiences of dismissal by her pediatrician, which leads her to independently diagnosis her child's behavior problems and gross motor delays and to seek out experts in these two separate areas accordingly,

> The concerns we had, I don't think she understood them. And that's when we finally, after a few years, just that was it, we switched. It was a lot of the things, the valid concerns that we had with our son, it was just, she brushed them off as "he's strong minded and strong willed." No! I know my son can be strong willed and I know he can be stubborn but there's something else here. Besides behavior stuff, I was really concerned with some other things. Like, I noticed he would use one side of his body more, and looking back he was late in everything – to roll-over, to crawl, to walk – everything. I now know these are typical gross motor delays, so I found an OT [occupational therapist] person to help with this, and I called a child psychologist to try to figure out the behavior problems – or just some advice or something, you know? I did this completely outside of our doctor's recommendations.

In the narratives above, caregivers demonstrate a learned skill-set as part of playing the role of lay diagnostician, which involves evaluating and interpreting symptoms, self-initiated and persistent help-seeking behaviors, and building trust in one's life world experiential knowledge and abilities. These skills function to increase individual knowledge, sense of control, and access to resources and organizations. Accordingly, this section provides further depth in conceptualizing the lay diagnostician as a key mechanism to combat institutional obstacles and the dissatisfaction felt within clinical interactions and the formal health care system.

When these parents' concerns are continually dismissed by their pediatricians, they turn to a diverse set of community players to "unblock" the path necessary to gain access and resources that only the official diagnosis will grant. In the following section, I unpack this nuanced process with particular attention to the role of select key individuals in mothers' narratives, termed "community catalysts."

BREAKING DOWN ADDITIONAL BARRIERS TO THE DIAGNOSIS: COMMUNITY CATALYSTS

This section demonstrates how exactly lay caregivers gain significant traction in their battles for recognition through a diagnosis; how they move from simply tracking concerning behaviors to obtaining an official medical diagnosis of autism. I show how caregivers navigate the winding diagnostic process with the help of a crucial "community catalyst," who serves the following functions: (1) challenges the dismissal by medical professionals by acknowledging, validating, and supporting mother's intuitive concerns and (2) acts as a spark that pushes the diagnostic journey onward by connecting them with a necessary, yet missing, piece of information or resource necessary to reach the diagnosis.

Community Catalysts: Lay Agents and Informal Networks

In Aimee's case, her child's day care worker serves this role as the most significant catalyst in her fight for the diagnosis. Aimee was notified that her daycare provider would no longer accept her 2.5-year-old son because of his violent behaviors (biting and pushing other children), and the daycare owner "insisted that something wasn't quite right." The insistence by her daycare worker validated Aimee's concerns that she had for years, yet went undiagnosed or medically legitimated. In her own words, Aimee describes her family's diagnosis story as a process from self-doubt and questioning of red flags to key moments of outside validation by her daycare provider, which led to a diagnostic evaluation:

> It was his daycare actually who insisted that something wasn't quite right. There was such a difference between my daughter at Sam's age, a difference. And then I thought his behaviors – up to two he was pretty typical, and then he just kind of quit playing with toys, and I thought, "Eh, he's just weird," you know, he was lining them up instead of playing with them. But, it didn't ring a bell. Huge temper tantrums, but I figured he's just spoiled, I mean he's a little one and the girls spoil him rotten. So I thought, "He's just kind of a brat." The aggression – then he started banging his head on things, and that's when his daycare said, "I can't keep him if you don't get him tested." So I called our pediatrician immediately.

Aimee continues to describe what happens next,

> I called his pediatrician and said, "My daycare says I have to get him tested for something, she doesn't know what's wrong." And he sent me the M-CHAT [The Modified Checklist for Autism in Toddlers-Revised (M-CHAT-R)] and I sent it back and he said, "Well, from this I should be referring you, but you were just here a month ago and everything was okay." And it was, sort of.

I inquired further about the inconsistencies found here, she replied

> Yeah, that's the thing that's super confusing. You can check "no" on some things, but they're all, like deceiving .... Yes, he did have the 35 required words, but I guess I didn't think about the fact that I hadn't heard them in weeks. So I just checked "yes" he knows 35 words .... And nothing prompted the pediatrician to be concerned either, he's a good guy, I like him.

Eventually, based on the M-CHAT autism screening results, Aimee's pediatrician refers her to the local hospital's autism clinic, where they conducted many tests and confirmed that, "Yep. He has autism." Aimee's narrative of the road to the diagnosis is puzzling, and yet common, in many instances – she lacks professional or expert validation of her concerns both before and after an official diagnostic measure confirms that her son may have autism and should be evaluated by a specialist. Both her intuitive fears and the concerns of an outside lay daycare workers are eventually confirmed though the autism clinic evaluation, but all the while, her son has been seen by her pediatrician on numerous visits without any hint of autism concern, and testing is misleading. Although her son was completely nonverbal at three years old, avoided eye-contact, and continually screamed and banged his head on things, it was not her pediatrician or any other medical professional that alerted Aimee that her son's behaviors are atypical; it was the daycare workers insistence on the fact that "something was just not right," that served as the mobilizing force in taking action to understand her son's symptoms and in receiving the diagnosis.

Additionally, specific family members and loosely-aquatinted peers with children on the spectrum – individuals who are able to recognize behaviors through the lens of autism – frequently served as community catalysts by validating caregivers' red-flag concerns and pushing the journey to the diagnosis onward. In almost 50% of the families in this study, the caregiver had a family member or friend with a child with autism who recognized the child's symptomatic behavior, validated parents' concerns, and advised them on what to do, who to contact, and where to go. For example, here Terri's sister played the important role of community catalyst in her story,

> My sister, Jess is the one who made me do the speech therapy. Like she was the one who was like, "You need to get into speech – he should be talking a lot more than he is." And she just kept on me, and so we did. And then, but as soon as I got this diagnosis of autism, and she was like, "No, no, no, no. He just needs speech." (*Rolls her eyes and giggles softly*). So it was like, you know, me sending them articles, or me sending them, videos of stuff that's kind of helped me/helped them realize that it is what it is, so.

Informal networks often served a vital function is gaining access to institutional bodies and process that grant services and the diagnostic evaluation, which often requires lengthy waiting-list periods and extensive red-tape and paperwork before being evaluated. Samantha describes how an informal conversation with a coworker led to her immediate entry into Alta California Regional Center (ACCRC), which is a "collaborative partner" who "links consumers to existing community resources on a needs basis, and one that also accept referrals from the community" (Alta California Regional Center, 2008). Previously, she was placed on a 30-day waitlist and was very concerned about how to survive these first 30 days. She states,

> So after the evaluation, I went home, called Alta, because that's the number they gave me, and they said that there is a waitlist, that within 30 days someone would call me. So then I called Warmline, it was a family resource center, and they connected me with someone whose child had autism, and they kind of gave me some ideas of things to do, you know, read this book, try this, so I read that book – you know, not really helpful! And then at work – I didn't go to work for a couple of days, but when I went, my coworker said, "I happen to know somebody in Alta," so I got in two days later to see her. She made a call. I don't know if I could have waited ... just a regional center worker, someone who sets you up with services, she made it all happen. I don't know if I could have made it 30 days.

When dismissed by pediatricians or primary care physicians, friends and family members, daycare workers, and coworkers act as vital nodes in each family's informal networks and, at times, as institutional gatekeepers, who can provide entrance into vital professional and non-professional networks of medical care and support. Furthermore, in other cases, it is the unique linkage of a lay individual and exceptional specialist who, as a pair, allows families to overcome major obstacles to the diagnosis.

The following section expands on this process and details the next steps in "life after the diagnosis," which emphasizes the search for specialized treatment and resources is similarly ambiguous and confusing – often times described as a "battle" – for which becoming a sophisticated expert caregiver is the primary coping mechanism.

LIFE AFTER THE DIAGNOSIS: BECOMING AN EXPERT CAREGIVER AND LAY EXPERT

After the diagnosis, the major coping mechanism and skill-set used to confront these institutional limits lie in the process of becoming an "expert patient," or more aptly, the "expert caregiver." To combat the uncertainty involved in many aspects of the autism diagnosis and prognosis, parents seek out information and resources in every way possible, and throughout this process they become exemplars of the expert caregiver and patient family, and the ultimate medical consumer, while simultaneously blurring professional-lay boundaries. In particular, in this section I detail the rationale and motivation that drive these practices, the actual form, mechanisms, and spaces in which they occur, and the resulting proficiency in comprehending and appropriating medical literature and knowledge, navigating bureaucratic health care systems, securing resources through professional agencies, and experimenting with self-designed treatment regimens.

Health Literacy

One of most prominent themes in the process of becoming an expert patient takes the form of health literacy. Health literacy is defined by the Institute of Medicine (2004) as, "the degree to which individuals have the capacity to obtain, process, and understand basic health information and services needed to make appropriate health decisions." Health literacy requires a complex group of reading, listening, analytical, and decision-making skills, and the ability to apply these skills to health situations. For example, it includes the ability to understand instructions on prescription drug bottles, medical education brochures, doctor's directions and consent forms, and the ability to negotiate complex health care systems (Institute of Medicine, 2004). The mothers in my sample all engage in diverse health literacy practices and learn to build these skills throughout the caring experiences, in varying degrees. Some caregivers exhibit exceptional levels of health literacy, while others employ more passive strategies or struggle with the limits of professional-lay boundaries.

For example, Susan, a part-time administrative assistant with an Associate's degree in computer science, exemplifies a remarkably high level of health literacy that extends beyond traditional carework and the illness experience, to include exceptional information-seeking, gathering, and analysis skills,

> I read everything! Medical clinical books, research studies, parent blogs, Jenny McCarthy's books. I put my kid in every study I can, I talk to the doctors, I seek out new people ... I go to every talk and lecture and event I can. I ask questions, I don't hold back. I've seen just about every specialist and autism-related doctor in the state! I ask other parents for advice, I just try to gather as much information as I can, and keep on it. Studies are coming out so fast, so I have to keep on top of the latest reports.

Like Susan, many caregivers funnel their time and energy into becoming autism experts, spending hours each day reading clinical books, research studies, textbooks, online blogs, conducting extensive web searches, and contacting support groups, service agencies, and professional experts throughout the world. These expert patients are incredibly well-informed, self-educated, and connected. Aimee represents this practice of maximizing her health literacy, in the interest of the well-being of her son,

> I spent forever on Google; just researching by myself .... You just keep looking. I mean I had books on the verbal behavior approach, and pivotal response therapy and I have every book there is, reading them and trying to figure out, "Would any of this really work?" And they're all so technical. That's why I'm drawn to the Denver model. You can't do that when you're cooking, cleaning, and changing his diaper. But the Early Start Denver model there's even things I could do while I'm changing his diaper.

During an incredibly scary, stressful, and exhausting time, information and connection provided a sense of structure and control, a way to minimize anxiety, fear, and uncertainty and maximize individual sense of control, agency, and decision-making capacity for caregivers. As Lisa describes,

> If I can just read everything and at least know about all of the different treatments, and supplements, and experts, and stories of recovery – everything that I can – I can handle this, I can make the right decisions, I can make informed decisions, and I can help my son .... Because that's all we are trying to do here, make the best decisions for our kids. No one else is going to do it, and no one will give you the perfect answer!

Similarly, Stephanie states,

> I listen to Autism Spectrum Radio. I listen to podcasts .... I listen to about three different podcasts that have, new and updated stuff, and I think that's easier for me to listen to other people's stories than to read them for some reason. But I do try to keep up on everything – it's just hard, because I feel like somebody's trying to sell you something, and you can't try everything, you can't do everything. And I was getting into the gluten/casein-free diet, and reading all the information on it, and then sending it to my family, and being like, "What do you guys think?" And they're like, "Do it." But, it's so much easier said than done!

Aimee, Lisa, Stephanie, and Susan each illuminate both exceptional healthy literacy practices in their own way, as well as empirical and institutional constraints they experience, which include (1) time, energy, and financial resources and (2) lay-professional boundaries and issues of institutional access. The majority of women in this study have at least one other child, are married, take care of a home and family, and many work at least part-time outside of the home. To become an exceptionally literate expert caregiver requires enormous amounts of time, energy, and financial resources – the books, expensive supplements, membership fees, and tangible resources all are costly, and not everyone can or wishes to engage to the same intensity or degree as Lisa or Terri. Becoming health literate also can be arduous, and frankly, depressing for many parents. Dawn, a mother of a recently diagnosed three-year-old girl, addresses this issue by purposefully integrating a sense of levity into her health literacy practices. She reads medical and scientific literature in order to keep abreast on the latest research findings and suggestions. However, she also follows a number of humor-filled blogs to bring some balance to her heavy technical reading:

> I only read the abstract, and then I tend to go to a forum where I can read peoples' experiences with it. You know, just kind of weigh what people have said and done. There's a lot of – there are a number of wonderful blogs that I read daily. I'm a subscriber to probably about 20 really good ones. I like the funny ones.

Each caregiver employs different health literacy strategies to address their unique social locations and needs, however, what everyone lacks and is searching for is professional advice and answers to various questions that remain unaddressed or impossible to answer.

What I find here, is that the majority of clinical studies and texts, and the latest scientific findings and premier research studies do not address or begin to tackle the questions and areas of need that autism caregivers are seeking – how does this information directly relate to my everyday life? Therefore, it is easier to understand why the autism illness experience requires extensive parent-led self-education, research and experimentation, and the confidence to ask questions, to discern information, and to act on their learned knowledge, all alongside, but not (always) fully within, the formal institution of medicine and health care.

Blurring Expert-Lay Boundaries

A significant aspect of becoming an expert caregiver involves the blurring of expert-lay boundaries because of the pervasive nature of carework involved with autism. A disproportionate burden of carework is placed on caregivers of a child with autism, which expands far beyond the lay private sphere into dynamics of the clinic (i.e., medical diagnosis, experimenting with treatments, and close patient surveillance), formal health care organization (i.e., seeking out referrals, specialists, and inclusion within research studies), and local advocacy organizations and events, with what feels like life-and-death consequences. The stakes are high, particularly when dealing with a contested illness with no set prognosis or treatment plan, and consequently, the professional-lay boundaries are blurred. A conversation with Aimee best demonstrates this complicated position in which caregivers sit between lay caregiver and medical expert, and the self-doubt involved:

> And then you – with the therapies and the treatments, you're always second guessing. A couple weeks ago I was thinking, "Maybe MAPS [The Medical Academy of Pediatric Special Needs program] isn't a great idea, he's been hitting more." And I'm thinking, "Okay, I haven't seen any really big improvements in the last few months, maybe it's time to call it quits." But I don't know if that's the right choice, so I'm afraid to make it. And I ask his teacher and his therapist, and I get opinions from 50 people to tell me whether or not this program is good for my kid. It's kind of – it's frustrating, because you just want someone to tell you the right answer, or – if this will help, yeah. Somebody tell me what will help, and I'll do it. But I don't like having to be the one in charge of something I don't understand. What I tend to do, I don't trust myself at all, so I overreach. I think, "More is better." The kind of, the ESDM [the Early Start Denver Model] thing, you know, "Okay I've learned how to do this, but I'd like more." So I insist we go, and now he's in Square One and Maps, but he isn't talking, so maybe we need speech. So I shove that in too, thinking maybe he needs it, even though no one can tell me he needs more. It turns out, it didn't work out …. But I'm always adding, rather than taking away, because I don't know if … once you take something away, maybe you've given up.

Aimee continues to discuss how she experiments with diet and supplement changes with little professional oversight or direction, with the goal to decrease her son's symptoms. Here, she also illuminates the high stakes that drive lay help-seeking behaviors and treatment experimentation,

> I read a list of foods that I should avoid. And I know, subconsciously, that I'm going to avoid those foods now, because maybe I'm wrong. The bio stuff could be right. Or perhaps the combination of all of things that, you know this could be the missing – the piece that will start some sort of significant change. And that's, I mean, that's just a huge experiment. It's just experimenting, taking away, adding things left and right. But with huge consequences, you know. The responsibility of my child's life! Because I hate the idea of not doing something that could have helped. And I harass people all the time, "What do you think of this?" We're talking *life or death decisions* here, *that's how it feels all the time anyway*.

Kristina similarly discusses her self-designed treatment plan for her son based on research and lay recommendations:

> My son can be really aggressive, so I've been looking into how to decrease the aggressive behaviors. I read a lot about a vitamin called L-carnosine for calming. So I bought it off Amazon. And the company I bought it from is called like "Autism Coach," so it's like for autistic children. But it's a liquid form that I put in its chocolate milk every morning. And I think that he's gotten less aggressive and helps with digestion and stomach problems. So, I know that there's a lot of kids on the spectrum that have problems with constipation and stuff, so I'd definitely recommend it ... but it's 50 dollars a bottle.

The health literacy strategies demonstrated by the caregivers above also detail various dynamics of the intensification of carework involved in the autism illness experience. By noting the expansive caring experience associated with autism, the new, various, and the divergent roles caregivers are expected to perform well, we are better able to understand why parents "throw" themselves into health literary practices. Health literary practices provide the tools necessary to be informed, educated caregivers and medical consumers who are able to complete the expansive carework that is required of them to maximize their child's well-being.

However, it is important to note the significant limits and constraints involved in becoming the expert caregiver and maximizing one's health literacy. In other words, even the most advanced and sophisticated collective of resources will not always be able to provide the resources or knowledge necessary on the next steps in one's autism journey. For example, a community catalyst may afford some caregivers to be exemplar lay diagnosticians, to diagnosis and understand their child in the most technically up-to-date framework; however, these resources may not help them later in their battle to secure therapies or accommodations in school for their child. Tracking and classifying a disorder are very different from the skills necessary to understand state disability rights laws and to navigate school district and health care bureaucracies. In other words, one's toolkit of resources and contacts do to not always translate into the next realms in the autism caring experiences, which leaves many parents on their own to seek out new resources and navigate new winding processes.

Also, even the ultimate expert patient is limited by his/her social location, cultural capital, degree of institutional access and formal ties, lack of professional credentials, and official membership in the formal institution of medicine. This begs the question, what exactly is the goal in becoming an expert patient or caregiver? Where is the definitive line between physician and patient, professional and lay caregiver? An expert patient is not a medical professional, the patient-physician role is clearly defined, yet the findings in this study show differing ways in which the lay-professional boundaries are simultaneously complicated and blurred.

The Appropriation of Expert Knowledge

A major dynamic in becoming the expert caregiver and employing one's health literacy involves the appropriation of expert knowledge. To circumvent and push back against professional/formal limits, caregivers practice the appropriation of expert knowledge as a means to minimize the distance between expert and non-expert, and to gain entrée into previously off-limits realms. The appropriation of expert knowledge can serve the following purposes for lay caregivers: (1) a means to understand and engage with research and literature (i.e., in case studies, research studies, and reading paperwork), (2) a way to gain legitimacy in the clinic and to engage in more democratic dialogue in doctor-patient interactions, or (3) to gain access to different treatment forms and mechanisms, with the goal to minimize symptoms and improve quality of life. In my interviews, I hear how lay women appropriate expert knowledge, how they cite research studies, statistics, use clinical language and jargon to describe and communicate their experiences and interactions to me, and the purposes this serves. Lay mothers become experts of different kinds, which is particularly salient in contested and uncertain disorders.

This process by which lay caregivers embody expert roles and scripts can be understood as engagement in "lay epidemiology" (Davidson, Smith, & Frankel, 1991), "popular epidemiology" (Brown, 2000), or "street science" (Corburn, 2005); a lay way of knowing, or citizen science, that is based in part on an appropriation of expert knowledge by non-experts. All of these concepts are different ways to capture the same fundamental process and goal, which is a push-back, even in the smallest ways, against top-down knowledge and hierarchical practices in the clinic, which do not adequately reflect or affect caregivers' experiences. When the experts are unable to provide the answers or the assistance that parents need, parents themselves become the experts, and a primary means to do so is through the adoption of expert knowledge and learned proficiency in medicalese.

Medicalese refers to the use of formal medical terminology and semantic qualifiers, or the ability to read, understand, and use medical jargon appropriately. For example, to explain what autism is, Allie cites almost verbatim its technical-medical characterization and one can see the appropriation of clinical language in her response:

> I constantly find myself explaining what autism is to other people. I've created these little scripts, you know, that I've pretty much memorized, based on what I've read. To other adults, I say my son has a complex neuro-developmental disorder, which includes repetitive behaviors, and communication and social impairments. But to kids, like in his school or on the playground, I usually say, "Jimmy has a different brain and he understands and processes things different."

Similarly, throughout our interview, Maya incorporates the latest statistics and research findings into her family's general narrative with autism. For example, when describing the rationale behind her remarkable health literacy skills she states,

> You know that now 1 out of 88 kids are diagnosed with autism in this country, right? I mean, this is a huge statistic and we need to be doing something about it. So, why do I do all of this research to educate myself, call experts, and browbeat my way into the top doctor's offices – most of the specialists have like 6 month waiting-lists, you know. One doctor that I wanted to see, it was going to be over a year to see him. I do it because I notice people take me more seriously now, when I can show that I read the research and know the words and can talk like them. I can call "bullshit" when I know they are not telling me the right thing or completely brushing me off. Like I know the treatment options out there, I know the statistics on what has worked and hasn't, so don't lie to me.

Here, Maya demonstrates how self-education and access to research and diverse forms of information function as a way to build confidence in experiential knowledge and decision-making capability, and results in feelings of greater control over the illness experience and one's life. Many caregivers assert pseudo-scientific knowledge in their interactions as a means to gain leverage with professionals and formal organizations (i.e., school boards, medical professionals, health care management organizations, etc.). In order words, the learned use of medicalese is a strategic way to blur professional-lay boundaries and to gain power in hierarchical spaces, in which lay caregivers are traditionally rendered subordinate and powerless.

An additional mechanism that challenges expert-lay boundaries and professional domains lies in the practice of caregiver-led research and experimentation with treatment regimes. Many caregivers describe their ongoing research on various alternative treatment options, most often in the form of supplements and diet changes. Charlotte believes strongly in the role of supplements and diet in treating her son's symptoms. Here, she describes the regime she designed and follows, and how she has come to this plan,

> I went to a few lectures by a local naturopathic doctor who believes strongly in the role of supplementation and diet. I thought, I mean, really, what do we have to lose? Nothing! Except that it's pretty expensive. So I started by keeping a diary of everything my son ate and drank and noting any triggers or flare-ups to try to assess allergies or what could be making things better or worse. I did this for a while, and then following the protocol, I started introducing one supplement – vitamins and stuff – at a time, noting any changes. And then another and another. When things got worse, I took him off it. I also noticed dairy and gluten did seem to aggravate symptoms sometimes, which is typical with these kids, so I took him off dairy, but gluten is too difficult for a picky eater. So, I'm still experimenting with this and changing doses and keeping my diary. These changes have definitely helped with his sleeping problems. I also notice less tantrums, he seems calmer.

Many others have discussed experimenting with non-prescription homeopathic supplements and over-the-counter vitamins to treat many of the symptoms involved in autism, such as anxiety, depression, sleeping problems, and gastrointestinal issues. Most all caregivers learn of these treatment forms through self-researched books, web-based searches, and autism-community listservs and referrals, not from formal literature or professional recommendations. For example, when I asked Isabelle where exactly she finds out about different treatment options, she responded, "I spent forever on Google." Isabelle expands more on her self-guided research and literacy practices,

> You know, by myself, just researching. Yeah, you just keep looking. I mean I had books on the verbal behavior approach, and pivotal response therapy and I have every book there is, reading them and trying to figure out, "Would any of this really work?"

However, as Charlotte notes, all of these books and in-home diet and supplementation treatment forms are not covered by insurance; they are expensive and require large amounts of time and energy by caregivers, with little guidance. Amy provides a critical perspective by honestly addressing the difficulty to maintain and keep-up some of these parent-led alternative therapies, with, sometimes, few results:

> In that waiting period where we had nothing going, because after Alta we had to wait three months to get into the program, we tried the GFCF diet because everyone was saying we should. I noticed no changes, but it was so hard to do, so I quit doing it. We kept him off milk because I noticed diaper rashes went away, and I'm lactose intolerant, so I thought, "OK." So he drinks almond milk, that's all we kept. There's also been periods where people have said, "Oh, these supplements." And I've bought them, and tried them, and noticed no change. Every now and then I still give him some just because there are good vitamins in it. I don't think that I believe all of that works, I just usually keep my opinions to myself when people are talking about it ... you're desperate enough to try it, and if there's any improvement in that period, then you're a believer.

Here, we see how through the process of becoming an expert caregiver, which emphasizes health literacy and the appropriation of expert knowledge, caregivers maximize their sense of control, agency, and power within the autism caring experience and also secure vital resources and services, which lessens the gap between expert and patient family.

THE EXPERT CAREGIVER TOOLBOX: HEALTH LITERACY, INFORMAL SOCIAL TIES AND COMMUNITY CATALYSTS

This chapter details the rationales, strategies, and key embodied processes through which health-related educational skills and resources are learned, practiced, and mobilized by lay caregivers. This process begins during the diagnostic journey, where caregivers first learn that because of the emergent nature of autism, their illness and caring experience is going to differ significant from normative illness trajectories. In doing so, they begin to build a network of contacts, skills and resources, particularly learned through becoming a lay diagnostician, with the goal to better understand their child's and seek treatment accordingly.

In becoming lay diagnosticians, caregivers learn how to actively research, name and frame, and seek treatment for a medical condition with help from various lay allies or community catalysts, such as friends, daycare workers, and family members. I identify the community catalyst as a key player or event in the diagnostic journey that confirms parents' red-flag concerns and mobilizes action and resources, sometimes this comes in the form of vital dyad. The emphasis on each family's interaction with different community catalysts also illuminates how the receipt of a diagnosis is fundamentally embedded in micro-level social dynamics – within the local community, lay networks, the workplace, childcare facilities, etc.

Through the distinct process of becoming lay diagnosticians and expert caregivers, specific skills and tools are learned which cumulatively grant expert proficiency in three key areas, which include (1) medical diagnosis, symptom surveillance, and treatment experimentation, (2) health literacy, and (3) the appropriation of expert knowledge and medicalese. Specifically, caregivers first learn to trust maternal instincts and abilities in the diagnosis process, and next through acquiring health literacy skills one's self-confidence and trust in life world knowledge is further strengthened, which affords caregivers' greater decision-making power and feelings of control.

Together, this allows lay caregivers the confidence, ability, and resources necessary to advocate for their child and family amidst extensive contestation and ambiguity.

Particularly in the cases of emergent illnesses, the majority of all vital needs, services, and resources, and means for achieving these necessities are completed through outside community-based modes and mechanisms. In other words, many parents get to the diagnosis through informal networks and non-linear and inefficient paths, such as a conversation with a loosely acquainted coworker, a day at the playground when another parent identifies symptoms, a daycare worker's observation, and month-long waiting periods sometimes for the wrong professional. Therefore, I argue for the importance of a community-based perspective of health care and patient education, one that is grounded within these micro-level social dynamics, and takes seriously locality, informal social ties, and lay-initiated educational mechanisms.

CONCLUSION

Information-seeking and education-based practices are agentic realms that allow lay parents small, yet significant, moments of power. Through gaining access to clinical studies and literature, by Googling everything and anything on autism, by attending professional lectures and asking questions to anyone that may listen, they are not just increasing their knowledge of the disorder or their child, they are becoming an expert caregiver in order to shape their experiences to achieve the best care and outcomes not just for their child, but also for the entire autism community. Information gathering and knowledge building is powerful, it allows each caregiver to guide and create their experiences with medical professionals, non-professionals, peers and family members, local communities, and with the disorder itself. In doing so, these practices shed light on the importance of amassing interesting combinations of knowledge, skills, and resources as a mechanism for caregiver education, which is vital to meeting the spectrum of needs required by children with autism.

Diseases and disorders that follow a more linear trajectory, that have a clear prognosis, treatment regimen, and stable institutionalized service bodies, involve a different caring experience. In normative illness experiences, there is less ambiguity and uncertainty in all realms – you know who to contact, where to go, what to do, what therapies to try, what specialists to see, and institutionalized policies and procedures exist to help patients receive aid. The roadmap for how to meet a patient's needs and how to care for him/her is relatively linear, defined, straight-forward, and, it simply, exists. In these cases, wide-ranging community-based resources and self-initiated lay individuals and networks may not play the same role in their illness experiences.

However, for families with autism, every step in the journey is full of questions and unknowns and there lacks the necessary infrastructure to meet their needs, before the diagnosis and after. Therefore, the pervasive nature of the autism caring experience is an excellent case on which to demonstrate the importance of caregiver education (and how it is gathered and mobilized) and local community-based social ties to the lives of parents caring for a child with a contested disorder, one that is rife with unknowns and inconsistencies in health care and delivery.

REFERENCES

Alta California Regional Center. (2008). *What is Alta California Regional Center?* Retrieved from http://www.altaregional.org/what-alta-regional-center

American Psychiatric Institution. (2013). Diagnostic and statistical manual of mental disorders, DSM-V (5th ed.). Washington, DC: American Psychiatric Association.

Balint, E. (1969). The possibilities of patient-centered medicine. *Journal of the Royal College of General Practitioners*, *17*, 269–276.

Brown, P. (2000). Popular epidemiology and toxic waste contamination: Lay and professional ways of knowing. In S. Kroll-Smith, P. Brown, & V. J. Gunter (Eds.), *Illness and the environment: A reader in contested medicine*. New York, NY: University Press.

Centers for Disease Control and Prevention. (2014). *Autism Spectrum Disorders (ASDs): Data and statistics*. Retrieved from http://www.cdc.gov/ncbddd/autism/data.htm

Corburn, J. (2005). *Street science: Community knowledge and environmental health justice*. Cambridge, MA: MIT Press.

Davison, G., Smith, D., & Frankel, S. (1991). Lay epidemiology and the prevention paradox: The implications of coronary candidacy for health education. *Sociology of Health & Illness*, *13*(1), 1–19.

Department of Health. (2001). *The expert patient: A new approach to chronic disease management for the 21st century*. London: Department of Health.

Dixon-Woods, M. (2001). Writing wrongs? An analysis of published discourses about the use of patient information leaflets. *Social Science & Medicine*, *52*, 1417–1432.

Fox, N. J., Ward, K. J., & O'Rourke, A. J. (2005). The 'expert patient': Empowerment or medical dominance? The case of weight loss, pharmaceutical drugs and the Internet. *Social Science & Medicine*, *60*, 1299–1309.

Henwood, F., Wyatt, S., Hart, A., & Smith, J. (2003). 'Ignorance is bliss sometimes': constraints on the emergence of the 'informed patient' in the changing landscapes of health information. *Sociology of Health & Illness*, *25*(6), 589–607.

Institute of Medicine. (2004). *Health literacy: A prescription to end confusion*. Washington, DC: National Academies Press

Kleinman, A. (1988). *The illness narratives: Suffering, healing, and the human condition*. New York, NY: Basic Books.

Lupton, D. (1997). Consumerism, reflexivity and the medical encounter. *Social Science & Medicine*, *45*(3), 373–381.

Massé, R., Legare, F., Cote, L., & Dodin, S. (2001). The limitations of a negotiation model for perimenopausal women. *Sociology of Health and Illness*, *23*(1), 44–64.

Mead, N., & Bower, P. (2000). Patient-centredness: A conceptual framework and review of the empirical literature. *Social Science & Medicine*, *51*(7), 1087–1110.

Shaw, J., & Baker, M. (2004). Expert patient: Dream or nightmare? *British Medical Journal*, *328*, 723–724.

Shaw, C., Brittain, K., Tansey, R., & Williams, K. (2008). How people decide to seek health-care: A qualitative study. *International Journal of Nursing Studies*, *45*, 1516–1524.

Stewart, M. (1984). What is a successful doctor-patient interview? A study of interactions and outcomes. *Social Science & Medicine*, *19*, 167–175.

Printed and bound by CPI Group (UK) Ltd, Croydon, CR0 4YY

15/09/2026

14962364-0002